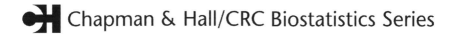 Chapman & Hall/CRC Biostatistics Series

Adaptive Design Methods in Clinical Trials

Chapman & Hall/CRC Biostatistics Series

Series Editor
Shein-Chung Chow, Ph.D.
Professor
Department of Biostatistics and Bioinformatics
Duke University School of Medicine
Durham, North Carolina, U.S.A.

Department of Statistics
National Cheng-Kung University
Tainan, Taiwan

1. *Design and Analysis of Animal Studies in Pharmaceutical Development,* Shein-Chung Chow and Jen-pei Liu
2. *Basic Statistics and Pharmaceutical Statistical Applications,* James E. De Muth
3. *Design and Analysis of Bioavailability and Bioequivalence Studies, Second Edition, Revised and Expanded,* Shein-Chung Chow and Jen-pei Liu
4. *Meta-Analysis in Medicine and Health Policy,* Dalene K. Stangl and Donald A. Berry
5. *Generalized Linear Models: A Bayesian Perspective,* Dipak K. Dey, Sujit K. Ghosh, and Bani K. Mallick
6. *Difference Equations with Public Health Applications,* Lemuel A. Moyé and Asha Seth Kapadia
7. *Medical Biostatistics,* Abhaya Indrayan and Sanjeev B. Sarmukaddam
8. *Statistical Methods for Clinical Trials,* Mark X. Norleans
9. *Causal Analysis in Biomedicine and Epidemiology: Based on Minimal Sufficient Causation,* Mikel Aickin
10. *Statistics in Drug Research: Methodologies and Recent Developments,* Shein-Chung Chow and Jun Shao
11. *Sample Size Calculations in Clinical Research,* Shein-Chung Chow, Jun Shao, and Hansheng Wang
12. *Applied Statistical Design for the Researcher,* Daryl S. Paulson
13. *Advances in Clinical Trial Biostatistics,* Nancy L. Geller
14. *Statistics in the Pharmaceutical Industry, 3rd Edition,* Ralph Buncher and Jia-Yeong Tsay
15. *DNA Microarrays and Related Genomics Techniques: Design, Analysis, and Interpretation of Experiments,* David B. Allsion, Grier P. Page, T. Mark Beasley, and Jode W. Edwards
16. *Basic Statistics and Pharmaceutical Statistical Applications, Second Edition,* James E. De Muth
17. *Adaptive Design Methods in Clinical Trials,* Shein-Chung Chow and Mark Chang

Chapman & Hall/CRC Biostatistics Series

Adaptive Design Methods in Clinical Trials

Shein-Chung Chow
Duke University School of Medicine
Durham, North Carolina, U.S.A.

National Cheng-Kung University
Tainan, Taiwan

Mark Chang
Millenium Pharmaceuticals
Cambridge, Massachusetts, U.S.A.

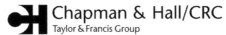

Chapman & Hall/CRC
Taylor & Francis Group
Boca Raton London New York

Chapman & Hall/CRC is an imprint of the
Taylor & Francis Group, an informa business

Chapman & Hall/CRC
Taylor & Francis Group
6000 Broken Sound Parkway NW, Suite 300
Boca Raton, FL 33487-2742

© 2007 by Taylor & Francis Group, LLC
Chapman & Hall/CRC is an imprint of Taylor & Francis Group, an Informa business

No claim to original U.S. Government works
Printed in the United States of America on acid-free paper
10 9 8 7 6 5 4 3 2 1

International Standard Book Number-10: 1-58488-776-1 (Hardcover)
International Standard Book Number-13: 978-1-58488-776-8 (Hardcover)

This book contains information obtained from authentic and highly regarded sources. Reprinted material is quoted with permission, and sources are indicated. A wide variety of references are listed. Reasonable efforts have been made to publish reliable data and information, but the author and the publisher cannot assume responsibility for the validity of all materials or for the consequences of their use.

No part of this book may be reprinted, reproduced, transmitted, or utilized in any form by any electronic, mechanical, or other means, now known or hereafter invented, including photocopying, microfilming, and recording, or in any information storage or retrieval system, without written permission from the publishers.

For permission to photocopy or use material electronically from this work, please access www.copyright.com (http://www.copyright.com/) or contact the Copyright Clearance Center, Inc. (CCC) 222 Rosewood Drive, Danvers, MA 01923, 978-750-8400. CCC is a not-for-profit organization that provides licenses and registration for a variety of users. For organizations that have been granted a photocopy license by the CCC, a separate system of payment has been arranged.

Trademark Notice: Product or corporate names may be trademarks or registered trademarks, and are used only for identification and explanation without intent to infringe.

Library of Congress Cataloging-in-Publication Data

Chow, Shein-Chung, 1955-
　　Adaptive design methods in clinical trials / Shein-Chung Chow and Mark Chang.
　　　　　p. cm. -- (Biostatistics ; 17)
　　Includes bibliographical references and index.
　　ISBN 1-58488-776-1
　　1. Clinical trials. 2. Adaptive sampling (Statistics). 3. Experimental design. 4. Clinical trials--Statistical methods. I. Chang, Mark. II. Title.

R853.C55.C53 2006
610.7'4--dc22
　　　　　　　　　　　　　　　　　　　　　　　　　　　　　　　　　　　　　2006048510

Visit the Taylor & Francis Web site at
http://www.taylorandfrancis.com

and the CRC Press Web site at
http://www.crcpress.com

Series Introduction

The primary objectives of the Biostatistics Book Series are to provide useful reference books for researchers and scientists in academia, industry, and government, and also to offer textbooks for undergraduate and/or graduate courses in the area of biostatistics. This book series will provide comprehensive and unified presentations of statistical designs and analyses of important applications in biostatistics, such as those in biopharmaceuticals. A well-balanced summary will be given of current and recently developed statistical methods and interpretations for both statisticians and researchers/scientists with minimal statistical knowledge who are engaged in the field of applied biostatistics. The series is committed to providing easy-to-understand, state-of-the-art references and textbooks. In each volume, statistical concepts and methodologies will be illustrated through real-world examples.

On March 16, 2004, the FDA released a report addressing the recent slowdown in innovative medical therapies being submitted to the FDA for approval, "Innovation/Stagnation: Challenge and Opportunity on the Critical Path to New Medical Products." The report describes the urgent need to modernize the medical product development process — the Critical Path — to make product development more predictable and less costly. Through this initiative, the FDA took the lead in the development of a national Critical Path Opportunities List, to bring concrete focus to these tasks. As a result, the FDA released a Critical Path Opportunities List that outlines 76 initial projects to bridge the gap between the quick pace of new biomedical discoveries and the slower pace at which those discoveries are currently developed into therapies two years later. The Critical Path Opportunities List consists of six broad topic areas: (i) development of biomarkers, (ii) clinical trial designs, (iii) bioinformatics, (iv) manufacturing, (v) public health needs, and (iv) pediatrics. As indicated in the Critical Path Opportunities Report, biomarker development and streamlining clinical trials are the two most important areas for improving medical product development. Streamlining clinical trials calls for advancing innovative trial designs such as adaptive designs to improve innovation in clinical development. These 76 initial projects are the most pressing scientific and/or technical hurdles causing major delays and other problems in the drug, device, and/or biologic development process. Among these six topics, biomarker development and streamlining clinical trials are the two most important areas for improving medical product development.

This volume provides useful approaches for implementation of adaptive design methods to clinical trials to pharmaceutical research and development. It covers statistical methods for various adaptive designs such as adaptive group sequential design, N-adjustable design, adaptive dose-escalation design, adaptive seamless phase II/III trial design (drop-the-losers design), adaptive randomization design, biomarker-adaptive design, adaptive treatment-switching design, adaptive-hypotheses design, and any combinations of the above designs. It will be beneficial to biostatisticians, medical researchers, pharmaceutical scientists, and reviewers in regulatory agencies who are engaged in the areas of pharmaceutical research and development.

Shein-Chung Chow

Preface

In recent years, the use of adaptive design methods in clinical trials has attracted much attention from clinical investigators and biostatisticians. Adaptations (i.e., modifications or changes) made to the trial and/or statistical procedures of on-going clinical trials based on accrued data have been in practice for years in clinical research and development. In the past several decades, we have adopted statistical procedures in the literature and applied them directly to the design of clinical trials originally planned by ignoring the fact that adaptations, modifications, and/or changes have been made to the trials. As pointed out by the United States Food and Drug Administration (FDA), these procedures, however, may not be motivated by best clinical trial practice. Consequently, they may not be the best tools to handle certain situations. Adaptive design methods in clinical research and development are attractive to clinical scientists and researchers due to the following reasons. First, they do reflect medical practice in the real world. Second, they are ethical with respect to both efficacy and safety (toxicity) of the test treatment under investigation. Third, they are not only flexible but also efficient in clinical development, especially for early phase clinical development. However, there are issues regarding the adjustments of treatment estimations and p-values. In addition, it is also a concern that the use of adaptive design methods in a clinical trial may have led to a totally different trial that is unable to address the scientific/medical questions the trial is intended to answer.

In practice, there existed no universal definition of adaptive design methods in clinical research until recently, when The Pharmaceutical Research and Manufacturers of America (PhRMA) gave a formal definition. Most literature focuses on adaptive randomization with respect to covariate, treatment, and/or clinical response; adaptive group sequential design for interim analysis; and sample size re-assessment. In this book, our definition is broader. Adaptive design methods include any adaptations, modifications, or changes of trial and/or statistical procedures that are made during the conduct of the trials. Although adaptive design methods are flexible and useful in clinical research, little or no regulatory guidances/guidelines are available. The purpose of this book is to provide a comprehensive and unified presentation of the principles and methodologies in adaptive design and analysis with respect to adaptations made to trial and/or statistical procedures based on accrued data of on-going clinical trials. In addition, this book is intended to give a well-balanced summary of current regulatory perspectives and recently developed statistical methods in this area. It is our goal to provide a complete, comprehensive, and updated reference and textbook in the area of adaptive design and analysis in clinical research and development.

Chapter 1 provides an introduction to basic concepts regarding the use of adaptive design methods in clinical trials and some statistical considerations of adaptive design methods. Chapter 2 focuses on the impact on target patient populations as the result of protocol amendments. Also included in this chapter is the generalization of statistical inference, which is drawn based on data collected from the actual patient population as the result of protocol amendments, to the originally planned target patient population. Several adaptive randomization procedures that are commonly employed in clinical trials are reviewed in Chapter 3. Chapter 4 studies the use of adaptive design methods in the case where hypotheses are modified during the conduct of clinical trials. Chapter 5 provides an overall review of adaptive design methods for dose selection, especially in dose finding and dose response relationship studies in early clinical development. Chapter 6 introduces the commonly used adaptive group sequential design methods in clinical trials. Blinded procedures for sample size re-estimation are given in Chapter 7. Statistical tests for seamless phase II/III adaptive designs and statistical inference for switching from one treatment to another adaptively, and the corresponding practical issues that may arise are studied in Chapter 8 and Chapter 9, respectively. Bayesian approaches for the use of adaptive design methods in clinical trials are outlined in Chapter 10. Chapter 11 provides an introduction to the methodology of clinical trial simulation for evaluation of the performance of the adaptive design methods under various adaptive designs that are commonly used in clinical development. Case studies regarding the implementation of adaptive group sequential design, adaptive dose-escalation design, and adaptive seamless phase II/III trial design in clinical trials are discussed in Chapter 12.

From Taylor & Francis, we would like to thank David Grubbs and Dr. Sunil Nair for providing us the opportunity to work on this book. We would like to thank colleagues from the Department of Biostatistics and Bioinformatics and Duke Clinical Research Institute (DCRI) of Duke University School of Medicine and Millennium Pharmaceuticals, Inc., for their support during the preparation of this book. We wish to express our gratitude to the following individuals for their encouragement and support: Roberts Califf, M.D. and John Hamilton, M.D. of

Duke Clinical Research Institute and Duke University Medical Center; Nancy Simonian, M.D., Jane Porter, M.S., Andy Boral, M.D. and Jim Gilbert, M.D. of Millennium Pharmaceuticals, Inc.; Greg Campbell, Ph.D. of the U.S. Food and Drug Administration; and many friends from academia, the pharmaceutical industry, and regulatory agencies.

Finally, the views expressed are those of the authors and not necessarily those of Duke University School of Medicine and Millennium Pharmaceuticals, Inc. We are solely responsible for the contents and errors of this edition. Any comments and suggestions will be very much appreciated.

Shein-Chung Chow, Ph.D.
Duke University School of Medicine, Durham, NC

Mark Chang, Ph.D.
Millennium Pharmaceuticals, Inc., Cambridge, MA

Contents

1	Introduction		1
	1.1	What Is Adaptive Design?	3
	1.2	Regulatory Perspectives	6
	1.3	Target Patient Population	8
	1.4	Statistical Inference	10
	1.5	Practical Issues	11
		1.5.1 Moving target patient population	12
		1.5.2 Adaptive randomization	13
		1.5.3 Adaptive hypotheses	14
		1.5.4 Adaptive dose-escalation trials	15
		1.5.5 Adaptive group sequential design	15
		1.5.6 Adaptive sample size adjustment	16
		1.5.7 Adaptive seamless phase II/III design	17
		1.5.8 Adaptive treatment switching	18
		1.5.9 Bayesian and hybrid approaches	18
		1.5.10 Clinical trial simulation	19
		1.5.11 Case studies	19
	1.6	Aims and Scope of the Book	20
2	**Protocol Amendment**		23
	2.1	Actual Patient Population	23
	2.2	Estimation of Shift and Scale Parameters	26
		2.2.1 The case where μ_{Actual} is random and σ_{Actual} is fixed	28
	2.3	Statistical Inference	31
		2.3.1 Test for equality	33
		2.3.2 Test for non-inferiority/superiority	34
		2.3.3 Test for equivalence	34
	2.4	Sample Size Adjustment	35
		2.4.1 Test for equality	35
		2.4.2 Test for non-inferiority/superiority	36
		2.4.3 Test for equivalence	37
	2.5	Statistical Inference with Covariate Adjustment	38
		2.5.1 Population and assumption	38

		2.5.2 Conditional inference	39
		2.5.3 Unconditional inference	40
	2.6	Concluding Remarks	43

3 Adaptive Randomization — 47
- 3.1 Conventional Randomization — 48
- 3.2 Treatment-Adaptive Randomization — 52
- 3.3 Covariate-Adaptive Randomization — 55
- 3.4 Response-Adaptive Randomization — 58
- 3.5 Issues with Adaptive Randomization — 70
- 3.6 Summary — 73

4 Adaptive Hypotheses — 75
- 4.1 Modifications of Hypotheses — 76
- 4.2 Switch from Superiority to Non-Inferiority — 78
- 4.3 Concluding Remarks — 87

5 Adaptive Dose-Escalation Trials — 89
- 5.1 Introduction — 89
- 5.2 CRM in Phase I Oncology Study — 91
- 5.3 Hybrid Frequentist-Bayesian Adaptive Design — 93
- 5.4 Simulations — 100
- 5.5 Concluding Remarks — 104

6 Adaptive Group Sequential Design — 107
- 6.1 Sequential Methods — 108
- 6.2 General Approach for Group Sequential Design — 112
- 6.3 Early Stopping Boundaries — 114
- 6.4 Alpha Spending Function — 122
- 6.5 Group Sequential Design Based on Independent p-Values — 123
- 6.6 Calculation of Stopping Boundaries — 125
- 6.7 Group Sequential Trial Monitoring — 128
- 6.8 Conditional Power — 133
- 6.9 Practical Issues — 135

7 Adaptive Sample Size Adjustment — 137
- 7.1 Sample Size Re-estimation without Unblinding Data — 138
- 7.2 Cui–Hung–Wang's Method — 140
- 7.3 Proschan–Hunsberger's Method — 142
- 7.4 Muller–Schafer Method — 146
- 7.5 Bauer–Köhne Method — 146

	7.6	Generalization of Independent p-Value Approaches	148
	7.7	Inverse-Normal Method	157
	7.8	Concluding Remarks	158

8 Adaptive Seamless Phase II/III Designs — 161
- 8.1 Why a Seamless Design Is Efficient — 161
- 8.2 Step-Wise Test and Adaptive Procedures — 162
- 8.3 Contrast Test and Naive p-Value — 163
- 8.4 Comparison of Seamless Designs — 165
- 8.5 Drop-the-Loser Adaptive Design — 167
- 8.6 Summary — 171

9 Adaptive Treatment Switching — 173
- 9.1 Latent Event Times — 174
- 9.2 Proportional Hazard Model with Latent Hazard Rate — 177
  - 9.2.1 Simulation results — 179
- 9.3 Mixed Exponential Model — 181
  - 9.3.1 Biomarker-based survival model — 182
  - 9.3.2 Effect of patient enrollment rate — 184
  - 9.3.3 Hypothesis test and power analysis — 187
  - 9.3.4 Application to trials with treatment switch — 189
- 9.4 Concluding Remarks — 193

10 Bayesian Approach — 195
- 10.1 Basic Concepts of Bayesian Approach — 195
  - 10.1.1 Bayes rule — 196
  - 10.1.2 Bayesian power — 200
- 10.2 Multiple-Stage Design for Single-Arm Trial — 201
  - 10.2.1 Classical approach for two-stage design — 202
  - 10.2.2 Bayesian approach — 203
- 10.3 Bayesian Optimal Adaptive Designs — 205
- 10.4 Concluding Remarks — 209

11 Clinical Trial Simulation — 211
- 11.1 Simulation Framework — 212
- 11.2 Early Phases Development — 213
  - 11.2.1 Dose limiting toxicity (DLT) and maximum tolerated dose (MTD) — 214
  - 11.2.2 Dose-level selection — 214

		11.2.3	Sample size per dose level	215
		11.2.4	Dose-escalation design	215
	11.3	Late Phases Development		215
		11.3.1	Randomization rules	216
		11.3.2	Early stopping rules	216
		11.3.3	Rules for dropping losers	216
		11.3.4	Sample size adjustment	217
		11.3.5	Response–adaptive randomization	217
		11.3.6	Utility-offset model	218
		11.3.7	Null-model versus model approach	219
		11.3.8	Alpha adjustment	219
	11.4	Software Application		220
		11.4.1	Overview of ExpDesign studio	220
		11.4.2	How to design a trial with ExpDesign studio	222
		11.4.3	How to design a conventional trial	222
		11.4.4	How to design a group sequential trial	223
		11.4.5	How to design a multi-stage trial	224
		11.4.6	How to design a dose-escalation trial	225
		11.4.7	How to design an adaptive trial	227
	11.5	Examples		227
		11.5.1	Early phases development	228
		11.5.2	Late phases development	230
	11.6	Concluding Remarks		235
12	**Case Studies**			**239**
	12.1	Basic Considerations		239
		12.1.1	Dose and dose regimen	240
		12.1.2	Study endpoints	240
		12.1.3	Treatment duration	240
		12.1.4	Logistical considerations	241
		12.1.5	Independent data monitoring committee	241
	12.2	Adaptive Group Sequential Design		241
		12.2.1	Group sequential design	241
		12.2.2	Adaptation	242
		12.2.3	Statistical methods	243
		12.2.4	Case study — an example	243
	12.3	Adaptive Dose-Escalation Design		244
		12.3.1	Traditional dose-escalation design	244
		12.3.2	Adaptation	245
		12.3.3	Statistical methods	245
		12.3.4	Case study — an example	245

12.4	Adaptive Seamless Phase II/III Design		247
	12.4.1	Seamless phase II/III design	247
	12.4.2	Adaptation	248
	12.4.3	Methods	248
	12.4.4	Case study — some examples	249
	12.4.5	Issues and recommendations	252

Bibliography   **255**

Index   **269**

CHAPTER 1

Introduction

In clinical research, the ultimate goal of a clinical trial is to evaluate the effect (e.g., efficacy and safety) of a test treatment as compared to a control (e.g., a placebo control, a standard therapy, or an active control agent). To ensure the success of a clinical trial, a well-designed study protocol is essential. A protocol is a plan that details how a clinical trial is to be carried out and how the data are to be collected and analyzed. It is an extremely critical and the most important document in clinical trials, since it ensures the quality and integrity of the clinical investigation in terms of its planning, execution, conduct, and the analysis of the data of clinical trials. During the conduct of a clinical trial, adherence to the protocol is crucial. Any protocol deviations and/or violations may introduce bias and variation to the data collected from the trial. Consequently, the conclusion drawn based on the analysis results of the data may not be reliable and hence may be biased or misleading. For marketing approval of a new drug product, the United States Food and Drug Administration (FDA) requires that at least two adequate and well-controlled clinical trials be conducted to provide substantial evidence regarding the effectiveness of the drug product under investigation (FDA, 1988). However, under certain circumstances, the FDA Modernization Act (FDAMA) of 1997 includes a provision (Section 115 of FDAMA) to allow data from a single adequate and well-controlled clinical trial to establish effectiveness for risk/benefit assessment of drug and biological candidates for approval. The FDA indicates that substantial evidence regarding the effectiveness and safety of the drug product under investigation can only be provided through the conduct of adequate and well-controlled clinical studies. According to the FDA 1988 guideline for *Format and Content of the Clinical and Statistical Sections of New Drug Applications*, an adequate and well-controlled study is defined as a study that meets the characteristics of the following: (i) objectives, (ii) methods of analysis, (iii) design, (iv) selection of subjects, (v) assignment of subjects, (vi) participants of studies, (vii) assessment of responses, and (viii) assessment of effect. In the study protocol, it is essential to clearly state the study objectives of the study. Specific hypotheses that reflect the study objectives should be provided in the study protocol. The study design must be valid in order to provide a fair and unbiased assessment of the treatment effect as compared to a control. Target patient population should be defined through the inclusion/exclusion criteria to assure the disease conditions under study. Randomization procedures must be employed to minimize potential bias and to ensure the comparability between treatment groups. Criteria for assessment of the response should be pre-defined and reliable. Appropriate statistical methods should be employed for assessment of the effect. Procedures such as blinding for minimization of bias should be employed to maintain the validity and integrity of the trial.

In clinical trials, it is not uncommon to adjust trial and/or statistical methods at the planning stage and during the conduct of clinical trials. For example, at the planning stage of a clinical trial, as an alternative to the standard randomization procedure, an *adaptive* randomization procedure based on treatment response may be considered for treatment allocation. During the conduct of a clinical trial, some adaptations (i.e., modifications or changes) to trial and/or statistical procedures may be made based on accrued data. Typical examples for adaptations of trial and/or statistical procedures of on-going clinical trials include, but are not limited to, the modification of inclusion/exclusion criteria, the adjustment of study dose or regimen, the extension of treatment duration, changes in study endpoints, and modification in study design such as group sequential design and/or multiple-stage flexible designs (Table 1.1). Adaptations to trial and/or statistical procedures of on-going clinical trials will certainly have an immediate impact on the target population and, consequently, statistical inference on treatment effect of the target patient population. In practice, adaptations or modifications to trial and/or statistical procedures of on-going clinical trials are necessary, which not only reflect real medical practice on the actual patient

Table 1.1 Types of Adaptation in Clinical Trials

Adaptation	Examples
Prospective (by design)	Interim analysis
	Stop trial early due to safety, futility/efficacy
	Sample size re-estimation, etc.
On-going (ad hoc)	Inclusion/exclusion criteria
	Dose or dose regimen
	Treatment duration, etc.
Retrospective*	Study endpoint
	Switch from superiority to non-inferiority, etc.

*Adaptation at the end of the study prior to database lock or unblinding.

INTRODUCTION

population with the disease under study, but also increase the probability of success for identifying the clinical benefit of the treatment under investigation.

The remainder of this chapter is organized as follows. In the next section, a definition regarding so-called adaptive design is given. Section 1.2 provides regulatory perspectives regarding the use of adaptive design methods in clinical research and development. Sections 1.3 and 1.4 describe the impact of an adaptive design on the target patient population and statistical inference following adaptations of trial and/or statistical procedures, respectively. Practical issues that are commonly encountered when applying adaptive design methods in clinical research and development are briefly outlined in Section 1.5. Section 1.6 presents the aims and scope of the book.

1.1 What Is Adaptive Design

On March 16, 2006, the FDA released a Critical Path Opportunities List that outlines 76 initial projects to bridge the gap between the quick pace of new biomedical discoveries and the slower pace at which those discoveries are currently developed into therapies. (See, e.g., http://www.fda.gov/oc/initiatives/criticalpath.) The Critical Path Opportunities List consists of six broad topic areas of (i) development of biomarkers, (ii) clinical trial designs, (iii) bioinformatics, (iv) manufacturing, (v) public health needs, and (iv) pediatrics. As indicated in the Critical Path Opportunities Report, biomarker development and streamlining clinical trials are the two most important areas for improving medical product development. The streamlining clinical trials call for advancing innovative trial designs such as adaptive designs to improve innovation in clinical development.

In clinical investigation of treatment regimens, it is not uncommon to consider adaptations (i.e., modifications or changes) in early phase clinical trials before initiation of large-scale confirmatory phase III trials. We will refer to the application of adaptations to clinical trials as *adaptive design methods* in clinical trials. The adaptive design methods are usually developed based on observed treatment effects. To allow wider flexibility, adaptations in clinical investigation of treatment regimen may include changes of sample size, inclusion/exclusion criteria, study dose, study endpoints, and methods for analysis (Liu, Proschan, and Pledger, 2002). Along this line, the PhRMA Working Group defines an *adaptive design* as a clinical study design that uses accumulating data to decide on how to modify aspects of the study as it continues, without undermining the validity and integrity of the trial (Gallo et al., 2006). As indicated by the PhRMA Working Group, the adaptation is a design feature aimed to enhance the trial, not a remedy for inadequate planning. In other words, changes should be made *by design* and not on an *ad hoc* basis. *By design* changes, however, do not reflect real clinical practice. In addition, they do not allow flexibility. As a result, in this book we will refer to an adaptive design of a clinical trial as a design that allows adaptations or modifications to some aspects (e.g., trial and/or statistical procedures) of the trial after its initiation without undermining the validity and integrity of the trial (Chow, Chang, and Pong, 2005). Adaptations or modifications of on-going clinical trials that are commonly made to trial procedures include eligibility criteria, study dose or regimen, treatment duration, study endpoints, laboratory testing procedures, diagnostic procedures, criteria for evaluability, assessment of clinical responses, deletion/addition of treatment groups, and safety parameters. In practice, during the conduct of the clinical trial, statistical procedures including randomization procedure in treatment allocation, study objectives/hypotheses, sample size reassessment, study design, data monitoring and interim analysis procedure, statistical analysis plan, and/or methods for data analysis are often adjusted in order to increase the probability of success of the trial by controlling the pre-specified type I error. Note that in many cases, an adaptive design is also known as a *flexible* design (EMEA, 2002).

Adaptive design methods are very attractive to clinical researchers and/or sponsors due to their flexibility, especially when there are priority changes for budget/resources and timeline constraints, scientific/statistical justifications for study validity and integrity, medical considerations for safety, regulatory concerns for review/approval, and/or business strategies for go/no-go decisions. However, there is little or no information available in regulatory requirements as to what level of flexibility in modifications of trial and/or statistical procedures of on-going clinical trials would be acceptable. It is a concern that the application of adaptive design methods may result in a totally different clinical trial that is unable to address the scientific/medical questions/hypotheses the clinical trial is intended to answer. In addition, an adaptive design suffers from the following disadvantages. First, it may result in a major difference between the actual patient population as the result of adaptations made to the trial and/or statistical procedures and the (original) target patient population. The actual patient population under study could be a moving target depending upon the frequency and extent of modifications (flexibility) made to study parameters. Second, statistical inferences such as confidence interval and/or p-values on the treatment effect of the test treatment under study may not be reliable. Consequently, the observed clinical results may not be reproducible. In recent years, the use of adaptive design methods in clinical trials has attracted much attention from clinical scientists and biostatisticians.

In practice, adaptation or modification made to the trial and/or statistical procedures during the conduct of a clinical trial based on accrued data is usually recommended by the investigator, the sponsor, or an independent datamonitoring committee. Although the adaptation or modification is flexible and attractive, it may introduce bias and consequently has an impact on statistical inference on the assessment of treatment effect for the target patient population under study. The complexity could be substantial depending upon the adaptation employed. Basically, the adaptation employed can be classified into three categories: prospective (by design) adaptation, concurrent (or on-going ad hoc) adaptation (by protocol amendment), and retrospective adaptation (after the end of the conduct of the trial, before database lock and/or unblinding). As it can be seen, the on-going ad hoc adaptation has higher flexibility, while prospective adaptation is less flexible. Both types of adaptation require careful planning. It should be noted that statistical methods for certain kinds of adaptation may not be available in the literature. As a result, some studies with complicated adaptation may be more successful than others.

Depending upon the types of adaptation or modification made, commonly employed adaptive design methods in clinical trials include, but are not limited to: (i) an adaptive group sequential design, (ii) an N-adjustable design, (iii) an adaptive seamless phase II/III design, (iv) a drop-the-loser design, (v) an adaptive randomization design, (vi) an adaptive dose-escalation design, (vii) a biomarker-adaptive design, (viii) an adaptive treatment-switching design, (ix) an adaptive-hypotheses design, and (x) any combinations of the above. An adaptive group sequential design is an adaptive design that allows for prematurely terminating a trial due to safety, efficacy, or futility based on interim analysis results, while an N-adjustable design is referred to as an adaptive design that allows for sample size adjustment or re-estimation based on the observed data at interim. A seamless phase II/III adaptive trial design refers to a program that addresses within a single trial objectives that are normally achieved through separate trials in phases IIb and III (Inoue, Thall, and Berry, 2002; Gallo et al., 2006). An adaptive seamless phase II/III design would combine two separate trials (i.e., a phase IIb trial and a phase III trial) into one trial and would use data from patients enrolled before and after the adaptation in the final analysis (Maca, et al., 2006). A drop-the-loser design is a multiple-stage adaptive design that allows dropping the inferior treatment groups. Adaptive randomization design refers to a design that allows modification of randomization schedules. Adaptive dose-escalation design is often used in early phase clinical development to identify the maximum tolerable dose, which is usually considered the optimal dose for later phase clinical trials. Biomarker-adaptive design is a design that allows for adaptations based on the response of biomarkers such as genomic markers. Adaptive treatment-switching design is a design that allows the investigator to switch a patient's treatment from an initial assignment to an alternative treatment if there is evidence of lack of efficacy or safety of the initial treatment. Adaptive-hypotheses design refers to a design that allows change in hypotheses based on interim analysis results. Any combinations of the above adaptive designs are usually referred to as multiple adaptive designs. In practice, depending upon the study objectives of clinical trials, a multiple adaptive design with several adaptations may be employed at the same time. In this case, statistical inference is often difficult if not impossible to obtain. These adaptive designs will be discussed further in later chapters of this book.

In recent years, the use of these adaptive designs has received much attention. For example, the *Journal of Biopharmaceutical Statistics* (JBS) published a special issue (Volume 15, Number 4) on Adaptive Design in Clinical Research in 2005 (Pong and Luo, 2005). This special issue covers many statistical issues related to the use of adaptive design methods in clinical research (see e.g., Chang and Chow, 2005; Chow, Chang, and Pong, 2005; Chow and Shao, 2005; Hommel, Lindig, and Faldum, 2005; Hung et al., 2005; Jennison and Turnbull, 2005; Kelly, Stallard, and Todd, 2005; Kelly et al., 2005; Li, Shih, and Wang, 2005; Proschan, 2005; Proschan, Leifer, and Liu, 2005; Wang and Hung, 2005). The PhRMA Working Group also published an executive summary on adaptive designs in clinical drug development to facilitate wide usage of adaptive designs in clinical drug development (Gallo et al., 2006). This book is intended to address concerns and/or practical issues that may arise when applying adaptive design methods in clinical trials.

1.2 Regulatory Perspectives

As pointed out by the FDA, modification of the design of an experiment based on accrued data has been in practice for hundreds, if not thousands, of years in medical research. In the past, we have had a tendency to adopt statistical procedures in the literature and apply them directly to the design of clinical trials (Lan, 2002). However, since these procedures were not motivated by clinical trial practice, they may not be the best tools to handle certain situations. The impact of any adaptations made to trial and/or statistical methods before, during, and after the conduct of trial could be substantial.

The flexibility in design and analysis of clinical trials in early phases of the drug development is very attractive to clinical researchers/scientists and the sponsors. However, its use in late phase II or phase III clinical investigations has led to regulatory concerns regarding its limitation of interpretation and extrapolation from trial results. As there is an increasing need for flexibility in design and analysis of clinical trials, the European Agency for the Evaluation of Medicinal Products (EMEA) published a concept paper on points to consider on methodological issues in confirmatory clinical trials with flexible design and analysis plan (EMEA, 2002, 2006). The EMEA's points to consider discuss prerequisites and conditions under which the methods could be acceptable in confirmatory phase III trials for regulatory decision making. Principal pre-requisite for all considerations is that methods under investigation can provide correct p-values, unbiased estimates, and confidence intervals for the treatment comparison(s) in an actual clinical trial. As a result, the use of an adaptive design not only raises the importance of well-known problems of studies with interim analyses (e.g., lack of a sufficient safety database after early termination and over-running), but also bears new challenges to clinical researchers.

From a regulatory point of view, blinded review of the database at interim analyses is a key issue in adaptive design. During these blinded reviews, often the statistical analysis plan is largely modified. At the same time, more study protocols are submitted, where little or no information on statistical methods is provided and relevant decisions are deferred to a statistical analysis or even the blinded review, which has led to a serious regulatory concern regarding the validity and integrity of the trial. In addition, what is the resultant actual patient population of the study after the adaptations of the trial procedures, especially when the inclusion/exclusion criteria are made, is a challenge to the regulatory review and approval process. A commonly asked question is whether the adaptive design methods have resulted in a totally different trial with a totally different target patient population. In this case, is the usual regulatory review and approval process still applicable? However, there is little or no information in regulatory guidances or guidelines regarding regulatory requirement or perception as to the degree of flexibility that would be accepted by the regulatory agencies. In practice, it is suggested that regulatory acceptance should be justified based on the validity of statistical inference of the target patient population.

It should be noted that although adaptations of trial and/or statistical procedures are often documented through protocol amendments, standard statistical methods may not be appropriate and may lead to invalid inference/conclusion regarding the target patient population. As a result, it is recommended that appropriate adaptive statistical methods be employed. Although several adaptive design methods for obtaining valid statistical inferences on treatment effects available in the literature (see, e.g., Hommel, 2001; Liu, Proschan, and Pledger, 2002) are useful, they should be performed in a completely objective manner. In practice, however, it can be very difficult to reach this objectivity in clinical trials due to external inferences and different interests from the investigators and sponsors.

As a result, it is strongly recommended that a guidance/guideline for adaptive design methods be developed by the regulatory authorities to avoid every intentional or unintentional manipulation of the adaptive design methods in clinical trials. The guidance/guideline should describe in detail not only the standards for use of adaptive design methods in clinical trials, but also the level of modifications in an adaptive design that is acceptable to the regulatory agencies. In addition, any changes in the process of regulatory review/approval should also be clearly indicated in such a guidance/guideline. It should be noted that the adaptive design methods have been used in the review/approval process of regulatory submissions for years, though it may not have been recognized until recently.

1.3 Target Patient Population

In clinical trials, patient populations with certain diseases under study are usually described by the inclusion/exclusion criteria. Patients who meet all inclusion criteria and none of the exclusion criteria are qualified for the study. We will refer to this patient population as the *target patient population*. For a given study endpoint such as clinical response, time to disease progression, or survival in the therapeutic area of oncology, we may denote the target patient population by (μ,σ), where μ is the population mean of the study endpoint and σ denotes the population standard deviation of the study endpoint. For a comparative clinical trial comparing a test treatment and a control, the effect size of the test treatment adjusted for standard deviation is defined as

$$\frac{\mu_T - \mu_C}{\sigma},$$

where μ_T and μ_C are the population means for the test treatment and the control, respectively. Based on the collected data, statistical inference such as confidence interval and p-value on the effect size of the test treatment can then be made for the target patient population.

In practice, as indicated earlier, it is not uncommon to modify trial procedures due to some medical and/or practical considerations during the conduct of the trial. Trial procedures of a clinical trial are referred to as operating procedures, testing procedures, and/or diagnostic procedures that are to be employed in the clinical trial. As a result, trial procedures of a clinical trial include, but are not limited to, the inclusion/exclusion criteria, the selection of study dose or regimen, treatment duration, laboratory testing, diagnostic procedures, and criteria for evaluability. In clinical trials, we refer to statistical procedures of a clinical trial as statistical procedures and/or statistical models/methods that are employed at planning, execution, and conduct of the trial as well as the analysis of the data. Thus, statistical procedures of a clinical trial include power analysis for sample size calculation at planning stage, randomization procedure for treatment allocation prior to treatment, modifications of hypotheses, change in study endpoint, and sample size re-estimation at interim during the conduct of the trial. As indicated in the FDA 1988 guideline and the International Conference on Harmonization (ICH) Good Clinical Practices (GCP) guideline (FDA, 1988; ICH, 1996), a well-designed protocol should detail how the clinical trial is to be carried out. Any deviations from the protocol and/or violations of the protocol will not only distort the original patient population under study, but will also introduce bias and variation to the data collected from the trial. Consequently, conclusions drawn based on statistical inference obtained from the analysis results of the data may not be applied to the original target patient population.

In clinical trials, the inclusion/exclusion criteria and study dose or regimen and/or treatment duration are often modified due to slow enrollment and/or safety concerns during the conduct of the trial. For example, at screening, we may disqualify too many patients with stringent inclusion/exclusion criteria. Consequently, the enrollments may be too slow to meet the timeline of the study. In this case, a typical approach is to relax the inclusion/exclusion criteria to increase the enrollment. On the other hand, the investigators may wish to have the flexibility to adjust the study dose or regimen to achieve optimal clinical benefit of the test treatment during the trial. The study dose may be reduced when there are significant toxicities and/or adverse experiences. In addition, the investigators may wish to extend the treatment duration to (i) reach best therapeutic effect or (ii) achieve the anticipated event rate based on accrued data during the conduct of trial. These modifications of trial procedures are commonly encountered in clinical trials.

Modifications of trial procedures are usually accomplished through protocol amendments, which detail rationales for changes and the impact of the modifications.

Any adaptations made to the trial and/or statistical procedures may introduce bias and/or variation to the data collected from the trial. Consequently, it may result in a similar but slightly different target patient population. We will refer to such a patient population as the *actual* patient population under study. As mentioned earlier, in practice, it is a concern whether adaptations made to the trial and/or statistical procedures could lead to a totally different trial with a totally different target patient population. In addition, it is of interest to determine whether statistical inference obtained based on clinical data collected from the actual patient population could be applied to the originally planned target patient population. These issues will be studied in the next chapter.

1.4 Statistical Inference

As discussed in the previous section, modifications of trial procedures will certainly introduce bias/variation to the data collected from the trial. The sources of these biases and variations can be classified into one of the following four categories: (i) expected and controllable, (ii) expected but not controllable, (iii) unexpected but controllable, and (iv) unexpected and not controllable. For example, additional bias/variation is expected but not controllable when there is a change in study dose or regimen and/or treatment duration. For changes in laboratory testing procedures and/or diagnostic procedures, bias/variation is expected but controllable by (i) having experienced technicians to perform the tests or (ii) conducting appropriate training for inexperienced technicians. Bias/variation due to patient non-compliance to trial procedures is usually unexpected but is controllable by improving the procedure for patients' compliance. Additional bias/variation due to unexpected and uncontrollable sources is usually referred to as the random error of the trial.

In practice, appropriate statistical procedures should be employed to identify and eliminate/control these sources of bias/variation whenever possible. In addition, after the adaptations of the trial procedures, especially the inclusion/exclusion criteria, the target patient population has been changed to the actual patient population under study. In this case, how to generalize the conclusion drawn based on statistical inference of the treatment effect derived from clinical data observed from the actual patient population to the original target patient population is a challenge to clinical scientists. It, however, should be noted that although all modifications of trial procedures and/or statistical procedures are documented through protocol amendments, it does not imply that the collected data are free of bias/variation. Protocol amendments should not only provide rationales for changes but also detail how the data are to be collected and analyzed following the adaptations of trial and/or statistical procedures. In practice, it is not uncommon to observe the following inconsistencies following major adaptations of trial and/or statistical procedures of a clinical trial: (i) a right test for wrong hypotheses, (ii) a wrong test for the right hypotheses, (iii) a wrong test for wrong hypotheses, and (iv) the right test for the right hypotheses but insufficient power. Each of these inconsistencies will result in invalid statistical inferences and conclusions regarding the treatment effect under investigation.

Flexibility in statistical procedures of a clinical trial is very attractive to the investigator and/or sponsors. However, it suffers the disadvantage of invalid statistical inference and/or misleading conclusion if the impact is not carefully managed. Liu, Proschan, and Pledger (2002) provided a solid theoretical foundation for adaptive design methods in clinical development under which not only a general method for point estimation, confidence interval, hypotheses testing, and overall p-value can be obtained, but also its validity can be rigorously established. However, they do not take into consideration the fact that the target patient population has become a moving target patient population as the result of adaptations made to the trial and/or statistical procedures through protocol amendments. This issue will be further discussed in the next chapter.

The ICH GCP guideline suggests that a thoughtful statistical analysis plan (SAP), which details statistical procedures (including models/methods), should be employed for data collection and analysis. Any deviations from the SAP and violations of the SAP could decrease the reliability of the analysis results, and consequently the conclusion drawn from these analysis results may not be valid.

In summary, the use of adaptive design methods in clinical trials may have an impact on the statistical inference on the target patient population under study. Statistical inference obtained based on data collected from the actual patient population as the result of modifications made to the trial procedures and/or statistical procedures should be adjusted before it can be applied to the original target patient population.

1.5 Practical Issues

As indicated earlier, the use of adaptive design methods in clinical trials has received much attention because it allows adaptations of trial and/or statistical procedures of on-going clinical trials. The flexibility for adaptations to study parameters is very attractive to clinical scientists and sponsors. However, from regulatory point of view, several questions have been raised. First, what level of adaptations to the trial and/or statistical procedures would be acceptable to the regulatory authorities? Second, what are the regulatory requirements and standards for review and approval process of clinical data obtained from adaptive clinical trials with different levels of adaptations to trial and/or statistical procedures of on-going clinical trials? Third, has the clinical trial become a totally different clinical trial after the adaptations to the trial and/or statistical procedures for addressing the study objectives of the originally planned clinical trial? These concerns are necessarily addressed by the regulatory authorities before the adaptive design methods can be widely accepted in clinical research and development.

In addition, from the scientific/statistical point of view, there are also some concerns regarding (i) whether the modifications to the trial procedures have resulted in a similar but different target patient population, (ii) whether the modifications of hypotheses have distorted the study objectives of the trial, (iii) whether the flexibility in statistical procedures has led to biased assessment of clinical benefit of the treatment under investigation. In this section, practical issues associated with the above questions that are commonly encountered in clinical trials when applying adaptive design methods of on-going clinical trials are briefly described. These issues include moving target patient population as the result of protocol amendments, adaptive randomization, adaptive hypotheses, adaptive dose-escalation trials, adaptive group sequential designs, adaptive sample size adjustment, adaptive seamless phase II/III trial design, dropping the losers adaptively, adaptive treatment switching, Bayesian and hybrid approaches, clinical trial simulation, and case studies.

1.5.1 Moving target patient population

In clinical trials, it is important to define the patient population with the disease under study. This patient population is usually described based on eligibility criteria, i.e., the inclusion and exclusion criteria. This patient population is referred to as the *target* patient population. As indicated in Chow and Liu (2003), a target patient population is usually roughly defined by the inclusion criteria and then fine-tuned by the exclusion criteria to minimize heterogeneity of the patient population. When adaptations are made to the trial and/or statistical procedures, especially the inclusion/exclusion criteria during the conduct of the trial, the mean response of the primary study endpoint of the target patient population may be shifted with heterogeneity in variability. As a result, adaptations made to trial and/or statistical procedures could lead to a similar but different patient population. We will refer to this resultant patient population as the *actual* patient population. In practice, it is a concern that a major (or significant) adaptation could result in a totally different patient population. During the conduct of a clinical trial, if adaptations are made frequently, the target patient population is in fact a *moving* target patient population (Chow, Chang, and Pong, 2005). As a result, it is difficult to draw an accurate and reliable statistical inference on the moving target patient population. Thus, in practice, it is of interest to determine the impact of adaptive design methods on the target patient population and consequently the corresponding statistical inference and power analysis for sample size calculation. More details are given in the next chapter.

1.5.2 Adaptive randomization

In clinical trials, randomization models such as the population model, the invoked population model, and the randomization model with the method of complete randomization and permuted-block randomization are commonly used to ensure a balanced allocation of patients to treatment within either a fixed total sample size or a pre-specified block size (Chow and Liu, 2003). The population model is referred to as the concept that clinicians can draw conclusions for the target patient population based on the selection of a representative sample drawn from the target patient population by some random procedure (Lehmann, 1975; Lachin, 1988). The invoked population model is referred to as the process of selecting investigators first and then selecting patients at each selected investigator's site. As it can be seen, neither the selection of investigators nor the recruitment of patients at the selected investigator's site is random. However, treatment assignment is random. Thus, the invoked randomization model allows the analysis of the clinical data as if they were obtained under the assumption that the sample is randomly selected from a homogeneous patient population. Randomization model is referred to as the concept of randomization or permutation tests based on the fact that the study site selection and patient selection are not random, but the assignment of treatments to patients is random. Randomization model/method is a critical component in clinical trials because statistical inference based on the data collected from the trial relies on the probability distribution of the sample, which in turn depends upon the randomization procedure employed.

In practice, however, it is also of interest to adjust the probability of assignment of patients to treatments during the study to increase the probability of success of the clinical study. This type of randomization is called adaptive randomization because the probability of the treatment to which a current patient is assigned is adjusted based on the assignment of previous patients. The randomization codes based on the method of adaptive randomization cannot be prepared before the study begins. This is because the randomization process is performed at the time a patient is enrolled in the study, whereas adaptive randomization requires information on previously randomized patients. In practice, the method of adaptive randomization is often applied with respect to treatment, covariate, or clinical response. Therefore, the adaptive randomization is known as treatment-adaptive randomization, covariate-adaptive randomization, or response-adaptive randomization. Adaptive randomization procedures could have an impact on sample size required for achieving a desired statistical power and consequently statistical inference on the test treatment under investigation. More details regarding the adaptive randomization procedures described above and their impact on sample size calculation and statistical inference is given in Chapter 3 of this book.

1.5.3 Adaptive hypotheses

Modifications of hypotheses during the conduct of a clinical trial commonly occur due to the following reasons: (i) an investigational method has not yet been validated at the planning stage of the study, (ii) information from other studies is necessary for planning the next stage of the study, (iii) there is a need to include new doses, and (iv) recommendations from a pre-established data safety monitoring committee (Hommel, 2001). In clinical research, it is not uncommon to have more than one set of hypotheses for an intended clinical trial. These hypotheses may be classified as primary hypotheses and secondary hypotheses depending upon whether they are the primary study objectives or secondary study objectives. In practice, a pre-specified overall type I error rate is usually controlled for testing the primary hypotheses. However, if the investigator is interested in controlling the overall type I error rate for testing secondary hypotheses, then techniques for multiple testing are commonly employed. Following the ideas of Bauer (1999), Kieser, Bauer, and Lehmacher (1999), and Bauer and Kieser (1999) for general multiple testing problems, Hommel (2001) applied the same techniques

INTRODUCTION   15

to obtain more flexible strategies for adaptive modifications of hypotheses based on accrued data at interim by changing the weights of hypotheses, changing a prior order, or even including new hypotheses. The method proposed by Hommel (2001) enjoys the following advantages. First, it is a very general method in the sense that any type of multiple testing problems can be applied. Second, it is mathematically correct. Third, it is extremely flexible, which allows not only changes to design, but also changes to the choice of hypotheses or weights for them during the course of the study. In addition, it also allows the addition of new hypotheses. Modifications of hypotheses can certainly have an impact on statistical inference for assessment of treatment effect. More discussions are given in Chapter 4 of this book.

1.5.4 Adaptive dose-escalation trials

In clinical research, the *response* in a dose response study could be a biological response for safety or efficacy. For example, in a dose-toxicity study, the goal is to determine the maximum tolerable dose (MTD). On the other hand, in a dose-efficacy response study, the primary objective is usually to address one or more of the following questions: (i) Is there any evidence of the drug effect? (ii) What is the nature of the dose-response? and (iii) What is the optimal dose? In practice, it is always a concern as to how to evaluate dose–response relationship with limited resources within a relatively tight time frame. This concern led to a proposed design that allows less patients to be exposed to the toxicity and more patients to be treated at potentially efficacious dose levels. Such a design also allows pharmaceutical companies to fully utilize their resources for development of more new drug products. In Chapter 5, we provide a brief background of dose escalation trials in oncology trials. We will review the continued reassessment method (CRM) proposed by O'Quigley, Pepe, and Fisher (1990) in phase I oncology trials. We will study the hybrid frequentist-Bayesian adaptive approach for both efficacy and toxicity (Chang, Chow, and Pong, 2005) in detail.

1.5.5 Adaptive group sequential design

In practice, flexible trials are usually referred to as trials that utilize interim monitoring based on group sequential and adaptive methodology for (i) early stopping for clinical benefit or harm, (ii) early stopping for futility, (iii) sample size re-adjustment, and (iv) re-designing the study in midstream. In practice, an adaptive group sequential design is very popular due to the following two reasons. First, clinical endpoint is a moving target. The sponsors and/or investigators may change their minds regarding clinically meaningful effect size after the trial starts. Second, it is a common practice to request a small budget at the design and then seek supplemental funding for increasing the sample size after seeing the interim data.

To protect the overall type I error rate in an adaptive design with respect to adaptations in some design parameters, many authors have proposed procedures using observed treatment effects. This leads to the justification for the commonly used two-stage adaptive design, in which the data from both stages are independent and the first data set is used for adaptation (see, e.g., Proschan and Hunsberger, 1995; Cui, Hung, and Wang, 1999; Liu and Chi, 2001). In recent years, the concept of two-stage adaptive design has led to the development of the adaptive group sequential design. The adaptive group sequential design is referred to as a design that uses observed (or estimated) treatment differences at interim analyses to modify the design and sample size adaptively (e.g., Shen and Fisher, 1999; Cui, Hung, and Wang, 1999; Posch and Bauer, 1999; Lehmacher and Wassmer, 1999).

In clinical research, it is desirable to speed up the trial and at the same time reduce the cost of the trial. The ultimate goal is to get the products to the marketplace sooner. As a result, flexible methods for adaptive group sequential design and monitoring are the key factors for achieving this goal. With the availability of new technology such as electronic data capture, adaptive group sequential design in conjunction with the new technology will provide an integrated solution to the logistical and statistical complexities of monitoring trials in flexible ways without biasing the final conclusions. Further discussion regarding the application of adaptive group sequential designs in clinical trials can be found in Chapter 6.

1.5.6 Adaptive sample size adjustment

As indicated earlier, an adaptive design is very attractive to the sponsors in early clinical development because it allows modifications of the trial to meet specific needs during the trial within limited budget/resources and target timelines. However, an adaptive design suffers from a loss of power to detect a clinically meaningful difference of the target patient population under the actual patient population due to bias/variation that has been introduced to the trial as the result of changes in study parameters during the conduct of the trial. To account for the expected and/or unexpected bias/variation, statistical procedures for sample size calculation are necessarily adjusted for achieving the desired power.

For example, if the study, regimen, and/or treatment duration have been adjusted during the conduct of the trial, not only the actual patient population may be different from the target patient population, but also the baseline for the clinically meaningful difference to be detected may have been changed. In this case, sample size required for achieving the desired power for correctly detecting a clinically meaningful difference based on clinical data collected from the actual patient population definitely needs adjustment.

It should be noted that procedures for sample size calculation based on power analysis of an adaptive design with respect to specific changes in study parameters are very different from the standard methods. The procedures for sample size calculation could be very complicated for a multiple adaptive design (or a combined adaptive design) involving more than one study parameter. In practice, statistical tests for a null hypothesis of no treatment difference may not be tractable under a multiple adaptive design. Chapter 7 provides several methods for adaptive sample size adjustment which are useful for multiple adaptive designs.

1.5.7 Adaptive seamless phase II/III design

A phase II clinical trial is often a dose-response study, where the goal is to find the appropriate dose level for the phase III trials. It is desirable to combine phase II and III so that the data can be used more efficiently and duration of the drug development can be reduced. A seamless phase II/III trial design refers to a program that addresses within a single trial objective what is normally achieved through separate trials in phases IIb and III (Gallo et al., 2006). An adaptive seamless phase II/III design is a seamless phase II/III trial design that would use data from patients enrolled before and after the adaptation in the final analysis (Maca et al., 2006). Bauser and Kieser (1999) provide a two-stage method for this purpose, where the investigators can terminate the trial entirely or drop a subset of regimens for lack of efficacy after the first stage. As pointed out by Sampson and Sill (2005), their procedure is highly flexible, and the distributional assumptions are kept to a minimum. This results in a usual design in a number of settings. However, because of the generality of the method, it is difficult, if not impossible, to construct confidence intervals. Sampson and Sill (2005) derived a uniformly most powerful conditionally unbiased test for normal endpoint. For other types of endpoints, no results match Sampson and Sill's results. Thus, it is suggested that computer trial simulation be used in such cases. More information is provided in Chapter 8.

1.5.8 Adaptive treatment switching

For evaluation of the efficacy and safety of a test treatment for progressive diseases such as oncology and HIV, a parallel-group active-control randomized clinical trial is often conducted. Under the parallel-group active-control randomized clinical trial, qualified patients are randomly assigned to receive either an active control (a standard therapy or a treatment currently available in the marketplace) or a test treatment under investigation. Patients are allowed to switch from one treatment to another, due to ethical consideration, if there is lack of responses or there is evidence of disease progression. In practice, it is not uncommon that up to 80% of patients may switch from one treatment to another. This certainly has an impact on the evaluation of the efficacy of the test treatment. Despite allowing a switch between two treatments, many clinical studies are to compare the test treatment with the active-control agent as if no patients had ever switched. Sommer and Zeger (1991) referred to the treatment effect among patients who complied with treatment as biological efficacy. Branson and Whitehead (2002) widened the concept of biological efficacy to encompass the treatment effect as if all patients adhered to their original randomized treatments in clinical studies allowing treatment switch.

The problem of treatment switching is commonly encountered in cancer trials. In cancer trials, most investigators would allow patients to get off the current treatment and switch to another treatment (either the study treatment or a rescue treatment) when there is progressed disease, due to ethical consideration. However, treatment switching during the conduct of the trial has presented a challenge to clinical scientists (especially biostatisticians) regarding the analysis of some primary study endpoints such as median survival time. Under certain assumptions, Shao, Chang, and Chow (2005) proposed a method for estimation of median survival time when treatment switching occurs during the course of the study. Several methods for adaptive treatment switching are reviewed in Chapter 9.

1.5.9 Bayesian and hybrid approaches

Drug development is a sequence of drug decision-making processes, where decisions are made based on the constantly updated information. The Bayesian approach naturally fits this mechanism. However, in the current regulatory setting, the Bayesian approach is not ready as the criteria for approval of a drug. Therefore, it is desirable to use Bayesian approaches to optimize the trial and increase the probability of success under current frequentist criterion for approval. In the near future, it is expected that drug approval criteria will become Bayesian. In addition, full Bayesian is important because it can provide more informative information and optimal criteria for drug approval based on risk-benefit ratio rather than subjectively (arbitrarily) set $\alpha = 0.05$, as frequentists did.

1.5.10 Clinical trial simulation

It should be noted that for a given adaptive design, it is very likely that adaptations will be made to more than one study parameter simultaneously during the conduct of the clinical trial. To assess the impact of changes in specific study parameters, a typical approach is to perform a sensitivity analysis by fixing other study parameters. In practice, the assessment of the overall impact of changes in each study parameter is almost impossible due to possible confounding and/or masking effects among changes in study parameters. As a result, it is suggested that a clinical trial simulation be conducted to examine the individual and/or overall impact of changes in multiple study parameters. In addition, the performance of a given adaptive design can be evaluated through the conduct of a clinical trial simulation in terms of its sensitivity, robustness, and/or empirical probability of reproducibility. It, however, should be noted that a clinical trial simulation are conducted in such a way that the simulated clinical data are able to reflect the real situation of the clinical trial after all of the modifications are made to the trial procedures and/or statistical procedures. In practice, it is then suggested that assumptions regarding the sources of bias/variation as the results of modifications of the on-going trial be identified and be taken into consideration when conducting the clinical trial simulation.

1.5.11 Case studies

As pointed out by Li (2006), the use of adaptive design methods provides a second chance to re-design the trial after seeing data internally or externally at interim. However, it may introduce so-called operational biases such as selection bias, method of evaluations, early withdrawal, modification of treatments, etc. Consequently, the adaptation employed may inflate type I error rate. Li (2006) suggested a couple of principles when implementing adaptive designs in clinical trials: (i) adaptation should not alter trial conduct, and (ii) type I error should be preserved. Following these principles, some studies with complicated adaptations may be more successful than others. The successful experience for certain adaptive designs in clinical trials is important to investigators in clinical research and development. For illustration purposes, some successful case studies including the implementation of an adaptive group sequential design (Cui, Hung, and Wang, 1999), an adaptive dose-escalation design (Chang and Chow, 2005), and adaptive seamless phase II/III trial design (Maca et al., 2006) are provided in the last chapter of this book.

1.6 Aims and Scope of the Book

This is intended to be the first book entirely devoted to the use of adaptive design methods in clinical trials. It covers all of the statistical issues that may occur at various stages of adaptive design and analysis of clinical trials. It is our goal to provide a useful desk reference and the state-of-the art examination of this area to scientists and researchers engaged in clinical research and development, those in government regulatory agencies who have to make decisions in the pharmaceutical review and approval process, and biostatisticians who provide the statistical support for clinical trials and related clinical investigation. More importantly, we would like to provide graduate students in the areas of clinical development and biostatistics an advanced textbook in the use of adaptive design methods in clinical trials. We hope that this book can serve as a bridge between the pharmaceutical industry, government regulatory agencies, and academia.

The scope of this book covers statistical issues that are commonly encountered when modifications of study procedures and/or statistical procedures are made during the course of the study. In this chapter, the definition, regulatory requirement, target patient population, statistical issues of adaptive design, and analysis for clinical trials have been discussed. In the next chapter, the impact of modifications made to trial procedures and/or statistical procedures on the target patient population, statistical inference, and power analysis for sample size calculation as the result of protocol amendments are discussed. In Chapter 3, various adaptive randomization procedures for treatment allocation will be discussed. Chapter 4 covers adaptive design methods for modifications of hypotheses including the addition of new hypotheses after the review of interim data. Chapter 5 provides an overall review of adaptive design methods for dose selection, especially in dose-finding and dose-response relationship studies in early clinical development. Chapter 6 introduces the commonly used adaptive group sequential design in clinical trials. Blinded procedures for sample size re-estimation are given in Chapter 7. Statistical tests for adaptive seamless phase II/III designs, and statistical inference for switching from one treatment to another

INTRODUCTION

adaptively and the corresponding practical issues that may arise are studied in Chapter 8 and Chapter 9, respectively. Bayesian and hybrid approaches for the use of adaptive design methods in clinical trials are outlined in Chapter 10. Chapter 11 provides an introduction to the methodology of clinical trial simulation for evaluation of the performance of the adaptive design methods under various adaptive designs that are commonly used in clinical development. Case studies regarding the implementation of adaptive group sequential design, adaptive dose-escalation design, and adaptive seamless phase II/III trial design in clinical trials are discussed in Chapter 12.

For each chapter, whenever possible, real examples from clinical trials are included to demonstrate the use of adaptive design methods in clinical trials including clinical/statistical concepts, interpretations, and their relationships and interactions. Comparisons regarding the relative merits and disadvantages of the adaptive design methods in clinical research and development are discussed whenever deemed appropriate. In addition, if applicable, topics for future research are provided. All computations in this book are performed using 8.20 of SAS. Other statistical packages such as S-plus can also be applied.

CHAPTER 2

Protocol Amendment

In clinical trials, it is not uncommon to modify the trial and/or statistical procedures of on-going trials due to scientific/statistical justifications, medical considerations, regulatory concerns, and/or business interest/decisions. When modifications of trial and/or statistical procedures are made, a protocol amendment is necessarily filed to individual institutional review boards (IRBs) for review/approval before implementation. As discussed in the previous chapter, major (or significant) adaptation of trial and/or statistical procedures of a on-going clinical trial could alter the target patient population of the trial and consequently lead to a totally different clinical trial that is unable to answer the scientific/medical questions the trial is intended to address. In this chapter, we will examine the impact of protocol amendments on the target patient population through the assessment of a shift parameter, a scale parameter, and a sensitivity index. The impact of protocol amendments on power for detecting a clinically significant difference and the corresponding statistical inference are also studied.

In the next section, a shift parameter, a scale parameter, and a sensitivity index that provide useful measures of change in the target patient population as the result of protocol amendments are defined. Section 2.2 provides estimates of the shift and scale parameters of the target patient population and the sensitivity index both conditionally and unconditionally, assuming that the resultant actual patient population after modifications is random. The impact of protocol amendments on statistical inference and power analysis for sample size calculation is discussed in Sections 2.3 and 2.4, respectively. Section 2.5 provides statistical inference for treatment effect when there are protocol amendments, assuming that changes in protocol are made based on one or a few covariates. A brief concluding remark is given in the last section of this chapter.

2.1 Actual Patient Population

As indicated earlier, in clinical trials it is not uncommon to modify trial and/or statistical procedures of on-going trials. However, it should be noted that any adaptation made to the trial and/or statistical procedures may introduce bias and/or variation to the data collected from the trial. Most importantly, it may result in a similar but slightly different target patient population. We will refer to such a patient population as the *actual* patient population under study. After a given protocol amendment, we denote the actual patient population by (μ_1, σ_1), where $\mu_1 = \mu + \varepsilon$ is the population mean of the primary study endpoint and $\sigma_1 = C\sigma$ ($C > 0$) denotes the population standard deviation of the primary study endpoint. In this chapter, we will refer to ε and C as the shift and scale parameters of the target patient population (μ, σ) after modification is made. As it can be seen, the difference between the *actual* patient population (μ_1, σ_1) and the original target patient population (μ, σ) can be characterized as follows:

$$\left|\frac{\mu_1}{\sigma_1}\right| = \left|\frac{\mu+\varepsilon}{C\sigma}\right| = \left|\frac{\Delta\mu}{\sigma}\right| = |\Delta|\left|\frac{\mu}{\sigma}\right|,$$

where

$$\Delta = \frac{1+\varepsilon/\mu}{C}$$

is a measure of change in the signal-to-noise ratio of the actual patient population as compared to the original target population. Chow, Shao, and Hu (2002) refer to Δ as the sensitivity index. As a result, the signal-to-noise ratio of the actual patient population can be expressed as the sensitivity index times the effect size (adjusted for standard deviation) of the original target patient population. For example, when $\varepsilon = 0$ and $C = 1$ (i.e., the modification made has no impact on the target patient population), then $\Delta = 1$ (i.e., there is no difference between the target patient population and the actual patient population after the modification). For another example, if $\varepsilon = 0$ and $C = 0.5$ (i.e., there is no change in mean but the variation has reduced by 50% as the result of the modification), then $\Delta = 2$, which is an indication of sensitivity (i.e., the actual effect size to be detected is much larger than the originally planned effect size under the target patient population) as the result of the modifications made.

In practice, each modification to the trial procedures may result in a similar but slightly different actual patient population. Denote by (μ_i, σ_i) the actual patient population after the ith modification of trial procedure, where $\mu_i = \mu + \varepsilon_i$ and $\sigma_i = C_i\sigma$, $i = 0, 1, \ldots, m$. Note that $i = 0$ reduces to the original target patient population (μ, σ). That is, when $i = 0$, $\varepsilon_0 = 0$ and $C_0 = 1$. After m protocol amendments (i.e., m modifications are made to the study protocol), the resultant actual patient population becomes (μ_m, σ_m), where $\mu_m = \mu + \sum_{i=1}^{m} \varepsilon_i$ and $\sigma_m = \prod_{i=1}^{m} C_i\sigma$. It should be noted that (ε_i, C_i), $i = 1, \ldots, m$ are in fact random variables. As a result, the resultant actual patient population

Table 2.1 Changes in Sensitivity Indices With Respect To ε/μ and C

	Inflation of Variability		Deflation of Variability	
ε/μ (%)	C (%)	Δ	C (%)	Δ
−20	100	0.800	—	—
−20	110	0.727	90	0.889
−20	120	0.667	80	1.000
−20	130	0.615	70	1.143
−10	100	0.900	—	—
−10	110	0.818	90	1.000
−10	120	0.750	80	1.125
−10	130	0.692	70	1.571
−5	100	0.950	—	—
−5	110	0.864	90	1.056
−5	120	0.792	80	1.188
−5	130	0.731	70	1.357
0	100	1.000	—	—
0	110	0.909	90	1.111
0	120	0.833	80	1.250
0	130	0.769	70	1.429
5	100	1.050	—	—
5	110	0.955	90	1.167
5	120	0.875	80	1.313
5	130	0.808	70	1.500
10	100	1.100	—	—
10	110	1.000	90	1.222
10	120	0.917	80	1.375
10	130	0.846	70	1.571
20	100	1.200	—	—
20	110	1.091	90	1.333
20	120	1.000	80	1.500
20	130	0.923	70	1.714

following certain modifications to the trial procedures is a *moving* target patient population rather than a fixed target patient population. It should be noted that the effect of ε_i could be offset by C_i for a given modification i as well as by (ε_j, C_j) for another modification j. As a result, estimates of the effects of $(\varepsilon_i, C_i), i = 1, \ldots, m$ are difficult, if not impossible, to obtain. In practice, it is desirable to limit the combined effects of $(\varepsilon_i, C_i), i = 0, \ldots, m$ to an acceptable range for a valid and unbiased assessment of treatment effect regarding the target patient population based on clinical data collected from the actual patient population. Table 2.1 provides changes in Δ with respect to various values

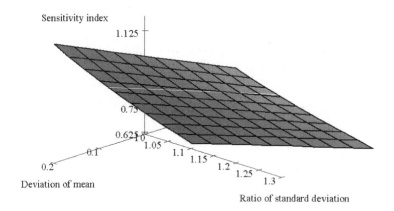

Figure 2.1 3-D Plot of Sensitivity Index Versus ε/μ and C.

of ε/μ and C. As it can be seen from Table 2.1, a shift in mean of target patient population (i.e., ε) may be offset by the scale parameter C, the inflation or reduction of the variability as the result of the modification made.

For example, a shift of 10% (-10%) in mean could be offset by a 10% inflation (reduction) of variability. As a result, Δ may not be sensitive due to the confounding (or masking) effect between ε and C. However, when $C(\varepsilon)$ remains unchanged, Δ is a reasonable measure for the sensitivity since Δ moves away from the unity (no change) as ε (C) increases. To provide a better understanding of the changes in Δ with respect to various values of ε/μ and C, a 3-dimensional plot is given in Figure 2.1. Figure 2.1 confirms that when $C(\varepsilon)$ remains unchanged, Δ moves away from the unity (i.e., there is no change in the target patient population) as ε (C) increases.

2.2 Estimation of Shift and Scale Parameters

The shift and scale parameters (i.e., ε and C) of the target population after a modification (or a protocol amendment) is made can be estimated by

$$\hat{\varepsilon} = \hat{\mu}_{Actual} - \hat{\mu},$$

and

$$\hat{C} = \hat{\sigma}_{Actual}/\hat{\sigma},$$

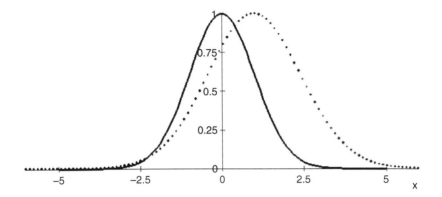

Figure 2.2 Plot of $N(x; \mu, \sigma^2)$ Versus $N(x; \mu_\mu, \sigma^2 + \sigma_\mu^2)$. Note that the solid line is for $N(x; \mu, \sigma^2)$ and the dot line is for $N(x; \mu_\mu, \sigma^2 + \sigma_\mu^2)$.

respectively, where $(\hat{\mu}, \hat{\sigma})$ and $(\hat{\mu}_{Actual}, \hat{\sigma}_{Actual})$ are some estimates of (μ, σ) and $(\mu_{Actual}, \sigma_{Actual})$, respectively. As a result, the sensitivity index can be estimated by

$$\hat{\Delta} = \frac{1 + \hat{\varepsilon}/\hat{\mu}}{\hat{C}}.$$

Estimates for μ and σ can be obtained based on data collected prior to any protocol amendments that are issued. Assume that the response variable x is distributed as $N(\mu, \sigma^2)$. Let x_{ji}, $i = 1, \ldots, n_j$; $j = 0, \ldots, m$ be the response of the ith patient after the jth protocol amendment. As a result, the total number of patients is given by

$$n = \sum_{j=0}^{m} n_j.$$

Note that n_0 is the number of patients in the study prior to any protocol amendments. Based on x_{0i}, $i = 1, \ldots, n_0$, the maximum likelihood estimates of μ and σ^2 can be obtained as follows:

$$\hat{\mu} = \frac{1}{n_0} \sum_{i=1}^{n_0} x_{0i}, \tag{2.1}$$

$$\hat{\sigma}^2 = \frac{1}{n_0} \sum_{i=1}^{n_0} (x_{0i} - \hat{\mu})^2. \tag{2.2}$$

To obtain estimates for μ_{Actual} and σ_{Actual}, for illustration purpose, we will only consider the case where μ_{Actual} is random and σ_{Actual} is fixed. For other cases such as (i) μ_{Actual} is fixed but σ_{Actual} is random, (ii) both μ_{Actual} and σ_{Actual} are random, (iii) μ_{Actual}, σ_{Actual} and n_j are all random, and (iv) μ_{Actual}, σ_{Actual}, n_j, and m are all random, estimates for μ_{Actual} and σ_{Actual} may be obtained following a similar idea.

2.2.1 The case where μ_{Actual} is random and σ_{Actual} is fixed

For convenience's sake, we set $\mu_{Actual} = \mu$ and $\sigma_{Actual} = \sigma$ for the derivation of estimates of ε and C. Assume that x conditional on μ, i.e., $x|_{\mu=\mu_{Actual}}$ follows a normal distribution $N(\mu, \sigma^2)$. That is,

$$x|_{\mu=\mu_{Actual}} \sim N(\mu, \sigma^2), \qquad (2.3)$$

where μ is distributed as $N(\mu_\mu, \sigma_\mu^2)$ and σ, μ_μ, and σ_μ are some unknown constants. Thus, the unconditional distribution of x is a mixed normal distribution given below

$$\int N(x; \mu, \sigma^2) N(\mu; \mu_\mu, \sigma_\mu^2) d\mu = \frac{1}{\sqrt{2\pi\sigma^2}} \frac{1}{\sqrt{2\pi\sigma_\mu^2}} \int_{-\infty}^{\infty} e^{-\frac{(x-\mu)^2}{2\sigma^2} - \frac{(\mu-\mu_\mu)^2}{2\sigma_\mu^2}} d\mu, \qquad (2.4)$$

where $x \in (-\infty, \infty)$. It can be verified that the above mixed normal distribution is a normal distribution with mean μ_μ and variance $\sigma^2 + \sigma_\mu^2$ (see proof given in the next section). In other words, x is distributed as $N(\mu_\mu, \sigma^2 + \sigma_\mu^2)$.

As it can be seen from Figure 2.2 when μ_{Actual} is random and σ_{Actual} is fixed, the shift from the target patient population to the actual population could be substantial, especially for large μ_μ and σ_μ^2.

Maximum Likelihood Estimation Given a protocol amendment j and independent observations x_{ji}, $i = 1, 2, \ldots, n_j$, the likelihood function is given by

$$l_j = \prod_{i=1}^{n_j} \left(\frac{1}{\sqrt{2\pi\sigma^2}} e^{-\frac{(x_{ij}-\mu_j)^2}{2\sigma^2}} \right) \frac{1}{\sqrt{2\pi\sigma_\mu^2}} e^{-\frac{(\mu_j-\mu_\mu)^2}{2\sigma_\mu^2}}, \qquad (2.5)$$

where μ_j is the population mean after the jth protocol amendment. Thus, given m protocol amendments and observations x_{ji}, $i = 1, \ldots, n_j$; $j = 0, \ldots, m$, the likelihood function can be written as

$$L = \prod_{j=0}^{m} l_j = (2\pi\sigma^2)^{-\frac{n}{2}} \prod_{j=0}^{m} \left[e^{-\sum_{i=1}^{n_j} \frac{(x_{ij}-\mu_j)^2}{2\sigma^2}} \frac{1}{\sqrt{2\pi\sigma_\mu^2}} e^{-\frac{(\mu_j-\mu_\mu)^2}{2\sigma_\mu^2}} \right]. \qquad (2.6)$$

Hence, the log-likelihood function is given by

$$LL = -\frac{n}{2}\ln\left(2\pi\sigma^2\right) - \frac{m+1}{2}\ln\left(2\pi\sigma_\mu^2\right) \tag{2.7}$$

$$-\frac{1}{2\sigma^2}\sum_{j=0}^{m}\sum_{i=1}^{n_j}(x_{ij}-\mu_j)^2 - \frac{1}{2\sigma_\mu^2}\sum_{j=0}^{m}(\mu_j-\mu_\mu)^2.$$

Based on (2.7), the maximum likelihood estimates (MLEs) of μ_μ, σ_μ^2, and σ^2 can be obtained as follows:

$$\tilde{\mu}_\mu = \frac{1}{m+1}\sum_{j=0}^{m}\tilde{\mu}_j, \tag{2.8}$$

where

$$\tilde{\mu}_j = \frac{1}{n_j}\sum_{i=1}^{n_j}x_{ji}, \tag{2.9}$$

$$\tilde{\sigma}_\mu^2 = \frac{1}{m+1}\sum_{j=0}^{m}(\tilde{\mu}_j - \tilde{\mu}_\mu)^2, \tag{2.10}$$

and

$$\tilde{\sigma}^2 = \frac{1}{n}\sum_{j=0}^{m}\sum_{i=1}^{n_j}(x_{ji} - \tilde{\mu}_j)^2. \tag{2.11}$$

Note that $\frac{\partial LL}{\partial \mu_j} = 0$ leads to

$$\tilde{\sigma}_\mu^2 \sum_{i=1}^{n_j} x_{ji} + \tilde{\sigma}^2 \tilde{\mu}_\mu - (n_j\tilde{\sigma}_\mu^2 + \tilde{\sigma}^2)\tilde{\mu}_j = 0.$$

In general, when $\tilde{\sigma}_\mu^2$ and $\tilde{\sigma}^2$ are compatible and n_j is reasonably large, $\tilde{\sigma}^2\tilde{\mu}_\mu$ is negligible as compared to $\tilde{\sigma}_\mu^2\sum_{i=1}^{n_j}x_{ji}$ and $\tilde{\sigma}^2$ is negligible as compared to $n_j\tilde{\sigma}_\mu^2$. Thus, we have the approximation (2.9), which greatly simplifies the calculation. Based on these MLEs, estimates of the shift parameter (i.e., ε) and the scale parameter (i.e., C) can be obtained as follows:

$$\tilde{\varepsilon} = \tilde{\mu} - \hat{\mu},$$

$$\tilde{C} = \frac{\tilde{\sigma}}{\hat{\sigma}},$$

respectively. Consequently, the sensitivity index can be estimated by simply replacing ε, μ, and C with their corresponding estimates $\tilde{\varepsilon}$, $\tilde{\mu}$, and $\tilde{C}$.

Remarks In the above derivation, we account for the sequence of protocol amendments assuming that the target patient population has been changed (or shifted) after each protocol amendment. Alternatively, if the cause of the shift in target patient population is not due to the sequence of protocol amendments but rather random protocol deviations or violations, we may obtain the following alternative (conditional) estimates.

Given m protocol deviations or violations and independent observations x_{ji}, $i = 1, \ldots, n_j$; $j = 0, \ldots, m$, the likelihood function can be written as

$$L = \prod_{j=0}^{m} \prod_{i=1}^{n_j} l_{ji}$$

$$= \prod_{j=0}^{m} \left[(2\pi\sigma^2)^{-\frac{n_j}{2}} e^{-\sum_{i=1}^{n_j} \frac{(x_{ij}-\mu_j)^2}{2\sigma^2}} (2\pi\sigma_\mu^2)^{-\frac{n_j}{2}} e^{-\frac{n_j(\mu_j-\mu_\mu)^2}{2\sigma_\mu^2}} \right].$$

Thus, the log-likelihood function is given by

$$LL = -\frac{n}{2}\ln(2\pi\sigma^2) - \frac{n}{2}\ln(2\pi\sigma_\mu^2) \qquad (2.12)$$
$$- \frac{1}{2\sigma^2}\sum_{j=0}^{m}\sum_{i=1}^{n_j}(x_{ij}-\mu_j)^2 - \frac{1}{2\sigma_\mu^2}\sum_{j=0}^{m}[n_j(\mu_j-\mu_\mu)^2].$$

As a result, the maximum likelihood estimates of μ_μ, σ_μ^2, and σ^2 are given by

$$\tilde{\mu}_\mu = \frac{1}{n}\sum_{j=0}^{m}\sum_{i=1}^{n_j} x_{ji} = \hat{\mu}, \qquad (2.13)$$

$$\tilde{\sigma}_\mu^2 = \frac{1}{n}\sum_{j=0}^{m}[n_j(\tilde{\mu}_j - \tilde{\mu}_\mu)^2], \qquad (2.14)$$

$$\tilde{\sigma}^2 = \frac{1}{n}\sum_{j=0}^{m}\sum_{i=1}^{n_j}(x_{ji} - \tilde{\mu}_j)^2, \qquad (2.15)$$

where

$$\tilde{\mu}_j \approx \frac{1}{n_j}\sum_{i=1}^{n_j} x_{ji}.$$

Similarly, under random protocol violations, the estimates of μ_μ, σ_μ^2, and σ^2 can also be obtained based on the unconditional probability distribution described in (2.4) as follows. Given m protocol amendments and observations x_{ji}, $i = 1, \ldots, n_j$; $j = 0, \ldots, m$, the likelihood function can be written as

$$L = \prod_{j=0}^{m}\prod_{i=1}^{n_j} \left(\frac{1}{\sqrt{2\pi(\sigma^2+\sigma_\mu^2)}} e^{-\frac{(x_{ji}-\mu_\mu)^2}{2(\sigma^2+\sigma_\mu^2)}} \right).$$

Hence, the log-likelihood function is given by

$$LL = -\frac{n}{2}\ln\left[2\pi(\sigma^2+\sigma_\mu^2)\right] + \sum_{j=0}^{m}\sum_{i=1}^{n_j} \frac{(x_{ji}-\mu_\mu)^2}{2(\sigma^2+\sigma_\mu^2)}. \quad (2.16)$$

Based on (2.16), the maximum likelihood estimates of μ_μ, σ_μ^2, and σ^2 can be easily found. However, it should be noted that the MLE for μ_μ and $\sigma_*^2 = (\sigma^2 + \sigma_\mu^2)$ are unique but the MLEs for σ^2 and σ_μ^2 are not unique. Thus, we have

$$\tilde{\mu} = \tilde{\mu}_\mu = \frac{1}{n}\sum_{j=0}^{m}\sum_{i=1}^{n_j} x_{ji},$$

$$\tilde{\sigma}^2 = \tilde{\sigma}_*^2 = \frac{1}{n}\sum_{j=0}^{m}\sum_{i=1}^{n_j}(x_{ji}-\tilde{\mu})^2.$$

In this case, the sensitivity index is equal to 1. In other words, random protocol deviations or violations (or the sequence of protocol amendments) do not have an impact on statistical inference on the target patient population. It, however, should be noted that the sequence of protocol amendments usually result in a moving target patient population in practice. As a result, the above estimates of μ_μ and σ_*^2 are often misused and misinterpreted.

2.3 Statistical Inference

To illustrate the impact on statistical inference regarding the target patient population after m protocol amendments, for simplicity, we will only focus on statistical inference on ε, C, and Δ for the case where μ_{Actual} is random and σ_{Actual} is fixed. For the cases where (i) μ_{Actual} is fixed and σ_{Actual} is random, (ii) both μ_{Actual} and σ_{Actual} are random, (iii) μ_{Actual}, σ_{Actual}, and n_j are all random, and (iv) μ_{Actual}, σ_{Actual}, n_j, and m are all random, the idea described in this section can be similarly applied.

First, we note that the test statistic is dependent on sampling procedure (it is a combination of protocol amendment and randomization). The following theorem is useful. We will frequently use the well-known fact that linear combination of independent variables with normal distribution or asymptotic normal distribution follows a normal distribution. Specifically,

Theorem 2.1 *Suppose that $X|_\mu \sim N(\mu, \sigma^2)$ and $\mu \sim N(\mu_\mu, \sigma_\mu^2)$, then*

$$X \sim N(\mu_\mu, \sigma^2 + \sigma_\mu^2) \tag{2.17}$$

Proof. *Consider the following characteristic function of a normal distribution $N(t; \mu, \sigma^2)$*

$$\phi_0(w) = \frac{1}{\sqrt{2\pi\sigma^2}} \int_{-\infty}^{\infty} e^{iwt - \frac{1}{2\sigma^2}(t-\mu)^2} dt = e^{iw\mu - \frac{1}{2}\sigma^2 w^2}. \tag{2.18}$$

For distribution $X|_\mu \sim N(\mu, \sigma^2)$ and $\mu \sim N(\mu_\mu, \sigma_\mu^2)$, the characteristic function after exchange the order of the two integrations is given by

$$\phi(w) = \int_{-\infty}^{\infty} e^{iw\mu - \frac{1}{2}\sigma^2 w^2} N(\mu; \mu_\mu, \sigma_\mu^2) d\mu = \int_{-\infty}^{\infty} e^{iw\mu - \frac{\mu - \mu_\mu}{2\sigma_\mu^2} - \frac{1}{2}\sigma^2 w^2} d\mu.$$

Note that

$$\int_{-\infty}^{\infty} e^{iw\mu - \frac{(\mu - \mu_\mu)^2}{2\sigma_\mu^2}} d\mu = e^{iw\mu - \frac{1}{2}\sigma^2 w^2}$$

is the characteristic function of the normal distribution. It follows that

$$\phi(w) = e^{iw\mu - \frac{1}{2}(\sigma^2 + \sigma_\mu^2)w^2},$$

which is the characteristic function of $N(\mu_\mu, \sigma^2 + \sigma_\mu^2)$. This completes the proof. □

Given protocol amendment j and that x_{ji}, $i = 1, 2, \ldots, n_j$ are independent and identically distributed (i.i.d.) normal $N(\mu_j, \sigma^2)$,

$$\tilde{\mu}_j = \frac{1}{n_j} \sum_{i=1}^{n_j} x_{ji}$$

is conditionally normally distributed with mean μ_j and variance $\frac{\sigma^2}{n_j}$, i.e.,

$$\tilde{\mu}_j \sim N\left(\mu_j, \frac{\sigma^2}{n_j}\right).$$

In addition,

$$\mu_j \sim N(\mu_\mu, \sigma_\mu).$$

Hence, from the above theorem, $\tilde{\mu}_j$ is normally distributed with mean μ_μ and variance $\frac{\sigma^2}{n_j} + \sigma_\mu^2$, i.e.,

$$\tilde{\mu}_j \sim N\left(\mu_\mu, \frac{\sigma^2}{n_j} + \sigma_\mu^2\right), \tag{2.19}$$

and
$$\tilde{\mu} \sim N\left(\mu_\mu, \frac{\sigma^2}{(m+1)^2}\sum_{j=0}^{m}\left(\frac{1}{n_j}\right) + \frac{\sigma_\mu^2}{m+1}\right), \quad (2.20)$$

where
$$\tilde{\mu} = \frac{1}{m+1}\sum_{j=0}^{m}\tilde{\mu}_j. \quad (2.21)$$

If n_j is random, i.e., n_j follows a distribution, say f_{n_j}, then, we have

$$\tilde{\mu} \sim \sum_{k}^{\infty} f_k N\left(\mu_\mu, \frac{\sigma^2}{(m+1)^2}\left(\frac{1}{k}\right) + \frac{\sigma_\mu^2}{m+1}\right). \quad (2.22)$$

Note that at the end of the study, σ^2 and σ_μ^2 can be replaced with their estimates if m and n_j are sufficiently large.

For two independent samples, we have
$$\tilde{\mu}_1 - \tilde{\mu}_2 \sim N(\mu_{\mu_1} - \mu_{\mu_2}, \sigma_p^2),$$
where
$$\sigma_p^2 = \frac{\sigma_1^2}{(m_1+1)^2}\sum_{j=0}^{m_1}\left(\frac{1}{n_{1j}}\right) + \frac{\sigma_{\mu_1}^2}{m_1+1} + \frac{\sigma_2^2}{(m_2+1)^2}\sum_{j=0}^{m_2}\left(\frac{1}{n_{2j}}\right) + \frac{\sigma_{\mu_2}^2}{m_2+1}, \quad (2.23)$$

and m_1 and m_2 are the number of modifications made to the two groups respectively.

2.3.1 Test for equality

To test whether there is a difference between the mean response of a test compound as compared to a placebo control or an active control agent, the following hypotheses are usually considered:
$$H_0: \mu_1 = \mu_2 \quad \text{vs} \quad H_a: \mu_1 \neq \mu_2.$$
Under the null hypothesis, the test statistic is given by
$$z = \frac{\tilde{\mu}_1 - \tilde{\mu}_2}{\tilde{\sigma}_p}, \quad (2.24)$$

where $\tilde{\mu}_1$ and $\tilde{\mu}_2$ can be estimated from (2.8) and (2.9) and σ_p^2 can be estimated using (2.23) with estimated variances from (2.10) and (2.11). Under the null hypothesis, the test statistic follows a standard normal distribution for large sample. Thus, we reject the null hypothesis at the α level of significance if $z > z_{\alpha/2}$.

2.3.2 Test for non-inferiority/superiority

As indicated by Chow, Shao, and Wang (2003), the problem of testing non-inferiority and (clinical) superiority can be unified by the following hypotheses:

$$H_0 : \mu_1 - \mu_2 \leq \delta \quad \text{vs} \quad H_a : \mu_1 - \mu_2 > \delta,$$

where δ is the non-inferiority or superiority margin. When $\delta > 0$, the rejection of the null hypothesis indicates the superiority of the test compound over the control. When $\delta < 0$, the rejection of the null hypothesis indicates the non-inferiority of the test compound against the control. Under the null hypothesis, the test statistic

$$z = \frac{\tilde{\mu}_1 - \tilde{\mu}_2 - \delta}{\tilde{\sigma}_p} \qquad (2.25)$$

follows a standard normal distribution for large sample. Thus, we reject the null hypothesis at the α level of significance if $z > z_\alpha$.

It should be noted that α level for testing non-inferiority or superiority should be 0.025 instead of 0.05 because when $\delta = 0$, the test statistic should be the same as that for testing equality. Otherwise, we may claim superiority with a small δ that is close to zero for observing an easy statistical significance. In practice, the choice of δ plays an important role for the success of the clinical trial. It is suggested that δ should be chosen in such a way that it is both statistically and clinically justifiable. The European Agency for the Evaluation of Medicinal Products recently issued a draft points to consider guideline on the choice of non-inferiority margin (EMEA, 2004). Along this line, Chow and Shao (2006) provided some statistical justification for the choice of δ in clinical trials.

2.3.3 Test for equivalence

For testing equivalence, the following hypotheses are usually considered:

$$H_0 : |\mu_1 - \mu_2| > \delta \quad \text{vs} \quad H_a : |\mu_1 - \mu_2| \leq \delta,$$

where δ is the equivalence limit. Thus, the null hypothesis is rejected and the test compound is concluded to be equivalent to the control if

$$\frac{\tilde{\mu}_1 - \tilde{\mu}_2 - \delta}{\tilde{\sigma}_p} \leq -z_\alpha \quad \text{or} \quad \frac{\tilde{\mu}_1 - \tilde{\mu}_2 - \delta}{\tilde{\sigma}_p} \geq z_\alpha. \qquad (2.26)$$

It should be noted that the FDA recommends an equivalence limit of (80%,125%) for bioequivalence based on geometric means using log-transformed data.

2.4 Sample Size Adjustment

2.4.1 Test for equality

The hypotheses for testing equality of two independent means can be written as

$$H_0 : \varepsilon = \mu_1 - \mu_2 = 0 \quad \text{vs} \quad H_a : \varepsilon \neq 0.$$

Under the alternative hypothesis that $\varepsilon \neq 0$, the power of the above test is given by

$$\Phi\left(\frac{\varepsilon}{\tilde{\sigma}_p} - z_{\alpha/2}\right) + \Phi\left(\frac{-\varepsilon}{\tilde{\sigma}_p} - z_{\alpha/2}\right) \approx \Phi\left(\frac{|\varepsilon|}{\tilde{\sigma}_p} - z_{\alpha/2}\right). \quad (2.27)$$

Since the true difference ε is an unknown, we can estimate the power by replacing ε in (2.27) with the estimated value $\tilde{\varepsilon}$. As a result, the sample size needed to achieve the desired power of $1 - \beta$ can be obtained by solving the following equation

$$\frac{|\varepsilon|}{\tilde{\sigma}_e \sqrt{\frac{2}{n}}} - z_{\alpha/2} = z_\beta, \quad (2.28)$$

where n is the sample size per group, and

$$\tilde{\sigma}_e = \sqrt{\frac{n}{2}\tilde{\sigma}_p^2} = \sqrt{\frac{\tilde{\sigma}^2}{(m+1)^2} \sum_{j=0}^{m} \left(\frac{n}{n_j}\right) + \frac{n\tilde{\sigma}_\mu^2}{(m+1)}} \quad (2.29)$$

for homogeneous variance condition and balance design. This leads to the sample size formulation

$$n = \frac{4(z_{1-\alpha/2} + z_{1-\beta})^2 \tilde{\sigma}_e^2}{\varepsilon^2}, \quad (2.30)$$

where ε, $\tilde{\sigma}^2$, $\tilde{\sigma}_\mu^2$, m, and $r_j = \frac{n_j}{n}$ are estimates at the planning stage of a given clinical trial. The sample size can be easily solved iteratively. Note that if $n_j = \frac{n}{m+1}$, then

$$n = \frac{4(z_{1-\alpha/2} + z_{1-\beta})^2 \left(\tilde{\sigma}^2 + \frac{n\tilde{\sigma}_\mu^2}{m+1}\right)}{\varepsilon^2}.$$

Solving the above equation for n, we have

$$n = \frac{1}{R} \frac{4(z_{1-\alpha/2} + z_{1-\beta})^2 (\tilde{\sigma}^2 + \tilde{\sigma}_\mu^2)}{\varepsilon^2} = \frac{1}{R} n_{classic}, \quad (2.31)$$

Table 2.2 Relative Efficiency

m	$\frac{\tilde{\sigma}_\mu^2}{\tilde{\sigma}^2}$	$\frac{\tilde{\sigma}_\mu^2}{\varepsilon^2}$	R
0	0.05	0.005	0.83
1	0.05	0.005	0.94
2	0.05	0.005	0.98
3	0.05	0.005	0.99
4	0.05	0.005	1.00

Note: $\alpha = 0.05$, $\beta = 0.1$.

where R is the relative efficiency given by

$$R = \frac{n_{classic}}{n} = \left(1 + \frac{\tilde{\sigma}_\mu^2}{\tilde{\sigma}^2}\right)\left(1 - \frac{4(z_{1-\alpha/2} + z_{1-\beta})^2}{\varepsilon^2} \frac{\tilde{\sigma}_\mu^2}{m+1}\right). \quad (2.32)$$

Table 2.2 provides various m and $\tilde{\sigma}_\mu^2$ with respect to R. As it can be seen from Table 2.2, an increase of m will result in a decrease of n. Consequently, there is a significant decrease of the desired power of the intended trial when no amendment $m = 0$ and $\tilde{\sigma}_\mu^2 = 0$, $R = 1$.

2.4.2 Test for non-inferiority/superiority

The hypotheses for testing non-inferiority or (clinical) superiority of a mean can be written as

$$H_0 : \varepsilon = \mu_1 - \mu_2 \leq \delta \quad \text{vs} \quad H_a : \varepsilon > \delta,$$

where δ is the non-inferiority or (clinical) superiority margin. Under the alternative hypothesis $\varepsilon > 0$, the power of the above test is given by

$$\Phi\left(\frac{\varepsilon - \delta}{\tilde{\sigma}_e \sqrt{\frac{2}{n}}} - z_{\alpha/2}\right). \quad (2.33)$$

The sample size required for achieving the desired power of $1 - \beta$ can be obtained by solving the following equation

$$\frac{\varepsilon - \delta}{\tilde{\sigma}_e \sqrt{\frac{2}{n}}} - z_{\alpha/2} = z_\beta. \quad (2.34)$$

This leads to

$$n = \frac{2(z_{1-\alpha} + z_{1-\beta})^2 \tilde{\sigma}_e^2}{(\varepsilon - \delta)^2}, \quad (2.35)$$

where $\tilde{\sigma}_e^2$ is given by (2.29), and ε, $\tilde{\sigma}^2$, $\tilde{\sigma}_\mu^2$, m, and $r_j = \frac{n_j}{n}$ are estimates at the planning stage of a given clinical trial. The sample size can be easily solved iteratively. If $n_j = \frac{n}{m+1}$, then the sample size can be explicitly written as

$$n = \frac{1}{R} \frac{(z_{1-\alpha} + z_{1-\beta})^2 \tilde{\sigma}^2}{(\varepsilon - \delta)^2}, \qquad (2.36)$$

where R is the relative efficiency given by

$$R = \frac{n}{n_{classic}} = \left(1 - \frac{(z_{1-\alpha} + z_{1-\beta})^2}{(\varepsilon - \delta)^2} \frac{\tilde{\sigma}_\mu^2}{m+1}\right). \qquad (2.37)$$

2.4.3 Test for equivalence

The hypotheses for testing equivalence can be written as

$$H_0 : |\varepsilon| = |\mu_1 - \mu_2| > \delta \quad \text{vs} \quad H_a : |\varepsilon| \leq \delta,$$

where δ is the equivalence limit. Under the alternative hypothesis that $|\varepsilon| \leq \delta$, the power of the of the test is given by

$$\Phi\left(\frac{\delta - \varepsilon}{\tilde{\sigma}_e \sqrt{\frac{2}{n}}} - z_\alpha\right) + \Phi\left(\frac{\delta + \varepsilon}{\tilde{\sigma}_e \sqrt{\frac{2}{n}}} - z_\alpha\right) - 1 \qquad (2.38)$$

$$\approx 2\Phi\left(\frac{\delta - |\varepsilon|}{\tilde{\sigma}_e \sqrt{\frac{2}{n}}} - z_\alpha\right) - 1.$$

As a result, the sample size needed in order to achieve the desired power of $1 - \beta$ can be obtained by solving the following equation

$$\frac{\delta - |\varepsilon|}{\tilde{\sigma}_e \sqrt{\frac{2}{n}}} - z_\alpha = z_{\beta/2}. \qquad (2.39)$$

This leads to

$$n = \frac{2(z_{1-\alpha} + z_{1-\beta/2})^2 \tilde{\sigma}_e^2}{(|\varepsilon| - \delta)^2}, \qquad (2.40)$$

where $\tilde{\sigma}_e^2$ is given by (2.29). If $n_j = \frac{n}{m+1}$, then the sample size is given by

$$n = \frac{1}{R} \frac{(z_{1-\alpha} + z_{1-\beta/2})^2 \tilde{\sigma}^2}{(|\varepsilon| - \delta)^2}, \qquad (2.41)$$

where R is the relative efficiency given by

$$R = \frac{n}{n_{classic}} = \left(1 - \frac{(z_{1-\alpha} + z_{1-\beta/2})^2}{(|\varepsilon| - \delta)^2} \frac{\tilde{\sigma}_\mu^2}{m+1}\right). \tag{2.42}$$

2.5 Statistical Inference with Covariate Adjustment

As indicated earlier, statistical methods of analyzing clinical data should be modified when there are protocol amendments during the trial, since any protocol deviations and/or violations may introduce bias to the conclusion drawn based on the analysis of data with no changes made to the study protocol. For example, the target patient population of the clinical trial is typically defined through the patient inclusion/exclusion criteria. If the patient inclusion/exclusion criteria are modified during the trial, then the resulting data may not be from the target patient population in the original protocol and, thus, statistical methods of analysis have to be modified to reflect this change. Chow and Shao (2005) modeled the population deviations due to protocol amendments using some covariates and developed a valid statistical inference which is outlined in this section.

2.5.1 Population and assumption

In this section, for convenience's sake, we denote the target patient population by $\mathcal{P}_0$. Parameters related to $\mathcal{P}_0$ are indexed by a subscript 0. For example, in a comparative clinical trial comparing a test treatment and a control, the effect size of the test treatment (or a given study endpoint) is $\mu_{0T} - \mu_{0C}$, where μ_{0T} and μ_{0C} are respectively the population means of the test treatment and the control for patients in $\mathcal{P}_0$.

Suppose that there are a total of K possible protocol amendments. Let $\mathcal{P}_k$ be the patient population after the kth protocol amendment, $k = 1, \ldots, K$. As indicated earlier, a protocol change may result in a patient population similar but slightly different from the original target patient population, i.e., $\mathcal{P}_k$ may be different from $\mathcal{P}_0$, $k = 1, \ldots, K$. For example, when patient enrollment is too slow due to stringent patient inclusion/exclusion criteria, a typical approach is to relax the inclusion/exclusion criteria to increase the enrollment, which results in a patient population larger than the target patient population. Because of the possible population deviations due to protocol amendments, standard statistical methods may not be appropriate and may lead to invalid inference/conclusion regarding the target patient population.

Let μ_k be the mean of the study variable related to the patient population $\mathcal{P}_k$ after the kth protocol amendment, $k = 1, \ldots, K$. Note that the subscript T or C to indicate the test treatment and the control is omitted for simplicity in general discussion. Suppose that, for each k, clinical data are observed from n_k patients so that the sample mean $\bar{y}_k$ is an unbiased estimator of μ_k, $k = 0, 1, \ldots, K$. Ignoring the difference among $\mathcal{P}_k$'s results in an estimator $\bar{y} = \sum_k n_k \bar{y}_k / \sum_k n_k$, which is an unbiased estimator of a weighted average of μ_k's, not the original defined treatment effect μ_0.

In many clinical trials, protocol changes are made by using one or a few covariates. Modifying patient inclusion/exclusion criteria, for example, may involve patient age or ethnic factors. Treatment duration, study dose/regimen, factors related to laboratory testing, or diagnostic procedures are other examples of such covariates. Let $\mathbf{x}$ be a (possibly multivariate) covariate whose values are distinct for different protocol amendments. Throughout this article we assume that

$$\mu_k = \beta_0 + \beta' \mathbf{x}_k, \quad k = 0, 1, \ldots, K, \qquad (2.43)$$

where β_0 is an unknown parameter, β is an unknown parameter vector whose dimension is the same as $\mathbf{x}$, β' denotes the transpose of β, and $\mathbf{x}_k$ is the value of $\mathbf{x}$ under the kth amendment (or the original protocol when $k = 0$). If values of $\mathbf{x}$ are different within a fixed population $\mathcal{P}_k$, then $\mathbf{x}_k$ is a characteristic of $\mathbf{x}$ such as the average of all values of $\mathbf{x}$ within $\mathcal{P}_k$.

Although $\mu_1, \ldots, \mu_K$ are different from μ_0, model (2.43) relates them with the covariate $\mathbf{x}$. Statistical inference on μ_0 (or more generally, any function of $\mu_0, \mu_1, \ldots, \mu_K$) can be made based on model (2.43) and data from $\mathcal{P}_k$, $k = 0, 1, \ldots, K$.

2.5.2 Conditional inference

We first consider inference conditional on a fixed set of $K \geq 1$ protocol amendments. Following the notation in the previous section, let $\bar{y}_k$ be the sample mean based on n_k clinical data from $\mathcal{P}_k$, which is an unbiased estimator of μ_k, $k = 0, 1, \ldots, K$. Again, a subscript T or C should be added when we consider the test treatment or the control. Under model (2.43), parameters β_0 and β can be unbiasedly estimated by

$$\begin{pmatrix} \hat{\beta}_0 \\ \hat{\beta} \end{pmatrix} = (\mathbf{X}'\mathbf{W}\mathbf{X})^{-1}\mathbf{X}'\mathbf{W}\bar{\mathbf{y}}, \qquad (2.44)$$

where $\bar{\mathbf{y}} = (\bar{y}_0, \bar{y}_1, \ldots, \bar{y}_K)'$, $\mathbf{X}$ is a matrix whose kth row is $(1, \mathbf{x}'_k)$, $k = 0, 1, \ldots, K$, and $\mathbf{W}$ is a diagonal matrix whose diagonal elements are $n_0, n_1, \ldots, n_K$. Here, we assume that the dimension of $\mathbf{x}$ is less or equal to K so that $(\mathbf{X'WX})^{-1}$ is well defined. To estimate μ_0, we may use the following unbiased estimator:

$$\hat{\mu}_0 = \hat{\beta}_0 + \hat{\beta}'\mathbf{x}_0.$$

For inference on μ_0, we need to derive the sampling distribution of $\hat{\mu}_0$. Assume first that, conditional on the given protocol amendments, data from each $\mathcal{P}_k$ are normally distributed with a common standard deviation σ. Since each $\bar{y}_k$ is distributed as $N(\mu_k, \sigma^2/n_k)$ and it is reasonable to assume that data from different $\mathcal{P}_k$'s are independent, $\hat{\mu}_0$ is distributed as $N(\mu_0, \sigma^2 c_0)$ with

$$c_0 = (1, \mathbf{x}_0)(\mathbf{X'WX})^{-1}(1, \mathbf{x}_0)'.$$

Let s_k^2 be the sample variance based on the data from $\mathcal{P}_k, k = 0, 1, \ldots, K$. Then, $(n_k - 1)s_k^2/\sigma^2$ has the chi-square distribution with $n_k - 1$ degrees of freedom and, consequently, $(N-K)s^2/\sigma^2$ has the chi-square distribution with $N - K$ degrees of freedom, where

$$s^2 = \sum_k (n_k - 1)s_k^2/(N - K)$$

and $N = \sum_k n_k$. Confidence intervals for μ_0 and testing hypotheses related to μ_0 can be carried out using the t-statistic $t = (\hat{\mu}_0 - \mu_0)/\sqrt{c_0 s^2}$.

When $\mathcal{P}_k$'s have different standard deviations and/or data from $\mathcal{P}_k$ are not normally distributed, we have to use approximation by assuming that all n_k's are large. By the central limit theorem, when all n_k's are large, $\hat{\mu}_0$ is approximately normally distributed with mean μ_0 and variance

$$\tau^2 = (1, \mathbf{x}_0)(\mathbf{X'WX})^{-1}\mathbf{X'W\Sigma X}(\mathbf{X'WX})^{-1}(1, \mathbf{x}_0)', \qquad (2.45)$$

where Σ is the diagonal matrix whose kth diagonal element is the population variance of $\mathcal{P}_k, k = 0, 1, \ldots, K$. Large sample statistical inference can be made by using the z-statistic $z = (\hat{\mu}_0 - \mu_0)/\hat{\tau}$ (which is approximately distributed as the standard normal), where $\hat{\tau}$ is the same as τ with the kth diagonal element of Σ estimated by $s_k^2, k = 0, 1, \ldots, K$.

2.5.3 Unconditional inference

In practice, protocol amendments are usually made in a random fashion; that is, the investigator of an on-going trial decides to make a protocol change with certain probability and, in some cases, changes are made based on the accrued data of the trial. Let $\mathcal{C}_K$ denote a particular set of K protocol amendments as described in the previous sections, and let $\mathcal{C}$ be the collection of all possible sets of protocol amendments. For example, suppose that there are a total of M possible protocol amendments

PROTOCOL AMENDMENT 41

indexed by $1, \ldots, M$. Let C_K be a subset of $K \leq M$ integers, i.e.,

$$C_K = \{i_1, \ldots, i_K\} \subset \{1, \ldots, M\}.$$

Then, C_K denotes the set of protocol amendments $i_1, \ldots, i_K$ and $\mathcal{C}$ is the collection of all subsets of $\{1, \ldots, M\}$. In a particular problem, C_K is chosen based on a (random) decision rule ξ (often referred to as adaptation rule) and $P(C_K) = P(\xi = C_K)$, the probability that C_K is the realization of protocol amendments, is between 0 and 1 and $\sum_{C_K \in \mathcal{C}} P(C_K) = 1$.

For a particular C_K, let z_{C_K} be the z-statistic defined in the previous section and let $\mathcal{L}(z_{C_K} | \xi = C_K)$ be the conditional distribution of z_ξ given $\xi = C_K$. Suppose that $\mathcal{L}(z_{C_K} | \xi = C_K)$ is approximately standard normal for almost every sequence of realization of ξ. We now show that $\mathcal{L}(z_\xi)$, the unconditional distribution of z_ξ, is also approximately standard normal. According to Theorem 1 in Liu, Proschan, and Hedger (2002),

$$\mathcal{L}(z_\xi) = E\left[\sum_{C_K \in \mathcal{C}} \mathcal{L}(z_{C_K} | \xi = C_K) I_{\xi = C_K}\right], \quad (2.46)$$

where $I_{\xi = C_K}$ is the indicator function of the set $\{\xi = C_K\}$ and the expectation E is with respect to the randomness of ξ. For every fixed real number t, by the assumption,

$$P(z_{C_K} \leq t | \xi = C_K) \to \Phi(t) \quad \text{almost surely,} \quad (2.47)$$

where Φ is the standard normal distribution function. Multiplying $I_{\xi = C_K}$ to both sides of (2.47) leads to

$$P(z_{C_K} \leq t | \xi = C_K) I_{\xi = C_K} \to \Phi(t) I_{\xi = C_K} \quad \text{almost surely.} \quad (2.48)$$

Since the left-hand side of (2.48) is bounded by 1, by the dominated convergence theorem,

$$E\left[P(z_{C_K} \leq t | \xi = C_K) I_{\xi = C_K}\right] \to E\left[\Phi(t) I_{\xi = C_K}\right]$$
$$= \Phi(t) E\left[I_{\xi = C_K}\right]$$
$$= \Phi(t) P(C_K).$$

It follows from (2.46) and (2.47) that

$$P(z_\xi \leq t) = \sum_{C_K \in \mathcal{C}} E\left[P(z_{C_K} \leq t | \xi = C_K) I_{\xi = C_K}\right]$$
$$\to \sum_{C_K \in \mathcal{C}} \Phi(t) P(C_K)$$
$$= \Phi(t).$$

Hence, large sample inference can be made using the z-statistic z_ξ.

It should be noted that the finite distribution of z_ξ given by (2.46) may be very complicated. Furthermore, assumption (2.47), i.e., $\mathcal{L}(z_{C_K}|\xi = C_K)$ is approximately standard normal for almost every sequence of realization of ξ, has to be verified in each application (via the construction of z_{C_K} and asymptotic theory such as the central limit theorem). Assumption (2.47) certainly holds when the adaptation rule ξ and z_{C_K} are independent for each $C_K \in \mathcal{C}$. For example, when protocol changes are modifying patient inclusion/exclusion criteria, the adaptation rule ξ is related to patient recruiting and, thus, is typically independent of the main study variable such as the drug efficacy. Another example is adjustments of study dose/regimen because of safety considerations, which may be approximately independent with the drug efficacy. Some other examples can be found in Liu, Proschan, and Hedger (2002).

Example 2.1 A placebo-control clinical trial was conducted to evaluate the efficacy of an investigational drug for treatment of patients with asthma. The primary study endpoint is the change in FEV1 (forced expired volume per second), which is defined to be the difference between the FEV1 after treatment and the baseline FEV1. During the conduct of the clinical trial, the protocol was amended twice due to slow enrollment. For each protocol amendment, a modification to the inclusion criterion regarding the baseline FEV1 was made. In the original protocol, patients were included if and only if their baseline FEV1 were between 1.5 Liters and 2.0 Liters. At the first and the second protocol amendments, the range of the baseline FEV1 in this inclusion criterion was changed to, respectively, 1.5 Liters to 2.5 Liters and 1.5 Liters to 3.0 Liters. Some summary statistics are given in Table 2.3.

We first consider the analysis conditional on the two protocol amendments, i.e., the sample size (number of patients) in each period of the trial (before or after protocol amendments) is treated as fixed.

Table 2.3 Summary Statistics in the Asthma Trial Example

	Baseline FEV1 Range	Number of Patients	Baseline FEV1 Mean	FEV1 Change Mean	FEV1 Change S.D.
	1.5 ~ 2.0	9	1.86	0.31	0.14
Test drug	1.5 ~ 2.5	15	2.30	0.42	0.14
	1.5 ~ 3.0	16	2.79	0.54	0.16
	1.5 ~ 2.0	8	1.82	0.16	0.15
Placebo	1.5 ~ 2.5	16	2.29	0.19	0.13
	1.5 ~ 3.0	16	2.84	0.20	0.14

Following the procedure described on the previous page with the mean of baseline FEV1 as the (one-dimensional) covariate $\mathbf{x}$ in assumption (2.43), we obtain estimates $\hat{\beta}_0 = -0.14$ and $\hat{\beta} = 0.25$ (according to formula (2.44)) for the test drug. Then, an estimate of μ_0, the population mean for the test drug under the original protocol, is $\hat{\mu}_0 = -0.14 + 0.25 \times 1.86 = 0.33$. An estimated τ according to formula (2.48) with elements of Σ estimated by sample variances is $\hat{\tau} = 0.04$. Similarly, for the placebo, the population mean under the original protocol is estimated as $0.099 + 0.038 \times 1.82 = 0.17$ with estimated τ to be 0.04. Thus, an estimate of the population mean difference (between the test drug and placebo under the original protocol) is $0.33 - 0.17 = 0.16$ with an estimated standard error $\sqrt{2} \times 0.04 = 0.057$. The approximate p-value for the one-sided null hypothesis that the test drug mean is no larger than the placebo mean is equal to 0.0021, and the approximate p-value for the two-sided null hypothesis that the test drug mean is the same as the placebo mean is 0.0042.

If we ignore the protocol amendments and combine all data, then our estimate of the mean difference between the test drug and placebo is 0.25, which is clearly biased. On the other hand, one may perform an analysis based on patients enrolled before the first protocol amendment, i.e., 9 patients in the test drug group and 8 patients in the placebo group. The resulting estimate of the mean difference between the test drug and placebo is 0.15 with an estimated standard error $\sqrt{2} \times 0.047 = 0.066$. The approximate p-value is 0.0116 for the one-sided null hypothesis and 0.0232 for the two-sided null hypothesis. The test drug effect seems less significant, but this is due to the use of data gathered before the first protocol amendment.

We now consider unconditional analysis. As we discussed above, if the adaptation rule is independent of the z-statistic for every possible way of making protocol amendments, then the z-statistic is still valid for unconditional analysis. In the asthma trial example, protocol amendments were made because of the slow enrollment and, hence, could be viewed as a process independent of the FEV1 change scores. Thus, the conclusions based on the conditional analysis and unconditional analysis in this example are the same.

2.6 Concluding Remarks

As indicated in this chapter, it is not uncommon to issue protocol amendments during the conduct of a clinical trial. The protocol amendments are necessary to describe what changes have been made and the rationales behind the changes to ensure the validity and integrity of the clinical trial. As the result of the modifications, the original target patient population under study could have become a similar but different patient population. If the modifications are made frequently during the conduct of the trial, the target patient population is in fact a moving target patient population. In practice, there is a risk that major (or significant) modifications made to the trial and/or statistical procedures could lead to a totally different trial, which cannot address the scientific/medical questions that the clinical trial is intended to answer. Thus, it is of interest to measure the impact of each modification made to the trial procedures and/or statistical procedure after the protocol amendment. In this chapter, it is suggested that independent estimates of ε, C and Δ, which are measures of the shift of mean response, cause the inflation/reduction of variability of the response and effect size of the primary study endpoint, respectively. The estimates of ε, C and Δ are useful in providing the signal regarding how the target patient population has been changed due to the protocol amendment. In practice, it should be noted that reliable estimates of ε, C and Δ may not be available for trials with small sample sizes. In other words, the estimates of ε, C and Δ may not be accurate and reliable because it is possible that only a few observations are available after the protocol amendment, especially when there are a number of protocol amendments. In addition, although we consider the case where the sample size after protocol amendment is random, the number of protocol amendments is also a random variable, which complicates the already complicated procedure for obtained accurate and reliable estimates of ε, C and Δ. In practice, it should be recognized that protocol amendments are not given gifts. Potential risks for introducing additional bias/variation as the result of modifications made should be carefully evaluated before addressing the issue of a protocol amendment. It is important to identify, control, and hopefully eliminate/minimize the sources of bias/variation. For good clinical and/or statistical practices, it is then strongly suggested that the protocol amendments be limited to a small number such as 2 or 3 in clinical trials.

In current practice, standard statistical methods are applied to the data collected from the actual patient population regardless the frequency of changes (protocol amendments) that have been made during the conduct of the trial, provided that the overall type I error is controlled at the pre-specified level of significance. This, however, has raised a serious regulatory/statistical concern as to whether the resultant statistical inference (e.g., independent estimates, confidence intervals, and p-values) drawn on the originally planned target patient population based on the clinical data from the actual patient population (as the result of the modifications made via protocol amendments) are accurate and reliable. As discussed in this chapter, the impact on statistical inference due to protocol amendments could be substantial, especially when there are major modifications, which have resulted in a significant shift in mean response and/or inflation of the variability of response of the study parameters. It is suggested that a sensitivity analysis with respect to changes in study parameters be performed to provide a better understanding on the impact of changes (protocol amendments) in study parameters on statistical inference. Thus, regulatory guidance on *what range of changes in study parameters are considered acceptable* is necessary. As indicated earlier, adaptive design methods are very attractive to the clinical researchers and/or sponsors due to their flexibility, especially in clinical trials of early clinical development. It, however, should be noted that there is a high risk that a clinical trial using adaptive design methods may fail in terms of its scientific validity and/or its limitation of providing useful information with a desired power, especially when the sizes of the trials are relatively small and there are a number of protocol amendments. In addition, statistically it is a challenge to clinical researchers when there are missing values. The causes of missing values could be related to or unrelated to the changes or modifications made in the protocol amendments. In this case, missing values must be handled carefully to provide an unbiased assessment and interpretation of the treatment effect.

For some types of protocol amendments, the method proposed by Chow and Shao (2005) gives valid statistical inference for characteristics (such as the population mean) of the original patient population. The key assumption in handling population deviation due to protocol amendments is assumption (2.43), which has to be verified in each application. Although a more complicated model (such as a non-linear model in **x**) may be considered, model (2.43) leads to simple derivations of sampling distributions of the statistics used in inference. The other difficult issue in handling protocol amendments (or, more generally, adaptive designs) is the fact that the decision rule for protocol amendments (or the adaptation rule) is often random and related to the main study variable through the accrued data of the on-going trial. Chow and Shao (2005) showed that if an approximate pivotal quantity conditional on each realization of the adaptation rule can be found, then it is also approximately pivotal unconditionally and can be used for unconditional inference. Further research on the construction of approximate pivotal quantities conditional on the adaptation rule in various problems is needed.

After some modifications are made to the trial and/or statistical procedures, not only the target patient population may have become a similar but different patient population, but also the sample size may not achieve the desired power for detection of a clinically important effect size of the test treatment at the end of the study. In practice, we expect to lose power when the modifications have led to a shift in mean response and/or inflation of variability of the response of the primary study endpoint. As a result, the originally planned sample size may have to be adjusted. In this chapter, it is suggested that the relative efficiency at each protocol amendment be taken into consideration for derivation of an adjusted factor for sample size in order to achieve the desired power. More details regarding the adjustment of sample size when various adaptive designs/methods are used in clinical trials are given in the subsequent chapters of this book.

CHAPTER 3

Adaptive Randomization

Randomization plays an important role in clinical research. For a given clinical trial, appropriate use of randomization procedure not only ensures that the subjects selected for the clinical trial are a truly representative sample of the target patient population under study, but also provides an unbiased and fair assessment regarding the efficacy and safety of the test treatment under investigation. As pointed out in Chow and Liu (2003), statistical inference of the efficacy and safety of a test treatment under study relies on the probability distribution of the primary study endpoints of the trial, which in turn depends on the randomization model/method employed for the trial. Inadequate randomization model/method may violate the primary distribution assumption and consequently distort statistical inference. As a result, the conclusion drawn based on the clinical data collected from the trial may be biased and/or misleading.

Based on the allocation probability (i.e., the probability of assigning a patient to a treatment), the randomization procedures that are commonly employed in clinical trials can be classified into four categories: conventional randomization, treatment-adaptive randomization, covariate-adaptive randomization, and response-adaptive randomization. The conventional randomization refers to any randomization procedures with a constant treatment allocation probability. Commonly used conventional randomization procedures include simple (or complete) randomization, stratified randomization, and cluster randomization. Unlike the conventional randomization procedures, treatment allocation probabilities for adaptive randomization procedures usually vary over time depending upon the cumulative information on the previously assigned patients. Similar to the conventional randomization procedures, treatment-adaptive randomization procedures can also be prepared in advance. For covariate-adaptive randomization and response-adaptive randomization procedures, the randomization codes are usually generated in a dynamically real-time fashion. This is because the randomization procedure is based on the patient information on covariates or response observed up to the time when the randomization is performed. Treatment-adaptive randomization and covariate-adaptive randomization are usually considered to reduce treatment imbalance or deviation from the target sample size ratio between treatment groups. On the other hand, response-adaptive randomization procedure emphasizes ethical consideration, i.e., it is desirable to provide patients with better/best treatment based on the knowledge about the treatment effect at that moment.

In practice, conventional randomization procedures could result in severe treatment imbalance at some time point during the trial or at the end of the trial, especially when there is a time-dependent heterogeneous covariance that relates to treatment responses. Treatment imbalance could decrease statistical power for demonstration of treatment effect of the intended trial and consequently the validity of the trial. In this chapter, we attempt to provide a comprehensive review of various randomization procedures from each category.

In the next section, the conventional randomization procedures are briefly reviewed. In Section 3.2, we introduce some commonly used treatment-adaptive randomization procedures in clinical trials. Several covariate-adaptive randomization procedures and response-adaptive randomization methods are discussed in Section 3.3 and Section 3.4, respectively. In Section 3.5, some practical issues in adaptive randomization are examined. A brief summary is given in the last section of this chapter.

3.1 Conventional Randomization

As mentioned earlier, the treatment allocation probability of conventional randomization procedures is a fixed constant. As a result, it allows the experimenters to prepare the randomization codes in advance. The conventional randomization procedures are commonly employed in clinical trials, particularly in double-blind randomized clinical trials. In what follows, we introduce some commonly employed conventional randomization procedures, namely, simple randomization, stratified randomization, and cluster randomization.

Simple randomization

Simple (or complete) randomization is probably one of the most commonly employed conventional randomization procedures in clinical trials. Consider a clinical trial for comparing the efficacy and safety of k treatments in treating patients with certain diseases. For a simple randomization, each patient is randomly assigned to each of the k treatment groups with a fixed allocation probability $p_i (i = 1, \ldots, k)$, where $\sum_{i=1}^{k} p_i = 1$. The allocation probabilities are often expressed as the ratio between the sample size (n_i) of the ith treatment group and the overall sample size $(n = \sum_{i=1}^{k} n_i)$, i.e., $p_i = \frac{n_i}{n}$, which is usually referred to as the *sample size ratio* of the ith treatment group. In the interest of treatment balance, an equal allocation probability for each treatment group (i.e., $p_i = p$ for all i) is usually considered, which has the following advantages. First, it has the most (optimal) statistical power for correct detection of a clinically meaningful difference under the condition of equal variances. Second, it is ethical in the sense of equal toxicity (Lachin, 1988). In practice, however, it may be of interest to have an unequal allocation between treatment groups. For example, it may be desirable to assign more patients to the treatment group than a placebo group. It, however, should be noted that a balanced design may not achieve the optimal power when there is heterogeneity in variance between treatment groups. The optimal power can only be achieved when the sample size ratio is proportional to the standard deviation of the group.

The simple (complete) randomization for a two-arm parallel group clinical trial can be easily performed assuming that the treatment assignments are independent Bernoulli random variable with a success probability of 0.5. In practice, treatment imbalance inevitably occurs even by chance alone. Since this treatment imbalance could result in a decrease in power for detecting a clinically meaningful difference, it is of interest to examine the probability of imbalance. Denote the two treatments under study by treatment A and treatment B, respectively. Let $D_n = N_A(n) - N_B(n)$ be the measure of the imbalance in treatment assignment at stage n, where $N_A(n)$ and $N_B(n)$ are the sample size of treatment A and treatment B at stage n, respectively. Then, the *imbalance* D_n is asymptotically normally distributed with mean 0 and variance n. Therefore, the probability of imbalance, for a real value $r > 0$, is given by (see, e.g., Rosenberger et al., 2002; Rosenberger and Lachin, 2002)

$$P(|D_n| > r) = 2\left[1 - \Phi\left(\frac{r}{\sqrt{n}}\right)\right]. \tag{3.1}$$

The sample size for a unbalanced design with homogeneous variance is given by

$$n = \frac{1}{R} \frac{2(z_{1-\alpha/2} + z_{1-\beta})\sigma^2}{\delta^2},$$

where the relative efficiency R is a function of sample size ratio $k = \frac{n_2}{n_1}$ between the two groups, i.e.,

$$R = \frac{4}{2 + k + 1/k}.$$

Table 3.1 Relative Efficiencies

Sample Size Ratio, k	Relative Efficiency, R	Pr(Efficiency< R)
1	1	1
1.5	0.96	0.11
2	0.889	0.01
2.5	0.816	0.001

Note: n = 64.

Let
$$r = n_2 - n_1 = \frac{k-1}{1+k}n.$$
Then
$$P(|D_n| > r) = 2\left[1 - \Phi\left(\frac{k-1}{1+k}\sqrt{n}\right)\right].$$

As it can be seen from Table 3.1, $\Pr(R < 0.96) = 11\%$ and $\Pr(R < 0.899) = 1\%$. Thus, $\Pr(0.899 < R < 0.96) = 10\%$.

Stratified randomization

As discussed above, simple (complete) randomization does not assure the balance between treatment groups. The impact of treatment imbalance could be substantial. In practice, treatment imbalance could become very critical, especially when there are important covariates. In this case, stratified randomization is usually recommended to reduce treatment imbalance. For a stratified randomization, the target patient population is divided into several homogenous strata, which are usually determined by some combinations of covariates (e.g., patient demographics or patient characteristics). In each stratum, a simple (complete) randomization is then employed. Similarly, treatment imbalance of stratified randomization for a clinical trial comparing two treatment groups can be characterized by the following probability of imbalance asymptotically (see, e.g., Hallstron and Davis, 1988)

$$P(|D| > r) = 2\left[1 - \Phi\left(\frac{r}{\sqrt{Var(D)}}\right)\right], \quad (3.2)$$

where
$$Var(D) = \frac{\sum_{i=1}^{s} b_i + s}{6},$$

s is the number of strata, b_i is the size of the ith block, and

$$D = \sum_{i=1}^{s} |N_i - 2A_i|,$$

in which N_i and A_i are the number of patients and the number of patients in treatment A within the ith stratum, respectively.

When the number of strata is large, it is difficult to achieve treatment balance across all stages. This imbalance will decrease the power of statistical analysis such as the analysis of covariance (ANCOVA).

Cluster randomization

In certain trials, the appropriate unit of randomization may be some aggregate of individuals. This form of randomization is known as cluster randomization or group randomization. Cluster randomization is employed by necessity in trials in which the intervention is by nature designed to be applied at the cluster level such as community-based interventions. In the simple cluster randomization, the degree of imbalance can be derived based on simple randomization, i.e.,

$$P(|D_{n_{cluster}}| > r) = 2\left[1 - \Phi\left(\frac{r}{\sqrt{n_{cluster}}}\right)\right],$$

where

$$D_{n_{cluster}} = N_{cluster\ A}(n_{cluster}) - N_{cluster\ B}(n_{cluster}).$$

The number of clusters is $N_{cluster} = N/k$ where k is the number of subjects within each cluster. Then

$$D_{n_{cluster}} = D_{n/k} = \frac{N_A(n/k)}{k} - \frac{N_B(n/k)}{k}.$$

Thus we have

$$P(|D_n|/k > r) = 2\left[1 - \Phi\left(\frac{r}{\sqrt{n}}\right)\right].$$

It can be written as

$$P(|D_n| > r) = 2\left[1 - \Phi\left(\frac{r}{k\sqrt{n}}\right)\right].$$

It should be noted that the analysis for a cluster-randomized trial is very different from that of an individual subject–based randomization trial. A cluster-randomization trial requires adequate numbers of both individual subjects and clusters.

Remarks For a given sample size, the statistically most powerful design is defined as a design with allocation probabilities proportional to the standard deviation of the group. For binary responses, Neyman's treatment allocation with the following allocation ratio leads to a most powerful design

$$r = n_a/n_b = \left(\frac{p_a}{p_b}\frac{1-p_a}{1-p_b}\right)^{\frac{1}{2}}, \qquad (3.3)$$

where p_a and p_b are the proportions for treatment A and treatment B, respectively. Note that for the most powerful design, the target imbalance is $r_0 \neq 0$ and the power of a design can be measured by the quantity

$$P(|D| > r - r_0).$$

3.2 Treatment-Adaptive Randomization

Treatment-adaptive randomization is also known as variance-adaptive randomization. The purpose of a treatment-adaptive randomization is to achieve a more balanced design or to reduce the deviation from the target treatment allocation ratio by utilizing a varied allocation probability. Commonly used treatment-adaptive randomization models in clinical research and development include *block randomization*, *a biased-coin model*, and various *urn models*. To introduce these randomization procedures, consider a two-arm parallel group randomized clinical trial comparing a test treatment (A) with a control (B).

Block randomization

In block randomization, the allocation probability is a fixed constant before any of the two treatment groups reach its target number. However, after the target number is reached in one of the two treatment groups, all the future patients in the trial will be assigned to the other treatment group. As a result, block randomization is a deterministic randomization procedure. It should be noted that although the block size of the block randomization can vary, a small block size will reduce the randomness. The minimum block size commonly chosen in clinical trials is two, which leads to an alternative assignment of the two treatments. In variance-adaptive randomization, the imbalance can be reduced or eliminated when the target number of patients is exactly randomized. Note that when there are two treatment groups, the block randomization is sometimes referred to as a *truncated binomial randomization*.

The allocation probability is defined as

$$P = \begin{cases} 0 & \text{if } N_A(j-1) = n/2, \\ 1 & \text{if } N_B(j-1) = n/2, \\ 0.5 & \text{otherwise,} \end{cases}$$

where $N_A(j-1)$ and $N_B(j-1)$ are the sample size of treatment A and treatment B at stage $j-1$, respectively and $n/2$ is the target number for each group.

Efron's biased coin model

Efron (1971) proposed a biased coin design to balance treatment assignment. The allocation rule to treatment A is defined as follows:

$$P(\delta_j | \Delta_{j-1}) = \begin{cases} 0.5 & \text{if } N_A(j) = N_B(j), \\ p & \text{if } N_A(j) < N_B(j), \\ 1-p & \text{if } N_A(j) > N_B(j), \end{cases}$$

where δ_j is a binary indicator for treatment assignment of the jth subject, i.e., $\delta_j = 1$ if treatment A is assigned and $\delta_j = 0$ if treatment B is assigned, and $\Delta_{j-1} = \{\delta_1, \ldots, \delta_{j-1}\}$ is the set of treatment assignment up to subject $j-1$. The imbalance is measured by

$$|D_n| = |N_A(n) - n|.$$

The limiting balance property can be obtained by random walk method as follows:

$$\lim_{m \to \infty} \Pr(|D_{2m}| = 0) = 1 - \frac{1-p}{p},$$

$$\lim_{m \to \infty} \Pr(|D_{2m}| = 1) = 1 - \frac{(1-p)^2}{p^2}.$$

Note that for an odd number of patients, the minimum imbalance is 1. It can be seen that as $p \to 1$, we achieve perfect balance. But such a procedure is deterministic.

Lachin's urn model

Lachin's urn model is another typical example of variance-adaptive randomization. The model is described as follows. Suppose that there are N_A white balls and N_B red balls in an urn initially. A ball is randomly drawn from the urn *without* replacement. If it is a white ball, the patient is assigned to receive treatment A; otherwise, the patient is assigned to receive treatment B. Therefore, if N_A and N_B are the target sample sizes for treatment groups A and B, respectively, the target sample size ratio (or balance) is always reached if the total planned number of patients is reached. The treatment allocation probability for treatment group A in a trial comparing two treatment groups is

$$P(A) = \frac{\frac{n}{2} - N_A(j-1)}{N_A + N_B - (j-1)}.$$

Although Lachin's urn model can result in a *perfect* balance design after all patients are randomized, the maximum imbalance occurs when half of the treatment allocations are completed, which is given by

$$P_{\max}(|D_n| > r) = 2\left[1 - \Phi\left(\frac{2r}{n}\sqrt{(n-1)}\right)\right].$$

Friedman-Wei's urn model

The Friedman-Wei's urn model is a popular model that can reduce possible treatment imbalance (see, e.g., Friedman, 1949; Wei, 1977; Rosenberger and Lachin, 2002). The Friedman-Wei's urn model is described below. Suppose that there is an urn containing a white balls and a red balls. For treatment assignment, a ball is drawn at random and then replaced. If the ball is white, then treatment A is assigned. On the other hand, if a red ball is drawn, then treatment B is assigned. Furthermore, b additional balls of the opposite color of the ball chosen are added to the urn. Note that a and b could be any reasonable nonnegative numbers. This drawing procedure is replaced for each treatment assignment. Denote a urn design by $UD(a, b)$. The allocation rule for $UD(a, b)$ can then be defined mathematically as follows:

$$P(\delta_j = 1|\Delta_{j-1}) = \frac{a + bN_B(j-1)}{2a + b(j-1)}. \tag{3.4}$$

Note that $UD(a, 0)$ is nothing but a simple or complete randomization.

Let D_n be the absolute difference in number of subjects between the two treatment groups after the nth treatment assignment. Then D_n forms a stochastic process with possible values $d \in \{0, 1, 2, \ldots, n\}$. At initial, $D_0 = 0$. The $(n+1)th$ stage transition probabilities are then given by (see also Wei, 1977)

$$\Pr(D_{n+1} = d - 1|D_n = d) = 1/2 + bd[2(2a + bn)], \tag{3.5}$$

$$\Pr(D_{n+1} = d + 1|D_n = d) = 1/2 - bd[2(2a + bn)],$$

$$\Pr(D_{n+1} = 1|D_n = 0) = 1,$$

where $n \geq d \geq 1$. Note that $P(d, n)$ is a monotonically increasing function with respect to d and a monotonically decreasing function with respect to n. $P(d, n)$ tends to 1/2 as n increases for a fixed $d > 0$. Therefore, the $UD(a, b)$ forces the trial to be more balanced when severe imbalance occurs. In addition, $UD(a, b)$ can also ensure the balance of a relatively small trial. It should be noted that $UD(a, b)$ behaves like the complete randomization design as n increases.

The transition probabilities in (3.1) can be used recursively to calculate the probability of an imbalance of degree d at any stage of the trial as

$$\Pr(D_{n+1} = d) = \Pr(D_{n+1} = d | D_n = d - 1) \Pr(D_{n+1} = d - 1)$$
$$+ \Pr(D_{n+1} = d | D_n = d + 1) \Pr(D_{n+1} = d + 1). \quad (3.7)$$

For a moderate or large n, the probability of imbalance is approximately the normal distribution, $D_n \sim N\left(0, \frac{n(a+b)}{3b-a}\right)$. As a result, the probability of imbalance for large sample size n can be expressed as

$$P(|D_n| > r) = 2\left\{1 - \Phi\left(r\sqrt{\frac{3b-a}{n(a+b)}}\right)\right\}. \quad (3.8)$$

Remarks The urn procedure is relative easy to implement. It forces a small-scale trial to be balanced but approaches complete randomization as the sample size increases. It has less vulnerability to selection bias than does the permuted-block design, biased-coin design, or random allocation rule. As n increases, the potential selection bias approaches to the complete randomization for which the expected selection bias is zero. The urn design can also be extended to the prospective stratification trial when the number of strata is either small or large.

The urn design can easily be generalized to the case of multiple-group comparisons (Wei, 1978; Wei, Smythe, and Smith 1986). We can even further generalize it using different a and b for difference groups in the urn model.

3.3 Covariate-Adaptive Randomization

The *covariate-adaptive randomization* is usually considered to reduce the covariate imbalance between treatment groups. Thus, the covariate-adaptive randomization is also known as *adaptive stratification*. Allocation probability for the covariate-adaptive randomization is modified over time during the trial based on the cumulative information about baseline covariates and treatment assignments. Covariate-adaptive randomization includes Zelen's model, Pocock-Simon's model, Wei's marginal urn design, minimization, and the Atkinson optimal model, which will be briefly described below.

Zelen's model

Zelen's model (Zelen, 1974) requires a simple randomization sequence. When the imbalance reaches a certain threshold, the next subject will be forced to be assigned to be the group with fewer subjects. Let $N_{ik}(n)$ be the number of patients in stratum $i = 1, 2, \ldots, s$ of the kth treatment $k = 1, 2$. When patient $n+1$ in stratum i is ready to be randomized, one computes $D_i(n) = N_{i1}(n) - N_{i2}(n)$. For an integer c, if $|D_i(n)| < c$, then the patient is randomized according to schedule; otherwise, the patient will be assigned to the group with fewer subjects, where the constant can be $c = 2, 3$, or 4 as Zelen suggested.

Pocock-Simon's model

Similar to the Zelen's model, Pocock and Simon (1975) proposed an alternative covariate-adaptive randomization procedure. We follow Rosenberger and Lachin's descriptions of the method (Rosenberger and Lachin, 2002). Let $N_{ijk}(n), i = 1, \ldots, I, j = 0, 2, \ldots, n_i$, and $k = 1, 2$ (1 = treatment A, 2 = treatment B) be the number of patients in stratum j of covariate i on treatment k after n patients have been randomized. Note that $\prod_{i=1}^{I} n_i = s$ is the total number of strata in the trial. Suppose the $(n + 1)$th patient to be randomized is a member of strata $r_1, \ldots, r_I$ of covariates $1, \ldots, I$. Let $D_i(n) = N_{ir_i1} - N_{ir_i2}$. Define the following weighted difference measure $D(n) = \sum_{i=1}^{I} w_i D_i(n)$, where w_i are weights chosen depending on which covariates are deemed of greater importance. If $D(n)$ is less than 1/2, then the weighted difference measure indicates that B has been favored thus far for that set, $r_1, \ldots, r_I$, of strata and the patient $n + 1$ should be assigned with higher probability to treatment A, and vice versa. If $D(n)$ is greater than $1/2$, Pocock and Simon (1975) suggested biasing a coin with

$$p = \frac{c^* + 1}{3}$$

and implementing the following rule: if $D(n) < 1/2$, then assign the next patient to treatment A with probability p; if $D(n) > 1/2$, then assign the next patient to treatment B with probability p; and if $D(n) = 1/2$, then assign the next patient to treatment A with probability $1/2$, where $c^* \in [1/2, 1]$.

Note that if $c^* = 1$, we have a rule very similar to Efron's biased coin design as described in the previous section. If $c^* = 2$, we have the deterministic minimization method proposed by Taves (1974) (see also Simon, 1979). Note that many other rules could also be derived following the Zelen's rule and Taves's minimization method with a biased coin

ADAPTIVE RANDOMIZATION

twist to give added randomization. Efron (1980) described one of such rules and applied it to a clinical trial in ovarian cancer research.

Pocock and Simon (1975) also generalized their covariate-adaptive randomization procedure to more than two treatments. They suggested the following allocation rule be applied:

$$p_k = c^* - \frac{2(Kc^* - 1)k}{K(K+1)}, \quad k = 1,\ldots, K,$$

where K is the number of treatments.

Wei's marginal urn design

In practice, when the number of covariates results in a large number of strata with small stratum sizes, the use of a separate urn in each stratum could result in treatment imbalance within strata. Wei (1978) proposed *marginal urn design* for solving the problem. Instead of using N urns, one for each unique stratum, he suggested using the urn with maximum imbalance to do the randomization each time. For a given new subject with covariate values $r(1), \ldots, r(I)$, treatment imbalance within each of the corresponding urns is calculated. The one with the greatest imbalance is used to generate the treatment assignment for the next subject. A ball from that urn is chosen with replacement. Meanwhile, b balls representing the opposite treatment are added to the urns corresponding to that patient's covariate values. Wei (1978) called this approach a *marginal urn design* because it tends to balance treatment assignments within each category of each covariate marginally, and thus also jointly (Rosenberger and Lachin, 2002).

Imbalance minimization model

Imbalance minimization allocation has been advocated as an alternative to the stratified randomization when there are large numbers of prognostic variables under the imbalance minimization model (Birkett, 1985). The allocation of a patient is determined as follows. A new patient is first classified according to the prognostic variables of interest. He/she is then tentatively assigned to each treatment group in turn, and a summary measure of the resulting treatment imbalance is calculated. The measure of imbalance is obtained by summing the absolute value of excess number of patients receiving one treatment rather than other treatment within every level of each prognostic variable. The two measures are compared, and final allocation is made to that group that minimizes that imbalance measurement. As indicated by Birkett (1985), the imbalance minimization would help gain the power.

Although minimization has been widely used in clinical trials, it is a concern that the potential risk of enabling the investigator to break the code due to the deterministic nature of the allocation may bias the enrollment of patients (Ravaris et al., 1976; Gillis and Ratkowsky, 1978; Weinthrau et al., 1977).

Atkinson optimal model

Atkinson (1982) considered a linear regression model to minimize the variance of treatment contrast in the presence of important covariates. The allocation rule is given by

$$p_k = \frac{d_A(k, \xi_n)}{\sum_{k=1}^{K} d_A(k, \xi_n)}, \qquad (3.9)$$

where

$$\xi_n = \arg\max_{\xi} \left\{ |A'M^{-1}(\xi)A|^{-1} \right\}, \qquad (3.10)$$

in which $M = X'X$ is the $p \times p$ dispersion matrix from n observations, and A is an $s \times p$ matrix of contrasts, $s < p$. More details regarding Atkinson's optimal model can be found in Atkinson and Donev (1992).

3.4 Response-Adaptive Randomization

Response-adaptive randomization is a randomization technique in which the allocation of patients to treatment groups is based on the response (outcome) of the previous patients. The purpose is to provide the patients better/best treatment based on the knowledge about the treatment effect at that moment. As a result, response-adaptive randomization takes the ethical concern into consideration. The well-known response-adaptive models include play-the-winner (PW) model, randomized play-the-winner (RPW) model, Rosenberger's optimization model, Bandit model, and optimal model with finite population. In what follows, these response-adaptive randomization models will be briefly described.

Play-the-winner model

Play-the-winner (PW) model can be easily applied to clinical trials comparing two treatments (e.g., treatment A and treatment B) with binary outcomes (i.e., *success* or *failure*). For PW model, it is assumed that the previous subject's outcome will be available before the next patient is randomized. The treatment assignment is based on treatment response of the previous patient. If a patient responds to treatment A, then the

ADAPTIVE RANDOMIZATION

next patient will be assigned to treatment A. Similarly, if a patient responds to treatment B, then the next patient will be assigned to treatment B. If the assessment of previous patient is not available, the treatment assignment can be based on the last available patient with response assessment or randomly assigned to treatment A or B. It is obvious that this model lacks randomness.

Randomized play-the-winner model

The randomized play-the-winner (RPW) model is a simple probabilistic model to sequentially randomize subjects in a clinical trial (see, e.g., Rosenberger, 1999; Coad and Rosenberger, 1999). RPW model is useful especially for clinical trials comparing two treatments with binary outcomes. For RPW, it is assumed that the previous subject's outcome will be available before the next patient is randomized. At the start of the clinical trial, an urn contains α_A balls for treatment A and α_B balls for treatment B, where α_A and α_B are positive integers. For convenience's sake, we will denote these balls by either type A or type B balls. When a subject is recruited, a ball is drawn and replaced. If it is a type A ball, the subject receives treatment A; if it is type B, the subject receives treatment B. When a subject's outcome is available, the urn is updated. A success on treatment A or a failure on treatment B will generate an additional b type B balls in the urn, where b is a positive integer. In this way, the urn builds up more balls representing the more successful (or less successful) treatment.

There are some interesting asymptotic properties with RPW. Let N_a/N be the proportion of subjects assigned to treatment A out of N subjects. Also, let $q_a = 1 - p_a$ and $q_b = 1 - p_b$ be the failure probabilities. Further, let F be the total number of failures. Then, we have (Wei and Durham, 1978)

$$\lim_{N \to \infty} \frac{N_a}{N_b} = \frac{q_b}{q_a}, \quad (3.11)$$

$$\lim_{N \to \infty} \frac{N_a}{N} = \frac{q_b}{q_a + q_b},$$

$$\lim_{N \to \infty} \frac{F}{N} = \frac{2 q_a q_b}{q_a + q_b}.$$

Note that for balanced randomization, $E(F/N) = (q_a + q_b)/2$.

Since treatment assignment is based on response of previous patients in RPW model, it is not optimized with respect to any clinical endpoint. It is reasonable to randomize treatment assignment based on some optimal criteria such as minimizing the expected numbers treatment failures. This leads to the so-called optimal designs.

Optimal RPW model

Adaptive designs have long been proposed for ethical reasons. The basic idea is to skew allocation probabilities to reflect the response history of patients, hopefully giving a greater than 50% chance of a patient's receiving the treatment performing better thus far in the trial. The optimal randomized play-winner model (ORPW) is to minimize the number of failures in the trial.

There are three commonly used efficacy endpoints in clinic trials, namely, simple proportion difference ($p_a - p_b$), the relative risk (p_a/p_b), and the odds ratio ($p_a q_b / p_b q_a$), where $q_a = 1 - p_a$ and $q_b = 1 - p_b$ are failure rates. These can be estimated consistently by replacing p_a with $\hat{p}_a$ and p_b with $\hat{p}_b$, where $\hat{p}_a$ and $\hat{p}_b$ are the proportions of observed successes in treatment groups A and B, respectively. Suppose that we wish to find the optimal allocation $r = n_a/n_b$ such that it minimizes the expected number of treatment failures $n_a q_a + n_b q_b$, which is mathematically given by

$$r^* = \arg\min_r \{n_a q_a + n_b q_b\} \qquad (3.12)$$

$$= \arg\min_r \left\{ \frac{r}{1+r} n q_a + \frac{1}{1+r} n q_b \right\}.$$

For simple proportion difference, the asymptotic variance is given by

$$\frac{p_a q_a}{n_a} + \frac{p_b q_b}{n_b} = \frac{(1+r)(p_a q_a + r\, p_b q_b)}{nr} = K, \qquad (3.13)$$

where K is some constant. Solving (3.13) for n yields

$$n = \frac{(1+r)(p_a q_a + r\, p_b q_b)}{rK}. \qquad (3.14)$$

Substituting (3.14) into (3.13), we obtain

$$r^* = \arg\min_r \left\{ \frac{(r\, p_a + q_b)(p_a q_a + r\, p_b q_b)}{rK} \right\}. \qquad (3.15)$$

Taking the derivative of (3.14) with respect to r and equating to zero, we have

$$r^* = \left(\frac{p_a}{p_b} \right)^{\frac{1}{2}}.$$

Note that r^* does not depend on K.

Note that the limiting allocation for the RPW rule ($\frac{q_b}{q_a}$) is not optimal for any of the three measures. It is also interesting to note that none of

ADAPTIVE RANDOMIZATION

Table 3.2 Asymptotic Variance with RPW

Measure	r^*	Asymptotic Variance
Proportion difference	$\left(\frac{p_a}{p_b}\right)^{\frac{1}{2}}$	$\frac{p_a q_a}{n_a} + \frac{p_b q_b}{n_b}$
Relative risk	$\left(\frac{p_a}{p_b}\right)^{\frac{1}{2}} \left(\frac{q_b}{q_a}\right)$	$\frac{p_a q_b^2}{n_a q_a^3} + \frac{p_b q_b}{n_b q_a^2}$
Odds ratio	$\left(\frac{p_b}{p_a}\right)^{\frac{1}{2}} \left(\frac{q_b}{q_a}\right)$	$\frac{p_a q_b^2}{n_a q_a^3 p_b^2} + \frac{p_b q_b}{n_b q_a^2 p_b^2}$

Source: Rosenberger and Lachin (2002), p. 176.

the optimal allocation rules yields Neyman allocation given by (Melfi and Page, 1998)

$$r^* = \left(\frac{p_a q_a}{p_b q_b}\right)^{\frac{1}{2}},$$

which minimizes the variance of the difference in sample proportions. Note that Neyman allocation would be unethical when $p_a > p_b$ (i.e., more patients receive the inferior treatment, Table 3.2).

Because the optimal allocation depends on the unknown binomial parameters, we must develop a sequential design that can approximate the optimal design. The rule for the proportion difference is to simply replace the unknown success probabilities in the optimal allocation rule by the current estimate of the proportion of successes (i.e., $\hat{p}_{a,n}$ and $\hat{p}_{b,n}$) observed in each treatment group thus far. This leads to the so-called sequential maximum likelihood procedure. Alternatively, we can use a Bayesian approach such as Bandit allocation rule, where different optimal criteria can be optionally utilized.

Bandit model

A bandit allocation rule is a Bayesian approach that utilizes prior information on unknown parameters in conjunction with incoming data to determine optimal treatment assignment at each stage of the trial (Hardwick and Stout, 1991, 1993, 2002). The weighting of returns is known as discounting, which consists of multiplying the payoff of each outcome by the corresponding element of a discount sequence. The properties of any given bandit allocation rule depend upon the associated discount sequence and prior distribution.

Consider a two-arm bandit (TAB) design for the two proportion difference. The procedure can be described as follows.

(1) Binary outcomes X_{ia} and X_{ib} for the two treatment groups are Bernoulli random variable:
$$X_{ia} \sim B(1, p_a), \qquad (3.16)$$
and
$$X_{ib} \sim B(1, p_b), \quad i = 1, 2, \ldots, n.$$

(2) Prior distribution is assumed to be a beta distribution:
$$p_a \sim Beta(a_0, b_0), \qquad (3.17)$$
and
$$p_b \sim Beta(c_0, d_0).$$

(3) At stage $m \leq n$, the posteriors of p_a and p_b are given by
$$(p_a|k, i, j) \sim Beta(a, b), \qquad (3.18)$$
and
$$(p_b|k, i, j) \sim Beta(c, d),$$
where
$$k = \sum_{i=1}^{m} \delta_{ia}, \quad i = \sum_{i=1}^{k} X_{ia}, \quad \text{and} \quad j = \sum_{i=1}^{m-k} X_{ia},$$
and
$$\begin{cases} a = i + a_0, \\ b = k - i - b, \\ c = j + c_0, \\ d = m - k - j + d_0. \end{cases} \qquad (3.19)$$

Thus, the posterior means of p_a and p_b at m stage are given by
$$E_m[p_a] = a/(a+b),$$
and
$$E_m[p_b] = c/(c+d),$$
where $E_m[.]$ denotes expectation under the model.

(4) Two commonly used discount sequences $\{1, \beta_1, \beta_2, \ldots, \beta_n\}$ are the n-horizon uniform sequence with all $\beta_i = 1$, and the geometric sequence with all $\beta_i = \beta (0 < \beta < 1)$.

(5) Allocation rule, δ, is defined to be a sequence $(\delta_1, \delta_2, \ldots, \delta_n)$ where $\delta_i = 1$ if the ith subject receives treatment A and $\delta_i = 0$ if the ith subject receives treatment B. It is required that the decision, δ_i at stage i be dependent only upon the information available at that time (not the

ADAPTIVE RANDOMIZATION

future). The two commonly used allocation rules are Uniform Bandit and Truncated Gittins Lower Bound.

The *truncation* here refers to a rule that if a state is reached such that the final decision cannot be influenced by any further outcomes, then the treatment with the best success rate will be used for all further subjects.

Uniform Bandit The n-horizon uniform TAB uses prior and accumulated information to minimize the number of failures *during* the trial. Let $F_m(i,j,k,l)$ denote the minimal possible expected number of failures remaining in the trial, if m patients have already been treated and there were i successes and j failures on treatment A, and k successes and l failures on treatment B. (Note that one parameter can be eliminated since $m = i + j + k + l$.) The algorithmic approach is based on the observation that if A were used on next patient, then the expected number of failures for patient $m + 1$ and through n would be

$$F_m^A(i,j,k,l) = E_m[p_a]F_{m+1}(i,j,k,l) + E_m[1-p_a](1 + F_{m+1}(i,j,k,l)), \quad (3.20)$$

If B were used, we would have

$$F_m^B(i,j,k,l) = E_m[p_b]F_{m+1}(i,j,k,l) + E_m[1-p_b](1 + F_{m+1}(i,j,k,l)). \quad (3.21)$$

Therefore, F satisfies the recurrence

$$F_m(i,j,k,l) = \min\{F_m^A(i,j,k,l), F_m^B(i,j,k,l)\}, \quad (3.22)$$

which can be solved by dynamic programming, starting with patient n and proceeding toward the first patient. The computation is at order of $O(n^4)$.

Gittins Lower Bound According to a theorem of Gittins and John (Berry and Fristedt, 1985), for bandit problems with geometric discount and independent arms, for each arm there exists an index with the property that, at given stage, it is optimal to select, at the next stage, the arm with the higher index. The index for an arm, the Gittins Index, is a function only of the posterior distribution and discount factor β. The existence of Gittins index removes many computation difficulties associated with other Bandit problems.

Remarks For small samples, the allocation rule can be implemented by means of dynamic programming (Hardwick and Stout, 1991). Sequential treatment allocation can also be done based on other optimal criteria. For example, Hardwick and Stout (2002) developed the allocation rule based on maximizing the likelihood of making the correct decision by utilizing a curtailed equal allocation rule with a minimal expected sample size. The optimization is given for any fixed $|p_a - p_b| = \Delta$ among the curtailed (pruned) equal allocation rule. The pruning refers to a rule whereby, if a state is reached such that the sign of the final observed difference in success rate for the two groups will not be influenced by any further outcomes, then the trial will be stopped. The pruning could result in an insufficient sample size or power for clinical trials.

Rosenberger et al.(2002) used computer simulations to compare the ORPW, Neyman allocation, the RPW rule, and equal allocation. They found out that the RPW rule tends to be highly variable for larger values of p_a and p_b. The adaptive structure of sequential designs includes dependencies that could result in extra-binomial variability. This increased variability will decrease power to some extent. ORPW reduces the expected number of failures from equal allocation and reduces the expected failures by around 3 or 4 when p_a and p_b are small to moderate. When p_a and p_b are large, there are more moderate reductions, and it is questionable whether adaptive designs would improve much over equal allocation when a test is based on proportion difference. For the RPW design, for example, if $p_a = 0.7$ and $p_b = 0.9$ with a sample size of 192, the RPW design has power 0.88 for z_1 with t expected 31.5 failures, while equal allocation design for 162 patients has power 0.90 with 32.4 failures.

The RPW rule does not require instantaneous outcomes, or even that they are available before randomization of the next subject. Investigators can update the urn when a subject's outcome is ascertained. The effect of this will "slow" the adaptation, and hence there will be less benefit to subjects, particularly those recruited early. If delay of the response is so significant, it could be practically impossible to implement the RPW rule.

Bandit model for finite population

The bandit allocation rule discussed in the previous section is optimal in the sense that it minimizes the number of failures in the trial. In what follows, we will discuss an optimal criterion in the scope of the entire patient population with the disease, and compare five different randomization procedures (Berry and Eick, 1995) with this criterion.

Suppose that the *"patient horizon"* is N. Each of the N patients is to be treated with one of two treatments, A and B. Treatment allocation is sequential for the first n patients and the response is dichotomous and immediate. Let $Z_j, j = 1, \ldots, N$, denote the response of patient j; $Z_j = 1$ if success and $Z_j = 0$ if failure. The probability of a success with treatment A is p_a and with B is p_b. We have that

$$E[Z_j | p_a, p_b] = \begin{cases} P[Z_j = 1 | p_a, p_b] = p_a, & \text{if patient } j \text{ receives treatment A} \\ P[Z_j = 1 | p_a, p_b] = p_b, & \text{if patient } j \text{ receives treatment B.} \end{cases}$$

Since treatment allocation for patients 1 to n is sequential, treatment assignment can depend upon the responses of all previously treated patients. However, treatment assignment for patients $n+1$ to N can depend only on the responses of patients 1 to n. In all the procedures we consider, these latter patients receive the treatment with the larger fraction of successes among the first n. (If the two observed success proportions are equal, then the treatment with the greater number of observations is given to patients $n+1$ to N.) Let D be the class of all treatment allocation procedures satisfying these restrictions.

The conditional worth (W) of procedure $\tau \in D$ (given p_a and p_b) is

$$W_\delta(p_a, p_b) = E_\delta \left[\sum_{j=1}^N Z_j | p_a, p_b \right], \qquad (3.23)$$

where the distribution of the Z_j's is determined by τ. This can be no greater than $N \max\{p_a, p_b\}$. The conditional expected successes lost (ESL) using τ is:

$$L_\tau(p_a, p_b) = N \max\{p_a, p_b\} - W_\tau(p_a, p_b). \qquad (3.24)$$

This function is obviously non-negative for all τ.

Allocation Procedures Barry and Eirick (1995) considered four adaptive procedures and compared them with a balanced randomized design or equal randomization (ER). All of these procedures are members of D. We describe the procedures on the basis of the way they allocate treatments to the first n patients. We assume for convenience that n is an even integer.

Procedure ER: Half of the first n patients are randomly assigned to treatment A and the other half to B. For comparison purposes, it does not matter whether patients are randomized in pairs, or in blocks of larger size.

Procedure JB (J. Bather): Treatments A and B are randomly assigned to patients 1 and 2 so that one patient receives each. Suppose that during the trial m patients have been treated, $2 \leq m < n$, and assume that s_a, f_a, s_b, f_b successes and failures have been observed on A and B, respectively ($s_a + f_a + s_b + f_b = m$). Define

$$\lambda(k) = (4 + \sqrt{k})/(15k). \qquad (3.25)$$

Let $\lambda_a = \lambda(s_a + f_a)$ and $\lambda_b = \lambda(s_b + f_b)$. Procedure JB randomizes between the respective treatments except that the randomization probabilities depend upon the previously observed response. Let

$$q = \frac{s_a}{s_a + f_a} - \frac{s_b}{s_b + f_b} + 2(\lambda_a - \lambda_b), \quad (3.26)$$

then under procedure JB, the next patient (patient $m + 1$) receives treatment A with probability

$$\frac{\lambda_a}{\lambda_a + \lambda_b} \exp(q/\lambda_a) \quad \text{for } q \leq 0$$

and

$$1 - \frac{\lambda_b}{\lambda_a + \lambda_b} \exp(q/\lambda_b) \quad \text{when } q > 0.$$

Procedure TAB is a two-armed bandit procedure where the first n patients are randomized based on the current probability distribution of (p_a, p_b), assuming a uniform prior density on (p_a, p_b):

$$\pi(p_a, p_b) = 1 \text{ on } (0, 1) \times (0, 1) \quad (3.27)$$

The next patient receives treatment A with probability equal to the current probability that $p_a > p_b$. This probability is

$$\int_0^1 \int_0^1 u^{s_a}(1-u)^{f_a} v^{s_b}(1-v)^{f_b} \, dudv$$

$$\{B(s_a + 1, f_a + 1)B(s_b + 1, f_b + 1)\}^{-1} \quad (3.28)$$

where $B(.,.)$ is the complete beta function:

$$B(a, b) = \int_0^1 u^{a-1}(1-u)^{b-1} du. \quad (3.29)$$

Procedure PW (Play-the-winner/Switch-from-loser): The first patient receives treatment A or B with a equal probability 0.5. For patients 2 to n, the treatment given to the previous patient is used again if it was successful; otherwise the other treatment is used.

Procedure RB (Robust Bayes): This strategy is optimal in the following two-arm bandit problem. Suppose that the uniform prior density of (p_a, p_b) is given, the discount sequence of $\beta = \{1, \beta_1, \beta_2, \ldots, \beta_n\}$ is defined by

$$\beta_i = \begin{cases} 1 & \text{for } 1 \leq i \leq n, \\ N - n & \text{for } i = n + 1, \\ 0 & \text{for } i > n + 1. \end{cases} \quad (3.30)$$

That means that all N patients have equal weights. The first n patients each have a weight of $N - n$. Procedure RB maximizes

$$\int_0^1 \int_0^1 W_\tau(p_a, p_b; \beta) \, dp_a dp_b \quad (3.31)$$

over all $\delta \in D$, where

$$W_\delta(p_a, p_b; \beta) = E_\delta \left[\sum_{j=1}^{N} \beta_j Z_j | p_a, p_b \right].$$

This maximum can be found using dynamic programming. The starting point is after the n patients in the trial have responded. The subsequent expected number of the successes is $N - n$ times the maximum of the current expected values of p_a and p_b. If both treatments are judged equally effective at any stage, then procedure RB randomizes the next treatment assignment.

Procedure RB comprises a dynamic programming process. The symmetry of the uniform prior distribution implies that the treatments are initially equivalent. For the first patient, one is chosen at random. If the first patient has a success, then the second patient receives the same treatment. If the first patient has a failure, then the second patient receives the other treatment. Thus, procedure RB imitates procedure PW for the first two treatment assignments. The same treatment is used as long as it is successful, again imitating PW. However, after a failure, switching to the other treatment may or may not be optimal. If the data sufficiently strongly favor the treatment that has just failed, then that treatment will be used again.

When following procedure RB, if the current probability of success for treatment A (which is the current expected value of p_a) is greater than that for treatment B, then treatment A may or may not be optimal for the next patient. If the current number of patients on treatment A, $s_a + f_a$ is smaller than the number of patients on B, $s_b + f_b$, then A is indeed optimal. However, if $s_a + f_a$ is greater than $s_b + f_b$, then, for sufficiently large N, treatment B is optimal irrespective of the current expected values of p_a and p_b. Procedure RB tends to assign the currently superior treatment, but less so for large N than for small N. As N increases, gathering information early on by balancing the treatment assignment is important. Thus, assignment to the two treatments tends to be more balanced when N is large than when it is small.

Some comparisons between these procedures are possible without detailed calculations. Procedure ER is designed to obtain information from the first n patients that will help patients outside the trial. Because it gives maximal information about $p_a - p_b$, its performance relative to the other procedures will improve as N increases.

Procedure RB is designed to perform well on the *average* for any $n, N, p_a,$ and p_b. Of the five procedures described, it alone specifically uses the value of N, giving it an advantage over the other procedures.

Procedure PW ignores most of the accumulating data; its treatment assignments are based not on sufficient statistics but only on the result for the previous patient. On the other hand, since PW tends to allocate patients to both of the treatments except when one or both p's is close to 1, it should perform well when N is large.

Procedures JB and TAB are quite similar. Both randomize allocations so that the currently superior treatment is more likely to be assigned.

As indicated above, RB maximizes (3.31) over all procedures in D. Thus, procedures PW, JB and TAB will not perform better than RB when averaged over p_a and p_b. However, they might outperform RB for some N and some moderately large set of (p_a, p_b). The computer simulations showed that they do not.

Remarks Berry and Eick (1995) conducted computer simulations comparing the five methods mentioned above with $N = 100$, 1000, 10,000 and 100,000. Their main conclusion is that a balanced randomized design is nearly optimal when the disease is relatively common, e.g., when N is moderately large (such as $N \geq 10,000$). However, when a substantial portion of patients are involved in the trial (as with a rare form of cancer), then adaptive procedures can perform substantially better than a balanced randomization. There are many relevant questions that need to be answered before these adaptive allocations can provide practical advantages. These questions include (i) How relevant is the condition? (ii) How effective are the treatments A and B? (iii) Are other effective treatments available? (iv) How long will it take to discover a new treatment that is clearly superior to both A and B? In addition, if a Bayesian approach is used, should p_a and p_b have different priorities because the control is using an approved drug?

Adaptive models for ordinal and continuous outcomes

Ordinal Outcome Ivan and Flournoy (2001) developed an urn model, called Ternary urn model, for categorical outcome. In this section, we will introduce an urn model for ordinal outcome. This model can fall into Rosenberger's treatment effect mapping model, whose allocation rule is given by

$$P(\delta_j | \Delta_{j-1}) = g(E_j),$$

where g is a function of treatment effect E_{j-1} at stage j.

We propose here a response-adaptive model with ordinal outcomes for multiple treatments. Suppose there are K treatment groups in the trial and the primary response is ordinal with M categories. Without

ADAPTIVE RANDOMIZATION

loss of generality, let $C_j(j = 1,..,M)$ be the integer scales for the ordinal response with a higher score indicating a desired outcome. The response-adaptive urn model is defined as follows. There are K types of balls in an urn, initially a_i balls of type i. The treatment assignment for a patient is determined by the ball type randomly drawn from the urn with replacement. If a ball of type k is drawn from the urn, the patient will be assigned treatment k. Then observe the response for all the patients treated. If a patient with treatment i had response C_j at stage n (n patients have been treated), then nC_j balls of type i will be added to the urn. Repeat this procedure for treatment assignment to all patients in the trial.

Normal Outcome Let Y_i be a continuous variable representing the response of the ith patient, treated with either A or B following the adaptive design. Assume responses to be instantaneous and normally distributed. Suppose μ_a and μ_b are population characteristics representing the treatment effects A and B, respectively (assume a larger value μ indicates a better result). For the ith patient, we define an indicator variable δ_i which takes the value 1 or 0 accordingly as the patient is treated by A or B. Then, the adaptive allocation rule is described as follows:

For the initial two patients, we randomly assign one to each treatment A or B. For patient $i + 1$ ($2 < i \leq n$), we assign him/her to treatment A with a probability of

$$P_a(\delta_{i+1}|\delta_1,\ldots,\delta_i, Y_1, \ldots, Y_i) = \left[\Phi\left(\frac{\hat{\mu}_a - \hat{\mu}_b}{\hat{\sigma}_p\sqrt{\frac{1}{i_a}+\frac{1}{i_b}}}\right)\right]^\alpha, \quad (3.32)$$

where α is constant that can be determined by optimal criteria later, $\Phi(\bullet)$ is the standard normal cumulative distribution function, i_a and i_b are number of patients in treatment A and B at state i, the pooled variance

$$\hat{\sigma}_p^2 = \frac{(i_a - 1)\hat{\sigma}_a^2 - (i_b - 1)\hat{\sigma}_b^2}{i_a - i_b - 2},$$

and $\hat{\mu}_a = \bar{Y}_a$ and $\hat{\mu}_b = \bar{Y}_b$. Note that Bandyopadhyay and Biswas (1997) suggested using the allocation probability $\Phi(\frac{\hat{\mu}_a - \hat{\mu}_b}{T})$, where T is a constant.

Survival Outcome Rosenber and Seshaiyer (1997) proposed a treatment effect mapping $g(S) = 0.5(1 + S)$, where S is the centered and scaled logrank test. We suggest using the optimal model proposed in the previous section since logrank test statistic is normally distributed.

3.5 Issues with Adaptive Randomization

Rosenberger and Lachin (2002) discussed the issues with adaptive design. They classified the bias into acrrual bias and selection bias as summarized below.

Accrual bias

RPW or other adaptive designs may lead to a unique type of bias, i.e., accrual bias, by which volunteers may wish to be recruited later in the study to take advantage of the benefit from previous outcomes. Earlier subjects are mostly to have higher probabilities of receiving the inferior treatment.

Accidental bias

Efron (1971) introduced the term accidental bias to describe the bias in estimation of treatment effect induced by an unobserved covariate. The bias in estimation of treatment, $(E(\hat{\alpha}) - \alpha)^2$, is minimized when treatment assignment is balanced, where α and $\hat{\alpha}$ are the true treatment effect and estimated treatment effect through linear regression, respectively. The bound of the bias due to unbalanced treatment assignments is controlled by the eigenvalue of covariance matrix of treatment assignment sequence. The eigenvalues for different randomization models are presented in Table 3.3.

Accidental bias does not appear to be a serious problem for any of the randomization models discussed so far, except for the truncated binomial design. More details regarding the accidental bias can be found in Rosenberger and Lachin (2002).

Table 3.3 Accidental Bias for Various Randomization Models

Model Name	Maximum Eigenvalue, $\lambda_{\max}$
Complete random	1
Lachin's allocation rule	$1+\frac{1}{n-1}$
Stratified Lachin's allocation rule	$1+\frac{1}{m-1}$
Truncated binomial model	$\sqrt{\pi n/3} \leq \lambda_{\max} \leq \sqrt{n/2}$
Friedman-Wei's urn model	$1+\frac{2}{3}\frac{\ln n}{n}+O(n^{-1})$

Note: n = sample size, and m = sample size with each stratum.

Selection bias

Selection bias refers to biases that are introduced into an unmasked study because an investigator may be able to guess the treatment assignment of future patients based on knowing the treatments assigned to the past patients. Patients usually enter a trial sequentially over time. Staggered entry allows the possibility for a study investigator to alter the composition of the groups by attempting to guess which treatment will be assigned next. Based on whichever treatment is guessed to be assigned next, the investigator can then choose the next patient scheduled for randomization to be one whom the investigator considers to be better suited for that treatment. One of the principal concerns in an unmasked study is that a study investigator might attempt to "beat the randomization" and recruit patients in a manner such that each patient is assigned to whichever treatment group the investigator feels is best suited to that individual patient (Rosenberger and Lachin, 2002).

Blackwell and Hodges (1957) developed a model for selection bias. Using this model the selection bias can be measured by the so-called *expected bias factor*,

$$E(F) = E(G - n/2), \qquad (3.33)$$

where G is total number of correct guesses (A better to B better), $n/2$ is the number of patients in each of the two groups.

Blackwell and Hodges (1957) showed that the optimal strategy for the experimenter upon randomizing the jth patient is to guess treatment A when $N_A(j-1) < N_B(j-1)$ and B when $N_A(j-1) > N_B(j-1)$. When there is a tie, the experimenter guesses with equal probability. This is called *convergence strategy*. The expected bias factors under convergence strategy for various randomization models are presented in Table 3.4.

Inferential analysis

Analyses based on a randomization model are completely different from traditional analyses using hypotheses tests of population parameters under the Neyman-Pearson paradigm. The most commonly used basis for the development of a statistical test is the concept of a population model, where it is assumed that the sample of patients is representative of a reference population and that the patient responses to treatment are independent and identically distributed from a distribution dependent on unknown population parameters. A null hypothesis under a population model is typically based on the equality of parameters from known distributions. Permutation tests or randomization tests are non-parametric tests. The null hypothesis of a permutation test is that the assignment of treatment A versus B has no effect on the responses of the

Table 3.4 Expected Selection Bias Factors Under Convergence Strategy

Model	Maximum Eigenvalue, λ_{max}
Complete random	0
Lachin's allocation rule	$\frac{2^{n-1}}{\binom{n}{n/2}} - \frac{1}{2}$
Stratified Lachin's allocation rule	$M\left(\frac{\frac{2^{m-1}}{m} - \frac{1}{2}}{\binom{m}{m/2}}\right)$
Truncated binomial model	$\frac{n}{2^{n+1}}\binom{n}{n/2}$
Friedman-Wei's urn model	$\sum_{i=1}^{n}\left[\frac{1}{2} + \frac{\beta E(|D_{i-1}|)}{2(2\alpha+\beta(i-1))}\right] - \frac{n}{2}$

Note: n = sample size, m = # of patients/block, and M = number of blocks.

n patients randomized in the study. The essential feature of a permutation test is that in a randomization null hypothesis, the set of observed responses is assumed to be a set of deterministic values that are unaffected by treatment. The observed difference between the treatment groups depends only upon the way in which the n patients were randomized. Permutation tests are assumption-free, but depend explicitly upon the particular randomization procedure used.

A number of questions arise about the permutation test. (1) What measure of extremeness, or test statistic, should be used? The most general family of permutation tests is the family of linear rank tests. Linear rank tests are used often in clinical trials, and the family includes such tests as the traditional Wilcoxon rank-sum test and the logrank test. (2) Which set of permutations of the randomization sequence should be used for comparison? (3) If the analysis of a clinical trial is based on a randomization model that does not in any way involve the notion of a population, how can results of the trial be generalized to determine the best care for future patients? However, this weakness exists in the population model too.

Power and sample size

For the urn $UD(\alpha, \beta)$ design, if the total sample size $n = 2m$ is specified, a perfectly balanced design with $n_a = n_b = m$ will minimize the quantity

$$\eta = [1/n_a + 1/n_b]$$

which is $\eta = 2/m$. If n is not known beforehand, it is interesting to know how many extra observations are needed for $UD(0, \beta)$ to reduce η to be less than or equal to $2/m$. That is, we continue taking observations until n_a and n_b satisfy

$$\frac{1}{n_a} + \frac{1}{n_b} \leq \frac{2}{m} \qquad (3.34)$$

If we write $n_a + n_b = 2m + \nu$, then ν is the number of additional observations required by the $UD(0, \beta)$ to satisfy this condition. It follows (Wei, 1978) that for any given ν and large m,

$$\Pr(\nu \leq z) \approx \Phi[(3z)^{1/2}] - \Phi[-(3z)^{1/2}]. \qquad (3.35)$$

For large m, $\Pr[\nu \leq 4]$ is approximately 0.9995, and thus the $UD(0, \beta)$ needs at most 4 extra observations to satisfy the above inequality, i.e., to yield the same efficiency as the perfectly balanced randomization allocation rule.

3.6 Summary

In this chapter, we have discussed several types of adaptive randomization. Theoretically, outcomes (efficacy or safety) with a response-dependent randomization are not independent. Therefore, the population-based inferential analysis method distinguishes the two types of adaptive designs. However, the randomization-based analysis (permutation test) can be used under both adaptive randomizations. When a test statistic for the non-adaptive randomized trial is going to be used for an adaptive randomization trial, the corresponding power/sample size calculation for the non-adaptive randomization trial can also be used. For small sample size, permutation can be used for the inferential analysis, confidence interval estimation, and power/sample size estimation. An adaptive randomization can be either optimal or intuitive. The outcome can be binary, ordinal, or continuous. The adaptive approach can be Bayesian or non-Bayesian. Our discussions have been focused on the cases with two treatment groups, but it can be easily expanded to multiple arms.

CHAPTER 4

Adaptive Hypotheses

Modifications of hypotheses of on-going clinical trials based on accrued data can certainly have an impact on statistical power for testing the hypotheses with the pre-selected sample size. Modifications of hypotheses of on-going trials commonly occur during the conduct of a clinical trial due to the following reasons: (i) an investigational method has not yet been validated at the planning stage of the study, (ii) information from other studies is necessary for planning the next stage of the study, (iii) there is a need to include new doses, and (iv) recommendations from a pre-established data (safety) monitoring committee (DMC) (Hommel, 2001). In addition, to increase the probability of success, the sponsors may switch a superiority hypothesis (originally planned) to a non-inferiority hypothesis. In this chapter, we will refer to adaptive hypotheses as modifications of hypotheses of on-going trials based on accrued data. Adaptive hypotheses can certainly affect the clinically meaningful difference (e.g., effect size, non-inferiority margin, or equivalence limit) to be detected, and consequently the sample size is necessarily adjusted for achieving the desired power.

In this chapter, we will examine the impact of a modification to hypotheses on the type I error rate, the statistical power of the test, and sample size for achieving the desired power. For a given clinical trial, the situations where hypotheses are modified as deemed appropriate by the investigator or as recommended by an independent data safety monitoring board (DSMB) after the review of interim data during the conduct of the clinical trial are described in the next section. In Section 4.2, the choice of non-inferiority margin, change in statistical inference, and impact on sample size calculation when switching from a superiority hypothesis to a non-inferiority hypothesis are discussed. Multiple hypotheses such as independent versus dependent and/or primary versus secondary hypotheses are discussed in Section 4.3. Also included in this section is a proposed decision theory approach for testing multiple hypotheses. A brief concluding remark is given in the last section.

4.1 Modifications of Hypotheses

In clinical trials with planned data monitoring for safety and interim analyses for efficacy, a recommendation for modifying or changing the hypotheses are commonly made after the review of interim data. The purpose for such a recommendation is to ensure the success of the clinical trials for identifying best possible clinical benefits to the patients who enter the clinical trials. In practice, the following situations are commonly encountered.

The first commonly seen situation for modifying hypotheses during the conduct of a clinical trial is switching a superiority hypothesis to a non-inferiority hypothesis. For a promising compound, the sponsor would prefer an aggressive approach for planning a superiority study. The study is usually powered to compare the promising compound with a placebo control or an active-control agent. However, the interim analysis results may not support superiority at interim analysis. In this case, instead of declaring the failure of the superiority trial, the independent data monitoring committee may recommend to switch from testing the superiority hypothesis to a non-inferiority hypothesis. The switch from a superiority hypothesis to a non-inferiority hypothesis will certainly increase the probability of success of the trial because the study objective has been modified to establish non-inferiority rather than show superiority. Note that the concept of switching a superiority hypothesis to a non-inferiority hypothesis is accepted by the regulatory agency such as the U.S. FDA, provided that the impact of the switch on statistical issues (e.g., the determination of non-inferiority margin) and inference (e.g., appropriate statistical methods) on the assessment of treatment effect are well justified. More details regarding the switch from a superiority hypothesis to a non-inferiority hypothesis are given in the next section.

Another commonly seen situation where the hypotheses are modified during the conduct of a clinical trial is the switch from a single hypothesis to a composite hypothesis or multiple hypotheses. A composite hypothesis is defined as a hypothesis that involves more than one study endpoint. These study endpoints may or may not be independent. In many clinical trials, in addition to the primary study endpoint, some clinical benefits may be observed based on the analysis/review of the interim data from secondary endpoints for efficacy and/or safety. It is then of particular interest to the sponsor to change testing a single hypothesis for the primary study endpoint to testing a composite hypothesis for the primary endpoint in conjunction with several secondary endpoints for clinical benefits or multiple hypotheses for the primary endpoint and the secondary endpoints. More details regarding testing multiple hypotheses are given in Section 4.3.

ADAPTIVE HYPOTHESES

Other situations where the hypotheses are modified during the conduct of a clinical trial include (i) change in hypotheses due to the switch in study endpoints, (ii) dropping ineffective treatment arms, and (iii) interchange between the null hypothesis and the alternative hypothesis. These situations are briefly described below.

In cancer trials, there is no universal agreement regarding which study endpoint should be used as the primary study endpoint for evaluation of the test treatment under investigation. Study endpoints such as response rate, time to disease progression, and survival are commonly used study endpoints for cancer clinical trials (see Williams, Pazdur, and Temple, 2004). A typical approach is to choose one study endpoint as the primary endpoint for efficacy. Power analysis for sample size calculation is then performed based on the primary endpoint, and other study endpoints are considered as secondary endpoints for clinical benefits. After the review of the interim data, the investigator may consider switching the primary endpoint to a secondary endpoint if no evidence of substantial efficacy in terms of the originally selected primary endpoint (e.g., response rate) is observed, but a significant improvement in efficacy is detected in one of the secondary endpoints (e.g., time to disease progression or median survival time).

For clinical trials comparing several treatments or several doses of the same treatment with a placebo or an active-control agent, a parallel-group design is usually considered. After the review of the interim data, it is desirable to drop the treatment groups or the dose groups which either show no efficacy or exhibit serious safety problems based on ethical consideration. It is also desirable to modify the dose and/or dose regimen for patients who are still on the study for best clinical results. As a result, hypotheses and the corresponding statistical methods for testing treatment effect are necessarily modified for a valid and fair assessment of the effect of the test treatment under investigation. More details regarding dropping the losers are discussed in Chapter 8.

In some cases, we may consider switching the null hypothesis and the alternative hypothesis. For example, a pharmaceutical company may conduct a bioavailability study to study the relative bioavailability of a newly developed formulation as compared to the approved formulation by testing the null hypothesis of bioinequivalence against the alternative hypothesis of bioequivalence. The idea is to reject the null hypothesis and conclude the alternative hypothesis. After the review of the interim data, the sponsor realizes that the relative bioavailabilities between the two formulations are not similar. As a result, instead of establishing bioequivalence, the sponsor may wish to demonstrate superiority in bioavailability for the new formulation.

4.2 Switch from Superiority to Non-Inferiority

As indicated in the previous section, it is not uncommon to switch from a superiority hypothesis (the originally planned hypothesis) to a non-inferiority hypothesis during the conduct of clinical trials. The purpose of this switching is to increase the probability of success. For testing superiority, if we fail to reject the null hypothesis of non-superiority, the trial is considered a failure. On the other hand, the rejection of the null hypothesis of inferiority provides the opportunity for testing superiority without paying any statistical penalty due to closed testing procedure.

When comparing a test treatment with a standard therapy or an active control agent, as indicated by Chow, Shao, and Wang (2003), the problem of testing non-inferiority and superiority can be unified by the following hypotheses:

$$H_0 : \epsilon \leq \delta \quad versus \quad H_a : \epsilon > \delta,$$

where $\epsilon = \mu_2 - \mu_1$ is the difference in mean responses between the test treatment (μ_2) and the active control agent (μ_1), and δ is the clinical superiority or non-inferiority margin. In practice, when $\delta > 0$, the rejection of the null hypothesis indicates *clinical* superiority over the reference drug product. When $\delta < 0$, the rejection of the null hypothesis implies non-inferiority against the reference drug product. Note that when $\delta = 0$, the above hypotheses are referred to as hypotheses for testing *statistical* superiority, which is usually confused with that of clinical superiority.

Non-inferiority margin

One of the major considerations in a non-inferiority test is the selection of the non-inferiority margin. A different choice of non-inferiority margin may affect the method of analyzing clinical data and consequently may alter the conclusion of the clinical study. As pointed out in the guideline by the International Conference on Harmonization (ICH), the determination of non-inferiority margins should be based on both statistical reasoning and clinical judgment. Despite the existence of some studies, there is no established rule or gold standard for determination of non-inferiority margins in active control trials.

According to the ICH E10 Guideline, a non-inferiority margin may be selected based on past experience in placebo control trials with valid design under conditions similar to those planned for the new trial, and the determination of a non-inferiority margin should not only reflect uncertainties in the evidence on which the choice is based, but also be suitably conservative. Furthermore, as a basic frequentist statistical principle, the hypothesis of non-inferiority should be formulated with population parameters, not estimates from historical trials. Along these lines, Chow and Shao (2006) proposed a method of selecting non-inferiority margins with some statistical justification. Chow and Shao proposed non-inferiority margin depends on population parameters including parameters related to the placebo control if it were not replaced by the active control. Unless a fixed (constant) non-inferiority margin can be chosen based on clinical judgment, a fixed non-inferiority margin not depending on population parameters is rarely suitable. Intuitively, the non-inferiority margin should be small when the effect of the active control agent relative to placebo is small or the variation in the population under investigation is large. Chow and Shao's approach ensures that the efficacy of the test therapy is superior to placebo when non-inferiority is concluded. When it is necessary/desired, their approach can produce a non-inferiority margin that ensures that the efficacy of the test therapy relative to placebo can be established with great confidence.

Because the proposed non-inferiority margin depends on population parameters, the non-inferiority test designed for the situation where the non-inferiority margin is fixed has to be modified in order to apply it to the case where the non-inferiority margin is a parameter. In what follows, Chow and Shao's method for determination of non-inferiority margin is described.

Chow and Shao's Approach Let θ_T, θ_A, and θ_P be the unknown population efficacy parameters associated with the test therapy, the active control agent, and the placebo, respectively. Also, let $\delta \geq 0$ be a non-inferiority margin. Without loss of generality, we assume that a large value of population efficacy parameter is desired. The hypotheses for non-inferiority can be formulated as

$$H_0 : \theta_T - \theta_A \leq -\delta \quad \text{versus} \quad H_a : \theta_T - \theta_A > -\delta. \tag{4.1}$$

If δ is a fixed pre-specified value, then standard statistical methods can be applied to testing hypotheses (4.1). In practice, however, δ is often unknown.

There exists an approach that constructs the value of δ based on a placebo-controlled historical trial. For example, δ = a fraction of the lower limit of the 95% confidence interval for $\theta_A - \theta_P$ based on some historical trial data (see, e.g., CBER/FDA Memorandum, 1999). Although this approach is intuitively conservative, it is not statistically valid because (i) if the lower confidence limit is treated as a fixed value, then the variability in historical data is ignored; and (ii) if the lower confidence limit is treated as a statistic, then this approach violates the basic frequentist statistical principle, i.e., the hypotheses being tested should not involve any estimates from current or past trials.

From a statistical point of view, the ICH E10 Guideline suggests that the non-inferiority margin δ should be chosen to satisfy at least the following two criteria:

Criterion 1. The ability to claim that the test therapy is non-inferior to the active-control agent and is superior to the placebo (even though the placebo is not considered in the active-control trial).

Criterion 2. The non-inferiority margin should be suitably conservative, i.e., variability should be taken into account.

A fixed δ (i.e., it does not depend on any parameters) is rarely suitable under criterion 1. Let $\Delta > 0$ be a *clinical* superiority margin if a placebo-controlled trial is conducted to establish the *clinical* superiority of the test therapy over a placebo control. Since the active control is an established therapy, we may assume that $\theta_A - \theta_P > \Delta$. However, when $\theta_T - \theta_A > -\delta$ (i.e., the test therapy is non-inferior to the active control) for a fixed δ, we cannot ensure that $\theta_T - \theta_P > \Delta$ (i.e., the test therapy is *clinically* superior to the placebo) unless $\delta = 0$.

Thus, it is reasonable to consider non-inferiority margins depending on unknown parameters. Hung et al. (2003) summarized the approach of using the non-inferiority margin of the form

$$\delta = \gamma(\theta_A - \theta_P), \tag{4.2}$$

where γ is a fixed constant between 0 and 1. This is based on the idea of preserving a certain fraction of the active control effect $\theta_A - \theta_P$. The smaller $\theta_A - \theta_P$ is, the smaller δ. How to select the proportion γ, however, is not discussed.

Following the idea of Chow and Shao (2006), we now derive a non-inferiority margin satisfying criterion 1. Let $\Delta > 0$ be a clinical superiority margin if a placebo control is added to the trial. Suppose that the non-inferiority margin δ is proportional to Δ, i.e., $\delta = r\Delta$, where r is a known value chosen in the beginning of the trial. To be conservative, r should be ≤ 1. If the test therapy is not inferior to the active-control agent and is superior over the placebo, then both

$$\theta_T - \theta_A > -\delta \quad \text{versus} \quad \theta_T - \theta_P > \Delta \tag{4.3}$$

should hold. Under the worst scenario, i.e., $\theta_T - \theta_A$ achieves its lower bound $-\delta$, the largest possible δ satisfying (4.3) is given by

$$\delta = \theta_A - \theta_P - \Delta,$$

which leads to

$$\delta = \frac{r}{1+r}(\theta_A - \theta_P). \tag{4.4}$$

From (4.2) and (4.4), $\gamma = r/(r+1)$. If $0 < r \leq 1$, then $0 < \gamma \leq \frac{1}{2}$.

ADAPTIVE HYPOTHESES

The above argument in determining δ takes Criterion 1 into account, but is not conservative enough, since it does not consider the variability. Let $\hat{\theta}_T$ and $\hat{\theta}_P$ be sample estimators of θ_T and θ_P, respectively, based on data from a placebo-controlled trial. Assume that $\hat{\theta}_T - \hat{\theta}_P$ is normally distributed with mean $\theta_T - \theta_P$ and standard error SE_{T-P} (which is true under certain conditions or approximately true under the central limit theorem for large sample sizes). When $\theta_T = \theta_A - \delta$,

$$P(\hat{\theta}_T - \hat{\theta}_P < \Delta) = \Phi\left(\frac{\Delta + \delta - (\theta_A - \theta_P)}{SE_{T-P}}\right) \quad (4.5)$$

where Φ denotes the standard normal distribution function. If δ is chosen according to (4.4) and $\theta_T = \theta_A - \delta$, then the probability that $\hat{\theta}_T - \hat{\theta}_P$ is less than Δ is equal to $\frac{1}{2}$. In view of Criterion 2, a value much smaller than $\frac{1}{2}$ for this probability is desired, because it is the probability that the estimated test therapy effect is not superior over that of the placebo.

Since the probability in (4.5) is an increasing function of δ, the smaller δ (the more conservative choice of the non-inferiority margin) is, the smaller the chance that $\hat{\theta}_T - \hat{\theta}_P$ is less than Δ. Setting the probability on the left-hand side of (4.5) to ϵ with $0 < \epsilon \leq \frac{1}{2}$, we obtain that

$$\delta = \theta_A - \theta_P - \Delta - z_{1-\epsilon}SE_{T-P},$$

where $z_a = \Phi^{-1}(a)$. Since $\Delta = \delta/r$, we obtain that

$$\delta = \frac{r}{1+r}(\theta_A - \theta_P - z_{1-\epsilon}SE_{T-P}). \quad (4.6)$$

Comparing (4.2) and (4.6), we obtain that

$$\gamma = \frac{r}{1+r}\left(1 - \frac{z_{1-\epsilon}SE_{T-P}}{\theta_A - \theta_P}\right),$$

i.e., the proportion γ in (4.2) is a decreasing function of a type of noise-to-signal ratio (or coefficient of variation).

As indicated by Chow and Shao (2006), the above non-inferiority margin (4.6) can also be derived from a slightly different point of view. Suppose that we actually conduct a placebo-controlled trial with superiority margin Δ to establish the superiority of the test therapy over the placebo. Then, the power of the large sample t-test for hypotheses $\theta_T - \theta_P \leq \Delta$ versus $\theta_T - \theta_P > \Delta$ is approximately equal to

$$\Phi\left(\frac{\theta_T - \theta_P - \Delta}{SE_{T-P}} - z_{1-\alpha}\right),$$

where α is the level of significance. Assume the worst scenario $\theta_T = \theta_A - \delta$ and that β is a given desired level of power. Then, setting the power to β leads to

$$\frac{\theta_A - \theta_P - \Delta - \delta}{SE_{T-P}} - z_{1-\alpha} = z_\beta,$$

i.e.,

$$\delta = \frac{r}{1+r}[\theta_A - \theta_P - (z_{1-\alpha} + z_\beta)SE_{T-P}]. \quad (4.7)$$

Comparing (4.6) with (4.7), we have

$$z_{1-\epsilon} = z_{1-\alpha} + z_\beta.$$

For $\alpha = 0.05$, the following table gives some examples of values of β, ϵ, and $z_{1-\epsilon}$.

β	ϵ	$z_{1-\epsilon}$
0.36	0.1000	1.282
0.50	0.0500	1.645
0.60	0.0290	1.897
0.70	0.0150	2.170
0.75	0.0101	2.320
0.80	0.0064	2.486

As a result, we arrive at the following conclusions with respect to the non-inferiority margin given by (4.6).

1. The non-inferiority margin (4.6) takes variability into consideration, i.e., δ is a decreasing function of the standard error of $\hat{\theta}_T - \hat{\theta}_P$. It is an increasing function of the sample sizes, since SE_{T-P} decreases as sample sizes increase. Choosing a non-inferiority margin depending on the sample sizes does not violate the basic frequentist statistical principle. In fact, it cannot be avoided when variability of sample estimators is considered. Statistical analysis, including sample size calculation in the trial planning stage, can still be performed. In the limiting case ($SE_{T-P} \to 0$), the non-inferiority margin in (4.6) is the same as that in (4.4).
2. The ϵ value in (4.6) represents a degree of conservativeness. An arbitrarily chosen ϵ may lead to highly conservative tests. When sample sizes are large (SE_{T-P} is small), one can afford a small ϵ. A reasonable value of ϵ and sample sizes can be determined in the planning stage of the trial.
3. The non-inferiority margin in (4.6) is non-negative if and only if $\theta_A - \theta_P \geq z_{1-\epsilon}SE_{T-P}$, i.e., the active control effect is substantial or the sample sizes are large. We might take our non-inferiority margin to be the larger of the quantity in (4.6) and 0 to force the non-inferiority margin to be nonnegative. However, it may be wise not to do so. Note that if θ_A is not substantially

larger than θ_P, then non-inferiority testing is not justifiable since, even if $\delta = 0$ in (4.1), concluding H_1 in (4.1) does not imply the test therapy is superior over the placebo. Using δ in (4.6), testing hypotheses (4.1) converts to testing the superiority of the test therapy over the active control agent when δ is actually negative. In other words, when $\theta_A - \theta_P$ is smaller than a certain margin, our test automatically becomes a superiority test and the property $P(\hat{\theta}_T - \hat{\theta}_P < \Delta) = \epsilon$ (with $\Delta = |\delta|/r$) still holds.

4. In many applications, there is no historical data. In such cases parameters related to placebo are not estimable and, hence, a non-inferiority margin not depending on these parameters is desired. Since the active control agent is a well-established therapy, let us assume that the power of the level α test showing that the active control agent is superior to placebo by the margin Δ is at the level η. This means that approximately,

$$\theta_A - \theta_P \geq \Delta + (z_{1-\alpha} + z_\eta)SE_{A-P}.$$

Replacing $\theta_A - \theta_P - \Delta$ in (4.6) by its lower bound given in the previous expression, we obtain the non-inferiority margin

$$\delta = (z_{1-\alpha} + z_\eta)SE_{A-P} - z_{1-\epsilon}SE_{T-P}.$$

To use this non-inferiority margin, we need some information about the population variance of the placebo group. As an example, consider the parallel design with two treatments, the test therapy and the active control agent. Assume that the same two-group parallel design would have been used if a placebo-controlled trial had been conducted. Then

$$SE_{A-P} = \sqrt{\sigma_A^2/n_A + \sigma_P^2/n_P}$$

and

$$SE_{T-P} = \sqrt{\sigma_T^2/n_T + \sigma_P^2/n_P},$$

where σ_k^2 is the asymptotic variance for $\sqrt{n_k}(\hat{\theta}_k - \theta_k)$ and n_k is the sample size under treatment k. If we assume $\sigma_P/\sqrt{n_P} = c$, then

$$\delta = (z_{1-\alpha} + z_\eta)\sqrt{\frac{\sigma_A^2}{n_A} + c^2} - z_{1-\epsilon}\sqrt{\frac{\sigma_T^2}{n_T} + c^2}. \quad (4.8)$$

Formula (4.8) can be used in two ways. One way is to replace c in (4.8) with an estimate. When no information from the placebo control is available, a suggested estimate of c is the smaller of the estimates of $\sigma_T/\sqrt{n_T}$ and $\sigma_A/\sqrt{n_A}$. The other way is to carry out a sensitivity analysis by using δ in (4.8) for a number of c values.

Statistical inference

When the non-inferiority margin depends on unknown population parameters, statistical tests designed for the case of constant non-inferiority margin may not be appropriate. Valid statistical tests for hypotheses (4.1) with δ given by (4.2) are derived in CBER/FDA Memorandum (1999), Holmgren (1999), and Hung et al. (2003), assuming that (i) γ is known and (ii) historical data from a placebo-controlled trial are available and the so-called "constancy condition" holds, i.e., the active control effects are equal in the current and the historical patient populations. In this section, we derive valid statistical tests for the non-inferiority margin given in (4.6) or (4.8). We use the same notations as described in the previous section.

Tests based on historical data under constancy condition We first consider tests involving the non-inferiority margin (4.6) in the case where historical data for a placebo-controlled trial assessing the effect of the active control agent are available and the constancy condition holds, i.e., the effect $\theta_{A0} - \theta_{P0}$ in the historical trial is the same as $\theta_A - \theta_P$ in the current active control trial, if a placebo control is added to the current trial. It should be emphasized that the constancy condition is a crucial assumption for the validity of the results.

Assume that the two-group parallel design is adopted in both the historical and current trials and that the sample sizes are respectively n_{A0} and n_{P0} for the active control and placebo in the historical trial and n_T and n_A for the test therapy and active control in the current trial. Without the normality assumption on the data, we adopt the large sample inference approach. Let $k = T, A, A0$ and $P0$ be the indexes, respectively, for the test and active control in the current trial and the active control and placebo in the historical trial. Assume that $n_k = l_k n$ for some fixed l_k and that, under appropriate conditions, estimators $\hat{\theta}_k$ for parameters θ_k satisfy

$$\sqrt{n_k}(\hat{\theta}_k - \theta_k) \to_d N(0, \sigma_k^2) \qquad (4.9)$$

as $n \to \infty$, where $\to_d$ denotes convergence in distribution. Also, assume that consistent estimators $\hat{\sigma}_k^2$ for σ_k^2 are obtained. The following result can be established.

Theorem 4.1 *We have*
$$\frac{\hat{\theta}_T - \hat{\theta}_A + \frac{r}{1+r}(\hat{\theta}_{A0} - \hat{\theta}_{P0} - z_{1-\epsilon}\widehat{SE}_{T-P}) - (\theta_T - \theta_A + \delta)}{\widehat{SE}_{T-C}} \to_d N(0, 1), \quad (4.10)$$

where
$$\widehat{SE}_{T-P} = \sqrt{\hat{\sigma}_T^2/n_T + \hat{\sigma}_{P0}^2/n_{P0}}$$

is an estimator of $SE_{T-P} = \sqrt{\sigma_T^2/n_T + \sigma_{P0}^2/n_{P0}}$ *and* $\widehat{SE}_{T-C}$ *is an estimator of* SE_{T-C}, *the standard deviation of* $\hat{\theta}_T - \hat{\theta}_A + \frac{r}{1+r}(\hat{\theta}_{A0} - \hat{\theta}_{P0})$, *i.e.,*

$$\widehat{SE}_{T-C} = \sqrt{\frac{\hat{\sigma}_T^2}{n_T} + \frac{\hat{\sigma}_A^2}{n_A} + \left(\frac{r}{1+r}\right)^2 \left(\frac{\hat{\sigma}_{A0}^2}{n_{A0}} + \frac{\hat{\sigma}_{P0}^2}{n_{P0}}\right)}.$$

Proof: From result (4.9), the independence of data from different groups, and the constancy condition,
$$\frac{\hat{\theta}_T - \hat{\theta}_A + \frac{r}{1+r}(\hat{\theta}_{A0} - \hat{\theta}_{P0}) - [\theta_T - \theta_A \frac{r}{1+r}(\theta_A - \theta_P)]}{SE_{T-C}} \to_d N(0, 1). \quad (4.11)$$

From the consistency of $\hat{\sigma}_k^2$ and the fact that $\sqrt{n} SE_{T-C}$ is a fixed constant,
$$\frac{\widehat{SE}_{T-P} - SE_{T-P}}{SE_{T-C}} = \frac{\sqrt{n}(\widehat{SE}_{T-P} - SE_{T-P})}{\sqrt{n} SE_{T-C}} = o_p(1)$$

and
$$\frac{\widehat{SE}_{T-C}}{SE_{T-C}} - 1 = \frac{\sqrt{n}(\widehat{SE}_{T-C} - SE_{T-C})}{\sqrt{n} SE_{T-C}} = o_p(1),$$

where $o_p(1)$ denotes a quantity converging to 0 in probability. Then
$$\frac{\hat{\theta}_T - \hat{\theta}_A + \frac{r}{1+r}(\hat{\theta}_{A0} - \hat{\theta}_{P0} - z_{1-\epsilon}\widehat{SE}_{T-P}) - (\theta_T - \theta_A + \delta)}{\widehat{SE}_{T-C}}$$

$$= \left\{\frac{\hat{\theta}_T - \hat{\theta}_A + \frac{r}{1+r}(\hat{\theta}_{A0} - \hat{\theta}_{P0}) - [\theta_T - \theta_A + \frac{r}{1+r}(\theta_A - \theta_P)]}{SE_{T-C}}\right.$$

$$\left. - \frac{r}{1+r} \frac{\widehat{SE}_{T-P} - SE_{T-P}}{SE_{T-C}}\right\} \frac{SE_{T-C}}{\widehat{SE}_{T-C}}$$

$$= \left\{\frac{\hat{\theta}_T - \hat{\theta}_A + \frac{r}{1+r}(\hat{\theta}_{A0} - \hat{\theta}_{P0}) - [\theta_T - \theta_A + \frac{r}{1+r}(\theta_A - \theta_P)]}{SE_{T-C}}\right.$$

$$\left. - o_p(1)\right\} [1 + o_p(1)]$$

and result (4.10) follows from result (4.11) and Slutsky's theorem.

Then, when the non-inferiority margin in (4.6) is adopted, the null hypothesis H_0 in (4.1) is rejected at approximately level α if

$$\hat{\theta}_T - \hat{\theta}_A + \frac{r}{1+r}(\hat{\theta}_{A0} - \hat{\theta}_{P0} - z_{1-\epsilon}\widehat{SE}_{T-P}) - z_{1-\alpha}\widehat{SE}_{T-C} > 0.$$

Impact on sample size

Using result (4.10), we can approximate the power of this test by

$$\Phi\left(\frac{\theta_T - \theta_A + \delta}{SE_{T-C}} - z_{1-\alpha}\right).$$

Using this formula, we can select the sample sizes n_T and n_A to achieve a desired power level (say β), assuming that n_{A0} and n_{P0} are given (in the historical trial). Assume that $n_T/n_A = \lambda$ is chosen. Then n_T should be selected as a solution of

$$\theta_T - \theta_A + \frac{r}{1+r}\left(\theta_A - \theta_P - z_{1-\epsilon}\sqrt{\frac{\sigma_T^2}{n_T} + \frac{\sigma_{P0}^2}{n_{P0}}}\right)$$

$$= (z_{1-\alpha} + z_\beta)\sqrt{\frac{\sigma_T^2}{n_T} + \frac{\lambda\sigma_A^2}{n_T} + \left(\frac{r}{1+r}\right)^2\left(\frac{\sigma_{A0}^2}{n_{A0}} + \frac{\sigma_{P0}^2}{n_{P0}}\right)}. \quad (4.12)$$

Although equation (4.12) does not have an explicit solution in terms of n_T, its solution can be numerically obtained once initial values for all parameters are given.

Remarks

The constancy condition The use of historical data usually increases the power of the test for hypotheses with a non-inferiority margin depending on parameters in the historical trial. On the other hand, using historical data without the constancy condition may lead to invalid conclusions. As indicated in Hung et al. (2003), checking the constancy condition is difficult. In this subsection we discuss a method of checking the constancy condition under an assumption much weaker than the constancy condition.

Note that the key is to check whether the active control effect $\theta_A - \theta_P$ in the current trial is the same as $\theta_{A0} - \theta_{P0}$ in the historical trial. If we assume that the placebo effects θ_P and θ_{P0} are the same (which is much weaker than the constancy condition), then we can check whether $\theta_A = \theta_{A0}$ using the data under the active control in the current and historical trials.

Tests without historical data We now consider tests when a non-inferiority margin (4.8) is chosen. Following the same argument as given in the proof of result (4.10), we can establish that

$$\frac{\hat{\theta}_T - \hat{\theta}_A + (z_{1-\alpha} + z_\eta)\widehat{SE}_{A-P} - z_{1-\epsilon}\widehat{SE}_{T-P} - (\theta_T - \theta_A + \Delta)}{\widehat{SE}_{T-A}} \to_d N(0, 1),$$
(4.13)

where

$$\widehat{SE}_{k-l} = \sqrt{\hat{\sigma}_k^2/n_k + \hat{\sigma}_l^2/n_l}.$$

Hence, when the non-inferiority margin in (4.8) is adopted, the null hypothesis H_0 in (4.1) is rejected at approximately level α if

$$\hat{\theta}_T - \hat{\theta}_A + (z_{1-\alpha} + z_\eta)\widehat{SE}_{A-P} - z_{1-\epsilon}\widehat{SE}_{T-A} - z_{1-\alpha}\sqrt{\frac{\hat{\sigma}_T^2}{n_T} + \frac{\hat{\sigma}_A^2}{n_A}} > 0.$$

The power of this test is approximately

$$\Phi\left(\frac{\theta_T - \theta_A + \delta}{SE_{T-A}} - z_{1-\alpha}\right).$$

If $n_T/n_A = \lambda$, then we can select the sample sizes n_T and n_A to achieve a desired power level (say β) by solving

$$\theta_T - \theta_A + (z_{1-\alpha} + z_\eta)\sqrt{\frac{\lambda\sigma_A^2}{n_T} + \frac{\sigma_P^2}{n_P}} - z_{1-\epsilon}\sqrt{\frac{\sigma_T^2}{n_T} + \frac{\sigma_P^2}{n_P}}$$

$$= (z_{1-\alpha} + z_\beta)\sqrt{\frac{\lambda\sigma_A^2}{n_T} + \frac{\sigma_T^2}{n_T}}.$$

4.3 Concluding Remarks

For large-scale clinical trials, a data safety monitoring committee (DMC) is usually established to monitor safety and/or perform interim efficacy analysis of the trial based on accrual data at some pre-scheduled time or when the trial has achieved a certain number of events. Based on the interim results, the DMC may recommend modification of study objectives and/or hypotheses. As an example, suppose that a clinical trial was designed as a superiority trial to establish the superiority of the test treatment as compared to a standard therapy or an active control agent. However, after the review of the interim results, it is determined that the trial will not be able to achieve the study objective of establishing superiority with the observed treatment effect size at interim.

The DMC does not recommend stopping the trial based on futility analysis. Instead, the DMC may suggest modifying the hypotheses for testing non-inferiority. This modification raises a critical statistical/clinical issue regarding the determination of a non-inferiority margin. Chow and Shao (2006) proposed a statistical justification for determining a non-inferiority margin based on accrued data at interim following ICH guidance.

CHAPTER 5

Adaptive Dose-Escalation Trials

In clinical research, the *response* in a dose response study could be a biological response for safety or efficacy. For example, in a dose-toxicity study, the goal is to determine the maximum tolerable dose (MTD). On the other hand, in a dose-efficacy response study, the primary objective is usually to address one or more of the following questions: (i) Is there any evidence of the drug effect? (ii) What is the nature of the dose response? and (iii) What is the optimal dose? In practice, it is always a concern as to how to evaluate the dose-response relationship with limited resources within a relatively tight time frame. This concern led to a proposed design that allows less patients to be exposed to the toxicity and more patients to be treated at potentially efficacious dose levels. Such a design also allows pharmaceutical companies to fully utilize their resources for development of more new drug products (see, e.g., Arbuck, 1996; Babb, Rogatko, and Zacks, 1998; Babb and Rogatko, 2001; Berry et al., 2002; Bretz and Hothorn, 2002).

The remainder of this chapter is organized as follows. In the next section, we provide a brief background of dose-escalation trials. The concepts of the continued reassessment method (CRM) in phase I oncology trials is reviewed in Section 5.2. In Section 5.3, we propose a hybrid frequentist-Bayesian adaptive approach. In Section 5.4, several simulations were conducted to evaluate the performance of the proposed method. The concluding remarks are presented in Section 5.5.

5.1 Introduction

For dose-toxicity studies, the traditional escalation rules (TER), which are also known as the "3 + 3" rules, are commonly used in the early phase of oncology studies. The "3 + 3" rule is to enter three patients at a new dose level and then enter another three patients when dose limiting toxicity (DLT) is observed. The assessment of the six patients is then performed to determine whether the trial should be stopped at the level or to increase the dose. Basically, there are two types of the "3 + 3" rules, namely the traditional escalation rule (TER) and strict traditional escalation rule (STER). TER does not allow dose de-escalation but STER does when two of three patients have DLTs. The "3 + 3" rules can be generalized to the "m + n" TER and STER escalation rules. Chang and Chow (2006a) provided a detailed description of general "m + n" designs with and without dose de-escalation. The corresponding formulas for sample size calculation can be found in Lin and Shih (2001).

Recently, many new methods such as the assessment of dose response using multiple-stage designs (Crowley, 2001) and the continued reassessment method (CRM) (see, e.g., O'Quigley, Pepe, and Fisher, 1990; O'Quigley and Shen, 1996; Babb and Rogatko, 2004) have been developed. For the method of CRM, the dose-response relationship is continually reassessed based on accumulative data collected from the trial. The next patient who enters the trial is then assigned to the potential MTD level. This approach is more efficient than that of the usual TER with respect to the allocation of the MTD. However, the efficiency of CRM may be at risk due to delayed response and/or a constraint on dose-jump in practice (Babb and Rogatko, 2004). In recent years, the use of adaptive design methods for characterizing dose-response curves has become very popular (Bauer and Rohmel, 1995). An adaptive design is a dynamic system that allows the investigator to optimize the trial (including design, monitoring, operating, and analysis) with cumulative information observed from the trial. For Bayesian adaptive design for dose-response trials, some researchers suggest the use of loss/utility function in conjunction with dose assignment based on minimization/maximization of loss/utility function (e.g., Gasparini and Eisele, 2000; Whitehead, 1997).

In this chapter, we use an adaptive method that combines CRM and utility-adaptive randomization (UAR) for multiple-endpoint trials (Chang, Chow, and Pong, 2005). The proposed UAR is similar to response-adaptive randomization (RAR). It is an extension of RAR to multi-endpoint case. In UAR scheme, the probability of assigning a patient to a particular dose level is determined by its normalized utility value (ranging from 0 to 1). The CRM could be a Bayesian, a frequentist, or a hybrid frequentist-Bayesian–based approach. This proposed method has the advantage of achieving the optimal design by means of the adaptation to the accrued data of an on-going trial. In addition, CRM could provide a better prediction of dose-response relationship by selecting an appropriate model as compared to the method simply based on the observed response. In practice, it is not uncommon that the observed response rate is lower in a higher-dose group than that in a lower-dose group provided that the high-dose group, in fact, has a higher response rate. The use of CRM is able to avoid this problem by using a monotonic function such as a logistic function in the model. The proposed adaptive method deals with multiple endpoints in two ways.

The first approach is to model each dose-endpoint relationship with or without constraints among the models. Each model is usually a monotonic function family such as logistic or some power function. The second approach is to combine the multiple endpoints into a single utility index, and then model the utility using a more flexible function family such as hyper-logistic function as proposed in this chapter.

5.2 CRM in Phase I Oncology Study

CRM is originally used in Phase I oncology trials (O'Quigley, Pepe, and Fisher, 1990). The primary goal of phase I oncology trials is not only to assess the dose-toxicity relationship, but also to determine MTD. Due to potential high toxicity of the study drug, in practice usually only a small number of patients (e.g., 3 to 6) are treated at each ascending dose level. The most common approach is the "3 + 3" TER with a prespecified sequence for dose escalation. However, this ad hoc approach is found to be inefficient and often underestimates the MTD, especially when the starting dose is too low. The CRM is developed to overcome these limitations. The estimation or prediction from CRM is weighted by a number of data points. Therefore, if the data points are mostly around the estimated value, then the estimation is more accurate. CRM assigns more patients near MTD; consequently, the estimated MTD is much more precise and reliable. In practice, this is the most desirable operating characteristic of the Bayesian CRM. In what follows, we will briefly review the CRM approach.

Dose-toxicity modeling

In most phase I dose response trials, it is assumed that there is monotonic relationship between dose and toxicity. This ideal relationship suggests that the biologically inactive dose is lower than the active dose, which is in turn lower than the toxic dose. To characterize this relationship, the choice of an appropriate dose-toxicity model is important. In practice, the logistic model is often utilized:

$$p(x) = [1 + b\exp(-ax)]^{-1}$$

where $p(x)$ is the probability of toxicity associated with dose x, and a and b are positive parameters to be determined. Practically, $p(x)$ is equivalent to toxicity rate or dose limiting toxicity (DLT) rate as defined by the Common Toxicity Criteria (CTC) of the United States National Cancer Institute. Denote θ the probability of DLT (or DLT rate) at MTD.

Then, the MTD can be expressed as

$$MTD = \frac{1}{a} \ln\left(\frac{b\theta}{1-\theta}\right).$$

If we can estimate a and b or their posterior distributions (for common logistic model, b is predetermined), we will be able to determine the MTD or provide predictive probabilities for MTD. The choice of toxicity rate at MTD, θ, depends on the nature of the DLT and the type of the target tumor. For an aggressive tumor and a transient and non-life-threatening DLT, θ could be as high as 0.5. For persistent DLT and less aggressive tumors, it could be as low as 0.1 to 0.25. A commonly used value is somewhere between 0 and 1/3 = 0.33 (Crowley, 2001).

Dose-level selection

The initial dose given to the first patients in a phase I study should be low enough to avoid severe toxicity but high enough for observing some activity or potential efficacy in humans. The commonly used starting dose is the dose at which 10% mortality (LD_{10}) occurs in mice. The subsequent dose levels are usually selected based on the following multiplicative set

$$x_i = f_{i-1} x_{i-1} \quad (i = 1, 2, \ldots k),$$

where f_i is called the dose escalation factor. The highest dose level should be selected such that it covers the biologically active dose, but remains lower than the toxic dose. In general, CRM does not require pre-determined dose intervals. However, the use of a pre-determined dose is often for practical convenience.

Reassessment of model parameters

The key is to estimate the parameter a in the response model. An initial assumption or a prior one about the parameter is necessary in order to assign patients to the dose level based the dose-toxicity relationship. This estimation of a is continually updated based on cumulative data observed from the trial. The estimation method can be a Bayesian or frequentist approach. For Bayesian approaches, it leads to the posterior distribution of a. For frequentist approaches such as maximum likelihood, estimate or least-square estimate are straightforward. Note that the Bayesian approach requires a prior distribution about parameter a. It it provides posterior distribution of a and predictive probabilities of MTD. The frequentist, Bayesian and a hybrid frequentist-Bayesian–based approaches in conjunction with the response-adaptive randomization will be further discussed in this chapter.

Assignment of next patient

The updated dose-toxicity model is usually used to choose the dose level for the next patient. In other words, the next patient enrolled in the trial is assigned to the current estimated MTD based on the dose-response model. Practically, this assignment is subject to safety constraints such as limited dose jump and delayed response. Assignment of patients to the most updated MTD is intuitive. It leads to the majority of the patients being assigned to the dose levels near MTD, which allows a more precise estimate of MTD with a minimum number of patients.

5.3 Hybrid Frequentist-Bayesian Adaptive Design

When Bayesian is used for multiple-parameter response model, some numerical irregularities cannot be easily resolved. In addition, Bayesian methods require an extensive computation for a multiple-parameter model. To overcome these limitations, a hybrid frequentist and Bayesian method is useful. The use of a utility-adaptive randomization allows the allocation of more patients to the superior dose levels and less patients to the inferior dose levels. This adaptive method is not only optimal ethically but also has a favorable benefit/risk ratio (such as benefit-safety and/or benefit-cost).

The adaptive model

In this section, we use the adaptive design as outlined in Figure 5.1 for dose-response trial or Phase II/III combined trials. Start with several dose levels with or without a placebo group, followed by the prediction of the dose-response relationship using Bayesian or other approaches based on accrued real-time data. The next patient is then randomized to a treatment group based on the utility-adaptive or response-adaptive randomization algorithm. We may allow the inferior treatment groups to be dropped when there are too many groups based on results from the analysis of the accrued data using Bayesian and/or frequentist approaches. It is expected that the predictive dose-response model in conjunction with a utility-adaptive randomization could lead to a design that assigns more patients to the superior arms and consequently a more efficient design. We will illustrate this point further via computer trial simulations. In the next section, technical details for establishing dose-response relationships using CRM in conjunction with utility-adaptive randomization are provided.

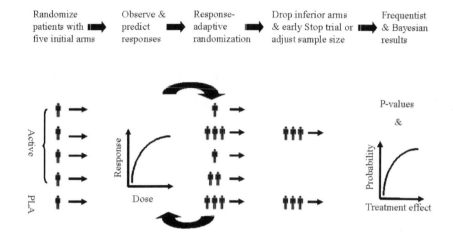

Figure 5.1 Bayesian adaptive trial.

Utility-based unified CRM adaptive approach

The utility-based unified CRM adaptive approach can be summarized by the following steps.

> Step 1: Construct utility function based on trial objectives;
> Step 2: Propose a probability model for dose–response relationship;
> Step 3: Construct prior probability distributions of the parameters in the response model;
> Step 4: Form the likelihood function based on incremental information on treatment response during the trial;
> Step 5: Reassess model parameters or calculate the posterior probability of the model parameters;
> Step 6: Update the expected utility function based on dose-response model;
> Step 7: Determine next action or make adaptations such as changing the randomization or drop inferior treatment arms;
> Step 8: Further collect trial data and repeat Steps 5 to 7 until stopping criteria are met.

Construction of utility function

Let $X = \{x_1, x_2, \ldots x_k\}$ be the action space where x_i is coded value for action of anything that would affect the outcomes or decision making, such as a treatment, a withdrawal of a treatment arm, a protocol amendment, stopping the trial, an investment of advertising for the prospective

ADAPTIVE DOSE-ESCALATION TRIALS

drug, or any combination of the above. x_i can be either a fixed dose or a variable of dose given to a patient. If action x_i is not taken, then $x_i = 0$. Let $y = \{y_1, y_2, \ldots y_m\}$ be the outcomes of interest, which can be efficacy or toxicity of a test drug, the cost of trial, etc. Each of these outcomes, y_i is a function of action $y_i(x)$, $x \in X$. The utility is defined as

$$U = \sum_{j=1}^{m} w_j = \sum_{j=1}^{m} w(y_j), \tag{5.1}$$

where U is normalized such that $0 \leq U \leq 1$ and w_j are pre-specified weights.

Probability model for dose response

Each of the outcomes can be modeled by the following generalized probability model:

$$\Gamma_j(\mathbf{p}) = \sum_{i=1}^{k} a_{ji} x_i, \ j = 1, \ldots, m \tag{5.2}$$

where

$$\mathbf{p} = \{p_1, \ldots, p_m\}, \quad p_j = P(y_j \geq \tau_j),$$

and τ_j is a threshold for jth outcome. The link function, $\Gamma_j(.)$, is a generalized function of all the probabilities of the outcomes. For simplicity, we may consider

$$\Gamma_j(p_j) = \sum_{i=1}^{k} a_{ji} x_i, j = 1, \ldots, m, \tag{5.3}$$

and

$$p_j(\mathbf{x}, \mathbf{a}) = \Gamma_j^{-1}\left(\sum_{i=1}^{k} a_{ji} x_i\right), \ j = 1, \ldots, m. \tag{5.4}$$

The essential difference between (5.4) and (5.5) is that the former models the outcomes jointly, while the latter models each outcome independently. Therefore, for (5.5), Γ_j^{-1} is simply the inverse function of Γ_j. However, for (5.4), Γ_j^{-1} is not a simple inverse function and sometimes the explicit solution may not exist. Γ_j can be used to model the constraints between outcomes, e.g., the relationship between the two blood pressures. Using the link functions could reduce some of the irregular models in the modeling process when there are multiple outcome endpoints.

For univariate case, logistic model is commonly used for monotonic response. However, for utility, we usually don't know whether it is

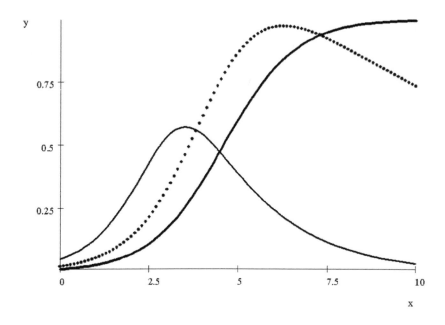

Figure 5.2 Curves of hyper-logistic function family.

monotonic or not. Therefore, we proposed the following model

$$p_j(\mathbf{x}, \mathbf{a}) = (a_{j1} \exp(a_{j2}x) + a_{j3} \exp(-a_{j4}x))^{-m}; \ (j = 1, \ldots m) \quad (5.5)$$

where a_{ji} and m are usually positive values and m is suggested to be 1. Note that when $a_{j1} = 1$, $a_{j2} = 0$, and $m = 1$, (5.7) degenerates to the common logistic model. When $a_{j1} = a_{j3} = 1$, $a_{j2} = 0$, and $a_{j4} = 2$, it reduces to the hyperbolic tangent model. Note that a_{ji} must be determined such that $0 \leq p_j(\mathbf{x}, \mathbf{a}) \leq 1$ for the dose range x under study. For convenience, we will refer to (5.7) as a hyper-logistic function.

The hyper-logistic function is useful especially in modeling utility index because it is not necessarily monotonic. However, the range of parameter should be carefully determined before modeling. It is suggested that corresponding various shapes be examined. Some different shapes that are generated by hyper-logistic function are presented in Figure 5.2.

A special case that is worth mentioning here is the following single-utility index (or combined outcomes) model, where the probability is based on utility rather than each outcome

$$p = P(U \geq \tau). \quad (5.6)$$

ADAPTIVE DOSE-ESCALATION TRIALS

Unlike the probability models defined based on individual outcomes such as single efficacy or safety outcome, the probability models defined based on utility are often single mode.

Prior distribution of parameter tensor **a**

The Bayesian approach requires the specification of prior probability distribution of the unknown parameter tensor a_{ji}.

$$\mathbf{a} \sim g_{j0}(\mathbf{a}), \quad j = 1, \ldots m, \tag{5.7}$$

where $g_{j0}(\mathbf{a})$ is the prior probability for the jth endpoint.

Likelihood function

The next step is to construct the likelihood function. Given n observations with y_{ji} associated with endpoint j and dose x_{m_i}, the likelihood function can be written as

$$f_{jn}(\mathbf{r}|\mathbf{a}) = \prod_{i=1}^{n} \left[\Gamma_j^{-1}(a_{jm_i}x_{m_i})\right]^{r_{ji}} \left[1 - \Gamma_j^{-1}(a_{jm_i}x_{m_i})\right]^{1-r_{ji}}, \quad j = 1, \ldots m, \tag{5.8}$$

where

$$r_{ji} = \begin{cases} 1, & \text{if } y_{ji} \geq \tau_j \\ 0, & \text{otherwise} \end{cases}, \quad j = 1, \ldots m. \tag{5.9}$$

Assessment of parameter **a**

The assessment of the parameters in the model can be carried out in different ways: Bayesian, frequentist, or hybrid approach. Bayesian and hybrid approaches are to assess the probability distribution of the parameter, while the frequentist approach is to provide a point estimate of the parameter.

Bayesian approach For the Bayesian approach, the posterior probability can be obtained as follows:

$$g_j(\mathbf{a}|\mathbf{r}) = \frac{f_{jn}(\mathbf{r}|\mathbf{a})g_{j0}(\mathbf{a})}{\int f_{jn}(\mathbf{r}|\mathbf{a})g_{j0}(\mathbf{a})\,d\mathbf{a}}, \quad j = 1, \ldots m. \tag{5.10}$$

We then update the probabilities of the outcome or the predictive probabilities

$$p_j = \int \Gamma_j^{-1}\left(\sum_{i=1}^{k} a_{ji}x_i\right) g_j(\mathbf{a}|\mathbf{r})\,d\mathbf{a}, \quad j = 1, \ldots m. \tag{5.11}$$

Note that the Bayesian approach is computationally intensive. Alternatively, we may consider a frequentist approach to simplify the calculation, especially when limited knowledge about the prior is available and non-informative prior is to be used.

Maximum likelihood approach The maximum likelihood estimates of the parameters are given by

$$a_{ji\ MLE} = \arg\max_{\mathbf{a}}\{f_{jn}(\mathbf{r}\,|\,\mathbf{a})\},\ j=1,\ldots m, \quad (5.12)$$

where $a_{ji\ MLE}$ is the parameter set for the jth outcome. After having obtained $a_{ji\ MLE}$, we can update the probability using

$$p_j(\mathbf{x},\mathbf{a}) = \Gamma_j^{-1}\left(\sum_{i=1}^k a_{ji\ MLE}\,x_i\right),\ j=1,\ldots m. \quad (5.13)$$

Least square approach The least square approach minimizes the difference between predictive probability and the observed rate or probability, which is given below.

$$\mathbf{a}_{jLSE} = \arg\min_{\mathbf{a}}\{L_j(\mathbf{a}))\},\ j=1,\ldots m, \quad (5.14)$$

where

$$L_j(\mathbf{a}) = \sum_{i=1}^k \left(p_j(x_i,\mathbf{a}) - \hat{p}_j(x_i,\mathbf{a})\right)^2.$$

We then update the probability

$$p_j(\mathbf{x},\mathbf{a}) = \Gamma_j^{-1}\left(\sum_{i=1}^k a_{ji\ LSE}\,x_i\right), \quad (5.15)$$

where $a_{ji\ LSE}$, the component of $\mathbf{a}$, is the parameter set for the jth outcome.

Hybrid frequentist-Bayesian approach Although Bayesian CRM allows the incorporation of prior knowledge about the parameters, some difficulties arise when it is used in a model with multiple parameters. The difficulties include (i) computational burden and (ii) numerical instability in evaluation posterior probability. A solution is to use the frequentist approach to estimate all the parameters and use the Bayesian approach to re-estimate the posterior distribution of some parameters. This hybrid frequentist-Bayesian approach allows the incorporation of prior knowledge about parameter distribution but avoids computational burden and numerical instability. Details regarding the hybrid method will be specified.

Determination of next action

As mentioned earlier, the actions or adaptations taken should be based on trial objectives or utility function. A typical action is a change of the randomization schedule. From the dose-response model, since each dose associates with a probability of response, the expected utility function is then given by $\bar{U} = \sum_{j=1}^{m} p_j(\mathbf{x}, \mathbf{a}) w_j$. Two approaches, deterministic and probabilistic, can be taken. The former refers to the optimal approach where actions can be taken to maximize the expected utility, while the latter refers to adaptive randomization where treatment assignment to the next patient is not fully determined by the algorithm.

Optimal approach As mentioned earlier, in the optimal approach, the dose level assigned to the next patient is based on optimization of the expected utility, i.e.,

$$x_{n+1} = \arg\max_{x_i} \bar{U} = \sum_{j=1}^{m} p_j w_j.$$

However, it is not feasible due to its difficulties in practice.

Utility-adaptive randomization approach Many of the response-adaptive randomizations (RAR) can be used to increase the expected response. However, these adaptive randomization are difficult to apply directly to the case of the multiple endpoints. As an alternative, the following utility-adaptive randomization algorithm is proposed. This utility-adaptive randomization, which combines the idea from randomized-play-winner (Rosenberger and Lachin, 2003) and Lachin's urn models, is based on the following. The target randomization probability to x_i group is proportional to the current estimation of utility or response rate of the group, i.e., $U(x_i) / \sum_{i=1}^{k} U(x_i)$, where K is the number of groups. When a patient is randomized into x_i group, the randomization probability to this group should be reduced. These lead to the following proposed randomization model:

Probability of randomizing a patient to group x_i is proportional to the corresponding posterior probability of the utility or response rate, i.e.,

$$\mathfrak{R}(x_i) = \frac{1}{c} \left(\frac{U(x_i)}{\sum_{i=1}^{k} U(x_i)} - \frac{n_i}{N} \right), \qquad (5.16)$$

where the normalization factor

$$c = \sum_{i} \left(\frac{U(x_i)}{\sum_{i=1}^{k} U(x_i)} - \frac{n_i}{N} \right),$$

n_i is the number of patients that have been randomized to the x_i group, and N is the total estimated number of patients in the trial. We will refer to this model as the *utility-offset model*.

Rules for dropping losers For ethical and economical reasons, we may consider to drop some inferior treatment groups. The issue is how to identify the inferior arms with certain statistical assurance. There are many possible rules for dropping an ineffective dose level. For example, just to name two, (i) maximum sample size ratio between groups that exceeds a threshold, R_n and the number of patients randomized exceeds a N_R; or (ii) the maximum utility difference, $U_{\max} - U_{\min} > \delta_u$ and its naive confidence interval width less than a threshold, δ_{uw}. The naive confidence interval is calculated as if U_{max} and U_{min} are observed responses with the corresponding sample size at each dose level. Note that the normalized utility index U ranges from 0 to 1. Note that, optionally, we may also choose to retain the control group or all groups for the purpose of comparison between groups.

Stopping rule Several stopping rules are available for stopping a trial. For example, we may stop the trial when

(i) General rule: total sample size exceeds N, a threshold, or
(ii) Utility rules: maximum utility difference $U_{max} - U_{min} > \delta_u$ and its naive confidence interval width is less than δ_{uw}, or
(iii) Futility Rules: $U_{max} - U_{min} < \delta_f$ and its naive confidence interval width is less than δ_{fw}.

5.4 Simulations

Design settings

Without loss of generality, a total of 5 dose levels is chosen for the trial simulations. The response rates, $p(U > u)$, associated with each dose level are summarized in Table 5.1. These response rates are not chosen from the hyper-logistic model, but arbitrarily in the interest of reflecting common practices.

Table 5.1 Assumed Dose-Response Relationship for Simulations

Dose Level	1	2	3	4	5
Dose	20	40	70	95	120
Target Response Rate	0.02	0.07	0.37	0.73	0.52

Response model

The probability model considered was $p(\mathbf{x}, \mathbf{a}) = P(U \geq u)$ under the hyper-logistic model with three parameters (a_1, a_3, a_4), i.e.,

$$p(\mathbf{x}, \mathbf{a}) = C \left(a_1 e^{0.03x} + a_3 e^{-a_4 x} \right)^{-1}, \tag{5.17}$$

where $a_1 \in [0.06, 0.1]$, $a_3 \in [150, 200]$. The use of scale factor C is a simple way to assure that $0 \leq p_j(\mathbf{x}, \mathbf{a}) \leq 1$ during in the simulation program.

Prior distribution

Two non-informative priors for parameter a_4 were used for the trial simulations. They are defined over $[0.05, 0.1]$ and $[0.01, 0.1]$, respectively.

$$a_4 \sim g_0(a_4) = \begin{cases} \frac{1}{b-a}, & a \leq a_4 \leq b \\ 0, & \text{otherwise.} \end{cases} \tag{5.18}$$

Reassessment method

In the simulations, the hybrid frequentist-Bayesian method was used. We first used the frequentist least squares method to estimate the 3 parameters a_i ($i = 1, 3, 4$), then used the estimated a_1, a_3, and the prior for a_4 in the model and Bayesian method to obtain the posterior probability distribution of parameter a_4 and the predictive probabilities.

Utility-adaptive randomization

Under the *utility-offset model* described earlier, the probability for randomizing a patient to the dose level x_i is given by

$$\Re(x_i) = \begin{cases} \frac{1}{K}, & \text{before an observed responder} \\ C \left(\frac{p(x_i)}{\sum_{i=1}^{k} p(x_i)} - \frac{n_i}{N} \right), & \text{after an observed responder,} \end{cases} \tag{5.19}$$

where $p(\mathbf{x}_i)$ is the response rate or the predictive probability in Bayesian sense, n_i is the number of patients that have been randomized to the x_i group, N is the total estimated number of patients in the trial, and K is number of dose groups.

Rules of dropping losers and stopping rule

In the simulations, no losers were dropped. The trial was stopped when the subjects randomized reached the prespecified maximum number.

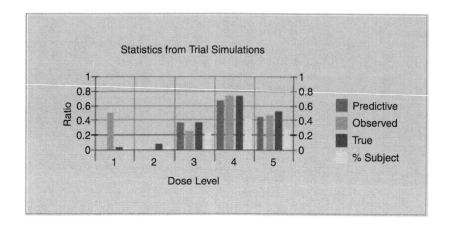

Figure 5.3 A typical example of simulation results.

Simulation results

Computer simulations were conducted to evaluate the operating characteristics. Four different sample sizes (i.e., N = 20, 30, 50, 100) and two different non-informative priors were used. The outcomes from a typical simulation are presented in Figure 5.3. It is shown that predicted response rates are still reasonably good even when the observed (simulated) response rates are showing the sine-shape. The average results from 1000 simulations per scenario are summarized in Table 5.2.

We can see that the number of patients randomized into each group is approximately proportional to the corresponding utility or rate in each dose group, which indicates that the utility-adaptive randomization is efficient in achieving the target patient allocations among treatment groups. Compared to traditional balanced design with multiple arms, the adaptive design smartly allocates majority patients to the desirable dose levels. In all cases, the predicted rates are similar to the simulated rates. This is reasonable since non-informative priors were used. The precision of the predictive rate at each dose level is measured by its standard deviation:

$$\delta_p = \sqrt{\frac{1}{N_s} \sum_{i=1}^{N_s} [\hat{p}_i(x) - \bar{p}(x)]^2}, \quad (5.20)$$

where N_s is the number of simulations, $\hat{p}_i(x)$ is the simulated response rate or predicted response rate, and $\bar{p}(x)$ is the mean response rate at dose level x. The hybrid method provides estimates with reasonable precision when there are 50 subjects (10 subjects per arm on average)

Table 5.2 Comparisons of Simulation Results[#]

Scenario	Dose Level	1	2	3	4	5
	Target rate	0.02	0.07	0.37	0.73	0.52
n* = 100	Simulated rate	0.02	0.07	0.36	0.73	0.52
	Predicted rate	0.02	0.07	0.41	0.68	0.43
	Standard deviation	0.00	0.01	0.08	0.07	0.03
	Number of subjects	1.71	4.78	25.2	41.8	26.6
n* = 50	Simulated rate	0.02	0.07	0.36	0.73	0.52
	Predicted rate	0.02	0.07	0.40	0.65	0.41
	Standard deviation	0.00	0.02	0.11	0.09	0.04
	Number of subjects	1.02	2.48	12.6	20.5	13.4
n* = 30	Simulated rate	0.02	0.05	0.36	0.73	0.51
	Predicted rate	0.02	0.07	0.40	0.63	0.40
	Standard deviation	0.00	0.02	0.13	0.11	0.05
	Number of subjects	1.00	1.62	7.50	11.9	8.00
n* = 20	Simulated rate	0.02	0.06	0.34	0.72	0.51
	Predicted rate	0.02	0.07	0.37	0.58	0.38
	Standard deviation	0.00	0.02	0.15	0.14	0.06
	Number of subjects	1.00	1.03	4.68	7.60	5.68
n** = 50	Simulated rate	0.02	0.07	0.36	0.73	0.51
	Predicted rate	0.02	0.07	0.41	0.65	0.41
	Standard deviation	0.00	0.02	0.11	0.09	0.04
	Number of subjects	1.02	2.53	12.7	20.5	13.3

[#] From simulation software: ExpDesign Studio by www.CTriSoft.net
* Uniform prior over [0.05, 0.1]; ** uniform prior over [0.01, 0.1].

or more. The precision reduces when sample size reduces, but the precision is not so bad even with only 20 patients. The relationships between number of subjects and precision for the most interested dose levels (level 3, 4, and 5) are presented in Figure 5.4. The predicted response rates seem not to be sensitive to the non-informative priors. The simulation results for the two non-informative priors are very similar. Note that precision very much depends upon the number of parameters used in the response model. The more parameters, the less precision. In the simulations a three-parameter hyper-logistic model was used. If a single-parameter model were used, the precision of the predicted response rates would be greatly improved.

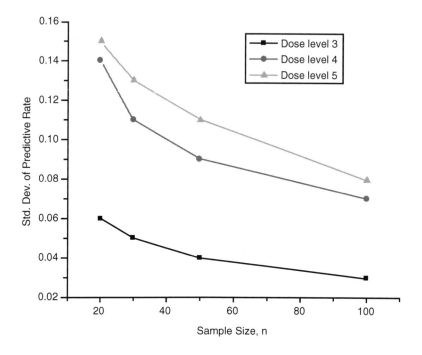

Figure 5.4 Relationship between sample size and standard deviation of predictive rate.

5.5 Concluding Remarks

The proposed utility-adaptive randomization has the desirable property that the proportion of subjects assigned to the treatment is proportional to the response rate or the predictive probability. Assigning more patients to the superior groups allows a more precise evaluation of the superior groups with relatively small number of patients. The hybrid CRM approach with hyper-logistic model gives reliable predictive results regarding dose response with a minimum number of patients. It is important to choose proper ranges for the parameters of the hyper-logistic model, which can be managed when one becomes familiar with the curves of hyper-logistic function affected by its parameters. In the case of low response rates, the sample size is expected to increase accordingly. The hybrid approach allows the users to combine the computational simplicity and numerical stability of frequentist method with the flexibility in priors and predictive nature of the Bayesian approach. The proposed method can be used in phase II/III combined study to accelerate the drug development process. However, there are some practical

ADAPTIVE DOSE-ESCALATION TRIALS 105

issues such as *how to perform a thorough review when the trial is ongoing*, which are necessarily considered for safety of the patients. Since the proposed Bayesian adaptive design is multiple-endpoint oriented, it can be used for various situations. For example, for ordinal responses (e.g., CTC grades), we can consider the different levels of responses as different endpoints, then model them separately, and calculate the expected utility based on the models. Alternatively, we can also form the utility first by assigning different weights to the response levels and then modeling the utility.

CHAPTER 6

Adaptive Group Sequential Design

In clinical trials, it is not uncommon to perform data safety monitoring and/or interim analyses based on accrued data up to a certain time point during the conduct of a clinical trial. The purpose is not only to monitor the progress and integrity of the trial, but also to take action regarding early termination (if there is evidence that the trial will put subjects in an unreasonable risk or the treatment is ineffective) or modifications to the study design in compliance with ICH GCP for data standards and data quality. In most clinical trials, the primary reasons for conducting interim analyses of accrued data are probably due to (Jennison and Turnbull, 2000): (i) ethical considerations, (ii) administrative reasons, and (iii) economic constraints. In practice, since clinical trials involve human subjects, it is ethical to monitor the trials to ensure that individual subjects are not exposed to unsafe or ineffective treatment regimens. When the trials are found to be negative (i.e., the treatment appears to be ineffective), there is an ethical imperative to terminate the trials early. Ethical consideration indicates that clinical data should be evaluated in terms of safety and efficacy of the treatment under study based on accumulated data in conjunction with updated clinical information from literature and/or other clinical trials.

From the administrative point of view, interim analyses are necessarily conducted to ensure that the clinical trials are being executed as planned. For example, it is always a concern whether subjects who meet the eligibility criteria are from the correct patient population (which is representative of the target patient population). Also, it is important to assure that the trial procedures, dose/dose regimen, and treatment duration adhere to the study protocol. An early examination of interim results can reveal the problems (such as protocol deviations and/or protocol violations) of the trials early. Immediate actions can be taken to remedy issues and problems detected by interim analyses. An early interim analysis can also verify critical assumptions made at the planning stage of the trials. If serious violations of the critical assumptions are found, modifications or adjustments must be made to ensure the quality and integrity of the trials.

The remainder of this chapter is organized as follows. In the next section, basic concepts of sequential methods in clinical trials are introduced. In Section 6.2, a unified approach for group sequential designs for normal, binary, and survival endpoints is introduced. In Section 6.3, the boundary function proposed by Wang and Tsiatis (1987) is considered for construction of the stopping boundaries based on equal information intervals. Also included in this section is the discussion of the use of unequal information intervals under a two-stage design which is of practical interest in clinical trials. Section 6.4 introduces a more flexible (adaptive) design, i.e., error-spending approach, where the information intervals and number of analyses are not pre-determined, but the error-spending function is pre-determined. The relationship between error-spending function and Wang and Tsiatis' boundary function is also discussed in this section. A proposed approach for formulating the group sequential design based on independent p-values from the sub-samples from different stages is described in Section 6.5. The formulation is valid regardless of the methods used for calculation of the p-values. Trial monitoring and conditional powers for assessment of futility for comparing means and comparing proportions are derived in Sections 6.7 and 6.8, respectively. Practical issues are given in the last section.

6.1 Sequential Methods

As pointed out by Jennison and Turnbull (2000), the concept of sequential statistical methods was originally motivated by the need to obtain clinical benefits under certain economic constraints. For a trial with a positive result, early stopping means that a new product can be exploited sooner. If a negative result is indicated, early stopping ensures that resources are not wasted. Sequential methods typically lead to saving in sample size, time, and cost when compared with the standard fixed sample procedures. Interim analyses enable management to make appropriate decisions regarding the allocation of limited resources for continued development of the promising treatment.

In clinical trials, sequential methods are used when there are formal interim analyses. An interim analysis is an analysis intended to assess treatment effect with respect to efficacy or safety at any time prior to the completion of a clinical trial. Because interim analysis results may introduce bias to subsequent clinical evaluation of the subjects who enter the trial, all interim analyses should be carefully planned in advance and described in the study protocol. Under special circumstances, there may be a need for an interim analysis that was not planned originally. In this case, a protocol amendment describing the rationale for such an interim analysis should be implemented prior to any clinical data being unblinded. For many clinical trials of investigational products, especially those that have public attention for major health significance, an external independent group or data monitoring committee (DMC) should be formed to perform clinical data monitoring for safety and interim analysis for efficacy. The U.S. FDA requires that the role/responsibility and function/activities of a DMC be clearly stated in the study protocol to maintain the integrity of the clinical trial (FDA, 2000, 2005; Offen, 2003).

Basic concepts

A (fully) sequential test is referred to as a test conducted based on accrued data after every new observation is obtained. A group sequential test, as opposed to a fully sequential test, is referred to as a test performed based on accrued data at some pre-specified intervals rather than after every new observation is obtained (Jennison and Turnbull, 2000).

Error-inflation For a conventional single-stage trial with one-sided $\alpha = 0.025$, the null hypothesis (H_0) is rejected if the statistic $z \geq 1.96$. For a sequential trial with K analyses, if at the k-th analysis ($k = 1, 2, \ldots, K$), if the absolute value of Z_k is sufficiently large, we will reject H_0 and stop the trial. It is not appropriate to simply apply a level-α one-sided test at each analysis since the multiple tests would lead to an inflation of the type-I error rate. In fact, the actual α level is given by $1-(1-\alpha)^k$. Thus, for $K = 5$, the actual α level is 0.071, nearly 3 times as big as that of the 0.025 significance level applied at each individual analysis.

Stopping boundary Stopping boundaries consist of a set of critical values that the test statistics calculated from actual data will be compared with to determine whether the trial should be terminated or continue. For example, Figure 6.1 provides a set of critical values as boundaries for stopping. In other words, if the observed sample mean at a given stage falls outside the boundaries, we will terminate the trial; otherwise, the trial continues.

Boundary scales Many different scales can be used to construct the stopping boundaries. The four commonly used scales are the standardized z-statistic, the sample-mean scale, the error-spending scale, and the sum-mean scale. In principle, these scales are equivalent to one another after appropriate transformation. Among the four scales, sample-mean scale and error-spending scale have most intuitive interpretations. As an example, consider the hypothesis for testing the difference between two-sample independent means. These scales are defined as follows:

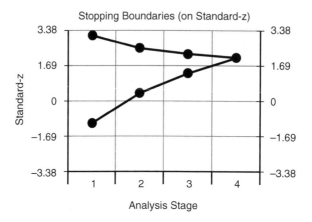

Figure 6.1 Stopping boundaries.

- Sample-mean scale: $\theta_k = \bar{x}_{Ak} - \bar{x}_{Bk}$.
- Standardized z-statistic: $Z_k = \theta_k \sqrt{I_k}$, where $I_k = \frac{n_k}{2\sigma^2}$ is the information level.
- Sum-mean scale: $D_k = \sum_{i=1}^{k} x_{Ai} - \sum_{i=1}^{k} x_{Bi}$.
- Error-spending scale: $\alpha(s_k)$, which is also known as probability scale.

When the number of interim analyses increases, there are too many possible designs with desired α and power. Hence, in practice, it is difficult to select a most appropriate design that can fit our need. Thus, it is suggested that a simple function to define the preferred stopping boundaries be used. Such a function with a few parameters such as the O'Brien-Fleming, Pocock, Lan-DeMets-Kim, or Wang and Tsiatis boundary functions are useful.

Optimal/flexible multiple-stage designs In early phase cancer trials, it is undesirable to stop a study early when the test drug is promising. On the other hand, it is desirable to terminate the study as early as possible when the test treatment is not effective due to ethical consideration. For this purpose, an optimal or flexible multiple-stage design is often employed to determine whether the test treatment holds sufficient promise to warrant further testing. In practice, optimal or flexible multiple-stage designs are commonly employed in phase II cancer trials with single arm. These multiple-stage designs include optimal multiple-stage designs such as minimax design and Simon's optimal two-stage design (Simon, 1989; Ensign et al., 1994) and flexible multiple-stage designs (see, e.g., Chen, 1997; Chen and Ng, 1998; Sargent and Goldberg, 2001).

The concept of an optimal two-stage design is to permit early stopping when a moderately long sequence of initial failure occurs, denoted by the number of subjects studied in the first and second stage by n_1 and n_2, respectively. Under a two-stage design, n_1 patients are treated at the first stage. If there are fewer than r_1 responses, then stop the trial. Otherwise, stage 2 is implemented by including the other n_2 patients. A decision regarding whether the test treatment is promising is then made based on the response rate of the $N = n_1 + n_2$ subjects. Let p_0 be the undesirable response rate and p_1 be the desirable response rate ($p_1 > p_0$). If the response rate of a test treatment is at the undesirable level, one may reject it as an ineffective compound with a high probability, and if its response rate is at the desirable level, one may not reject it as a promising compound with a high probability. As a result, under a two-stage trial design, it is of interest to test the following hypotheses:

$$H_0 : p \leq p_0 \quad \text{versus} \quad H_a : p \geq p_1.$$

Rejection of H_0 (or H_a) means that further (or not further) study of the test treatment should be carried out. Note that under the above hypotheses, the usual type I error is the false positive in accepting an ineffective drug and the type II error is the false negative in rejecting a promising compound. An alternative to the optimal two-stage design described above is so-called flexible two-stage design (Chen and Ng, 1998). The flexible two-stage design simply assumes that the sample sizes are uniformly distributed on a set of k consecutive possible values.

For comparison of multiple arms, Sargent and Goldberg (2001) proposed a flexible optimal design that allows clinical scientists to select the treatment to proceed for further testing based on other factors when the difference in the observed response rates between treatment arms falls into the interval of $[-\delta, \delta]$, where δ is a pre-specified quantity. The proposed rule is that if the observed difference in the response rates of the treatments is larger than δ, then the treatment with the highest observed response rate is selected. On the other hand, if the observed difference is less than or equal to δ, other factors may be considered in the selection. It should be noted that under this framework, it is not essential that the very best treatment is definitely selected; rather it is important that a substantially inferior treatment is not selected when a superior treatment exists.

Remarks Note that in a classic design with a fixed sample size, either a one-sided α of 0.025 or a two-sided α of 0.05 can be used because they will lead to the same results. However, in group sequential trials, two-sided tests should not be used based on the following reasons. For a trial that is designed to allow early stopping for efficacy, when the test drug is significantly worse than the control, the trial may continue to claim efficacy instead of stopping. This is due to the difference in continuation region between a one-sided and a two-sided test, which will have an impact on the differences in the consequent stopping boundaries between the one-sided and the two-sided test. As a result, it is suggested that the relative merits and disadvantages for the use of a one-sided test and a two-sided test should be carefully evaluated. It should be noted that if a two-sided test is used, the significance level α could be inflated (for futility design) or deflated (for efficacy design).

6.2 General Approach for Group Sequential Design

Jennison and Turnbull (2000) introduced a unified approach for group sequential trial design. This unified approach is briefly described below. Consider a group sequential study consisting of up to K analyses. Thus, we have a sequence of test statistics $\{Z_1, \ldots, Z_K\}$. Assume that these statistics follow a joint canonical distribution with information levels $\{I_1, \ldots, I_k\}$ for the parameter. Thus, we have

$$Z_k \sim N(\theta \sqrt{I_k}, 1), 1, \ldots, K,$$

where $Cov(Z_{k_1}, Z_{k_2}) = \sqrt{I_{k_1} I_{k_2}}$, $1 \leq k_1 \leq k_2 \leq K$.

Table 6.1 provides formulas for sample size calculations for different types of study endpoints in clinical trials, while Table 6.2 summarizes unified formulation for different types of study endpoints under a group sequential design. As an example, for the logrank test in a time-to-event analysis, the information can be expressed as

$$I_k = \frac{r}{(1+r)^2} d_k = \frac{r}{(1+r)^2} \frac{N_k}{\sigma^2},$$

where d_k is the expected number of deaths, N_k is the expected number of patients, and r is the sample size ratio.

Let T_0 and T_{max} be the accrual time and the total follow-up time, respectively. Then, under the condition of exponential survival distribution, we have

$$d_{ik} = \frac{N_{ik}}{T_0} \left(T_o - \frac{1}{\lambda_i e^{\lambda_i T}} \left(e^{\lambda_i T_o} - 1 \right) \right), \quad T > T_o; \quad i = 1, 2; \; k = 1, \ldots, K,$$

where d_{ik} is the number of deaths in group i at stage k, and N_{ik} is the number of patients in group i at stage k.

$$\sigma^2 = \frac{N_{1k} + N_{2k}}{d_{1k} + d_{2k}} = \frac{1+r}{\xi_1 + r\xi_2},$$

ADAPTIVE GROUP SEQUENTIAL DESIGN

Table 6.1 Sample Sizes for Different Types of Endpoints

Endpoint	Sample Size	Variance
One mean	$n = \frac{(z_{1-\alpha}+z_{1-\beta})^2 \sigma^2}{\varepsilon^2};$	
Two means	$n_1 = \frac{(z_{1-\alpha}+z_{1-\beta})^2 \sigma^2}{(1+1/r)^{-1}\varepsilon^2};$	
One proportion	$n = \frac{(z_{1-\alpha}+z_{1-\beta})^2 \sigma^2}{\varepsilon^2};$	$\sigma^2 = p(1-p)$
Two proportions	$n_1 = \frac{(z_{1-\alpha}+z_{1-\beta})^2 \sigma^2}{(1+1/r)^{-1}\varepsilon^2};$	$\sigma^2 = \bar{p}(1-\bar{p});$ $\bar{p} = \frac{n_1 p_1 + n_2 p_2}{n_1 + n_2}.$
One survival curve	$n = \frac{(z_{1-\alpha}+z_{1-\beta})^2 \sigma^2}{\varepsilon^2};$	$\sigma^2 = \lambda_0^2 \left(1 - \frac{e^{\lambda_0 T_0}-1}{T_0 \lambda_0 e^{\lambda_0 T_s}}\right)^{-1}$
Two survival curves	$n_1 = \frac{(z_{1-\alpha}+z_{1-\beta})^2 \sigma^2}{(1+1/r)^{-1}\varepsilon^2};$	$\sigma^2 = \frac{r\sigma_1^2 + \sigma_2^2}{1+r},$ $\sigma_i^2 = \lambda_i^2 \left(1 - \frac{e^{\lambda_i T_0}-1}{T_0 \lambda_i e^{\lambda_i T_s}}\right)^{-1}$

Note: $r = \frac{n_2}{n_1}$. $\lambda_0 =$ expected hazard rate, $T_0 =$ uniform patient accrual time and $T_s =$ trial duration. Logrank-test is used for comparison of the two survival curves.

Table 6.2 Unified Formulation for Sequential Design

Single mean	$Z_k = (\bar{x}_k - \mu_0)\sqrt{I_k}$	$I_k = \frac{n_k}{\sigma^2}$
Paired means	$Z_k = \bar{d}_k \sqrt{I_k}$	$I_k = \frac{n_k}{\sigma^2}$
Two means	$Z_k = (\bar{x}_{Ak} - \bar{x}_{Bk})\sqrt{I_k}$	$I_k = \left(\frac{\sigma_A^2}{n_{Ak}} + \frac{\sigma_B^2}{n_{Bk}}\right)^{-1}$
One proportion	$Z_k = (p_k - p_0)\sqrt{I_k}$	$I_k = \frac{n_k}{\sigma^2},\ \sigma^2 = \bar{p}(1-\bar{p})$
Two proportions	$Z_k = (p_{Ak} - p_{Bk})\sqrt{I_k}$	$I_k = \frac{1}{\sigma^2}\left(\frac{1}{n_{Ak}} + \frac{1}{n_{Bk}}\right)^{-1},$ $\sigma^2 = \bar{p}(1-\bar{p})$
One survival curve	$Z_k = S_k/\sqrt{I_k}$	$I_k = d_k = \frac{N_k}{\sigma^2},$ σ^2 is given in (6.1)
Two survival curves	$Z_k = S_k/\sqrt{I_k}$	$I_k = \frac{r d_k}{(1+r)^2} = \frac{r N_k}{(1+r)^2 \sigma^2},$ σ^2 is given in (6.1)

where

$$\xi_i = 1 - \frac{e^{\lambda_i T_o} - 1}{T_o \lambda_i e^{-\lambda_i T}}.$$

Note that in practice, we may first choose c and α in the stopping boundaries using the conditional probabilities and then perform sample size calculation based on the determined boundaries and the corresponding conditional probabilities for achieving the desired power.

6.3 Early Stopping Boundaries

In clinical trials, it is desirable to stop the trial early if the treatment under investigation is ineffective. On the other hand, if a strong (or highly significant) evidence of efficacy is observed, we may also terminate the trial early. In what follows, we will discuss boundaries for early stopping of a given trial due to (i) efficacy, (ii) futility, and (iii) efficacy or futility assuming that there are a total of K analyses in the trial.

Early efficacy stopping

For the case of early stopping for efficacy, we consider testing the one-sided null hypothesis that $H_0 : \mu_A \leq \mu_B$, where μ_A and μ_B could be means, proportions, or hazard rates for treatment groups A and B, respectively. Figure 6.2 illustrates stopping boundaries for efficacy based on standard Z score. The decision rules for early stopping for efficacy are then given by

$$\begin{cases} \text{If } Z_k < \alpha_k, & \text{continue on next stage}; \\ \text{If } Z_k \geq \alpha_k, & (k = 1, \ldots K - 1), \text{ stop reject } H_0, \end{cases}$$

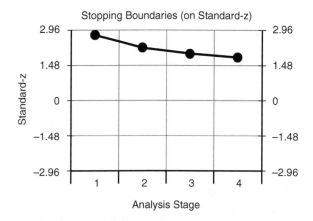

Figure 6.2 Stopping boundary for efficacy.

ADAPTIVE GROUP SEQUENTIAL DESIGN

and
$$\begin{cases} \text{If } Z_K < \alpha_K, \text{ stop accept } H_0; \\ \text{If } Z_K \geq \alpha_K, \text{ stop reject } H_0. \end{cases}$$

In addition to Pocock's test and O'Brien and Fleming's test, Wang and Tsiatis (1987) proposed a family of two-sided tests indexed by the parameter of Δ, which is also based on the standardized test statistic Z_k. Wang and Tsiatis' test includes Pocock's and O'Brien-Fleming's boundaries as special cases. As a result, in this section, we will simply focus on the method proposed by Wang and Tsiatis (1987). Wang and Tsiatis' boundary function is given by

$$a_k > \alpha_K \left(\frac{k}{K}\right)^{\Delta - 1/2}, \tag{6.1}$$

where α_K is function of K, α, and Δ.

Note that sample sizes N_0 in Table 6.3b (also, Table 6.4b, 6.5b) are generated using ExpDesign Studio$^{(R)}$ based on effect size $\delta_0 = 0.1$. Therefore, for an effect size δ, the sample size is given by $N = N_0 \left(\frac{0.1}{\delta}\right)^2$.

Example 6.1 (normal endpoint) Suppose that an investigator is interested in conducting a clinical trial with 5 analyses for comparing a test drug (T) with a placebo (P). Based on information obtained from a pilot study, data from the test drug and the placebo seem to have a common variance, i.e., $\sigma^2 = \sigma_1^2 = \sigma_2^2 = 4$ with $\mu_T - \mu_P = 1$. Assuming these observed values are true, it is desirable to select a maximum sample size such that there is a 85% $(1 - \beta = 0.85)$ power for detecting such a difference between the test drug and the placebo at the 2.5% (one-sided $\alpha = 0.025$) level of significance. The W-T stopping boundary with $\Delta = 0.3$ is used.

The stopping boundaries are given in Table 6.3a. From Table 6.3a, $\alpha_5 = 2.1697$. Since the effect size $\delta = \frac{\mu_T - \mu_P}{\sigma} = 0.5$, the required sample size for a classic design when there are no planned interim analyses is

$$N_{\text{fixed}} = 3592 \left(\frac{0.1}{0.5}\right)^2 = 144.$$

The maximum sample is given by

$$N_{\text{max}} = 3898 \left(\frac{0.1}{0.5}\right)^2 = 156,$$

while the expected sample size under the alternative hypothesis is

$$N = 2669 \left(\frac{0.1}{0.5}\right)^2 = 107.$$

Table 6.3a Final Efficacy Stopping Boundary α_K

Δ	K				
	1	2	3	4	5
0	1.9599	1.9768	2.0043	2.0242	2.0396
0.1		1.9936	2.0258	2.0503	2.0687
0.2		2.0212	2.0595	2.0870	2.1085
0.3		2.0595	2.1115	2.1452	2.1697
0.4		2.1115	2.1850	2.2325	2.2662
0.5		2.1774	2.2891	2.3611	2.4132
0.6		2.2631	2.4270	2.5403	2.6245
0.7		2.3642	2.6061	2.7807	2.9185
0.8		2.4867	2.8297	3.0900	3.3074
0.9		2.6306	3.1022	3.4820	3.8066
1.0		2.7960	3.4268	3.9566	4.4252

Note: Equal info intervals, one-sided $\alpha = 0.025$.

Table 6.3b Maximum Sample Size and Expected Sample Size Under H_a

Δ	K				
	1	2	3	4	5
0	3592	3616/3161	3652/2986	3674/2884	3689/2828
0.1		3644/3080	3685/2920	3713/2829	3732/2774
0.2		3691/3014	3739/2855	3771/2768	3794/2717
0.3		3758/2966	3829/2804	3870/2720	3898/2669
0.4		3850/2941	3962/2773	4031/2695	4078/2649
0.5		3968/2937	4161/2780	4285/2715	4374/2682
0.6		4128/2965	4436/2828	4662/2792	4834/2785
0.7		4316/3012	4809/2923	5195/2933	5520/2975
0.8		4548/3088	5288/3063	5914/3135	6487/3249
0.9		4821/3188	5881/3242	6860/3400	7788/3593
1.0		5130/3307	6586/3454	8011/3696	9427/3974

Note: Equal info intervals, one-sided $\alpha = 0.025$, power = 85% and effect size = 0.1.

Early futility stopping

For the case of early stopping for futility, similarly, we consider testing the one-sided null hypothesis that $H_o : \mu_A \leq \mu_B$, where μ_A and μ_B could be means, proportions, or hazard rates for treatment groups A and B, respectively. Figure 6.3 illustrates stopping boundaries for early futility

Table 6.4a Final Symmetric Futility Stopping Boundary β_K

			K		
Δ	1	2	3	4	5
0	1.9599	1.9546	1.9431	1.9316	1.9224
0.1		1.9500	1.9339	1.9201	1.9098
0.2		1.9419	1.9224	1.9063	1.8926
0.3		1.9316	1.9063	1.8857	1.8696
0.4		1.9155	1.8834	1.8581	1.8374
0.5		1.8972	1.8535	1.8202	1.7938
0.6		1.8765	1.8191	1.7754	1.7398
0.7		1.8512	1.7777	1.7238	1.6790
0.8		1.8237	1.7364	1.6698	1.6169
0.9		1.7950	1.6916	1.6169	1.5572
1.0		1.7651	1.6480	1.5641	1.4998

Note: Equal info intervals, one-sided $\alpha = 0.025$.

Table 6.4b Maximum Sample Size and Expected Sample Size Under H_o

			K		
Δ	1	2	3	4	5
0	3592	3608/2616	3636/2433	3656/2287	3672/2202
0.1		3626/2496	3658/2305	3683/2178	3705/2096
0.2		3655/2396	3700/2174	3734/2053	3759/1974
0.3		3701/2321	3770/2054	3817/1924	3855/1845
0.4		3761/2267	3874/1960	3956/1815	4020/1728
0.5		3845/2241	4024/1901	4165/1742	4285/1648
0.6		3950/2238	4223/1880	4454/1713	4662/1618
0.7		4073/2254	4459/1889	4805/1723	5131/1632
0.8		4207/2285	4726/1923	5196/1761	5651/1675
0.9		4352/2327	4999/1971	5594/1813	6167/1732
1.0		4500/2376	5266/2026	5963/1868	6632/1788

Note: Equal info intervals, one-sided $\alpha = 0.025$ and $\delta = 0.1$. Power $= 85\%$.

based on Z score. The decision rules for early stopping for futility are then given by

$$\begin{cases} \text{If } Z_k < \beta_k, & (k = 1, \ldots K-1), \text{ stop and accept } H_o; \\ \text{If } Z_k \geq \beta_k, & \text{continue on next stage,} \end{cases}$$

and

$$\begin{cases} \text{If } Z_K < \beta_K, & \text{stop and accept } H_o; \\ \text{If } Z_K \geq \beta_K, & \text{stop reject } H_o. \end{cases}$$

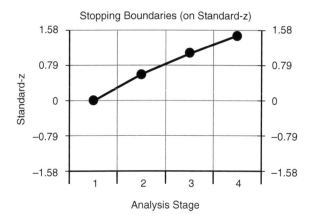

Figure 6.3 Stopping boundary for futility.

We propose an inner futility stopping boundary that is symmetric to the Wang-Tsiatis' efficacy stopping boundary on the z-scale and triangular boundary, which are given below, respectively:

- Symmetric boundary:

$$\beta_k > 2\beta_K \sqrt{\frac{k}{K}} - \beta_K \left(\frac{k}{K}\right)^{\Delta-1/2}. \quad (6.2)$$

- Triangular boundary:

$$\beta_k = \beta_K \frac{k - k_0}{K - k_0}, where k_0 = \left[\frac{K}{2}\right] + 1. \quad (6.3)$$

where $[x]$ is the integer part of x.

Example 6.2 (binary endpoint) Suppose that an investigator is interested in conducting a group sequential trial comparing a test drug with a placebo. The primary efficacy study endpoint is a binary response. Based on information obtained in a pilot study, the response rates for the test drug and the placebo are given by 20% ($p_1 = 0.20$) and 30% ($p_2 = 0.30$), respectively. Suppose that a total of 2 ($K = 2$) analyses are planned. It is desirable to select a maximum sample size in order to have an 85% ($1 - \beta = 0.85$) power at the 2.5% (one-sided $\alpha = 0.025$) level of significance. The effect size is

$$\delta = \frac{p_2 - p_1}{\sqrt{\bar{p}(1 - \bar{p})}} = \frac{0.3 - 0.2}{\sqrt{0.25(1 - 0.25)}} = 0.23094.$$

ADAPTIVE GROUP SEQUENTIAL DESIGN

If a symmetric inner boundary boundaries are used with $\Delta = 0.6$, it is an optimal design with the minimum expected sample size under the null hypothesis. From Table 6.5a, $\beta_2 = 1.8765$, and from (6.2), we have

$$\beta_1 = 2\beta_K \sqrt{\frac{k}{K}} - \beta_K \left(\frac{k}{K}\right)^{\Delta-1/2}$$
$$= 2(1.8765)\sqrt{1/2} - 1.8765\,(1/2)^{0.6-0.5}$$
$$= 0.902\,94.$$

From Table 6.5b, the sample size needed for a fixed sample size design is

$$N_{\text{fixed}} = 3592 \left(\frac{0.1}{0.23094}\right)^2 = 674.$$

The maximum sample size and the expected sample size under the null hypothesis are

$$N_{\max} = 3950 \left(\frac{0.1}{0.23094}\right)^2 = 742$$

and

$$N_{\exp} = 2238 \left(\frac{0.1}{0.23094}\right)^2 = 420.$$

Early efficacy-futility stopping

For the case of early stopping for efficacy or futility, similarly, we consider testing the one-sided null hypothesis that $H_o : \mu_A \leq \mu_B$, where μ_A and μ_B could be means, proportions, or hazard rates for treatment groups A and B, respectively. Figure 6.4 illustrates stopping boundaries for early efficacy/futility stopping. The decision rules for early stopping for efficacy or futility are then given by

$$\begin{cases} \text{If } Z_k < \beta_k, & (k=1,\ldots K), \text{ stop and accept } H_o; \\ \text{If } Z_k \geq \alpha_k, & (k=1,\ldots K), \text{ stop and reject } H_o. \end{cases}$$

The stopping boundaries are the combination of the previous efficacy and futility stopping boundaries, i.e.,
Symmetric boundary

$$\begin{cases} \alpha_k = \alpha_K (k/K)^{\Delta-1/2} \\ \beta_k = 2\beta_K \sqrt{\frac{k}{K}} - \beta_K (\frac{k}{K})^{\Delta-1/2} \end{cases} \quad (6.4)$$

Triangle boundary

$$\begin{cases} \alpha_k = \alpha_K (k/K)^{\Delta-1/2} \\ \beta_k = \beta_K \frac{k-k_0}{K-k_0}, \end{cases} \quad (6.5)$$

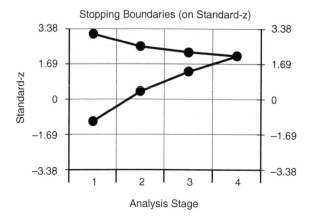

Figure 6.4 Stopping boundary for efficacy or futility.

where the starting inner boundary is given by $k_0 = \left[\frac{K}{2}\right] + 1$.

Example 6.3.3 (survival endpoint) Suppose that an investigator is interested in conducting a survival trial with 3 ($K = 3$) analyses at the 2.5% level of significance (one-sided $\alpha = 0.025$) with an 85% ($1-\beta = 0.85$) power. Assume that median survival time is 0.990 year ($\lambda_1 = 0.7/Year$) for group 1, 0.693 year ($\lambda_2 = 1/Year$) for group 2. $T_0 = 1$ year and study duration $T_s = 2$ years. Using

$$\sigma_i^2 = \lambda_i^2 \left(1 - \frac{e^{\lambda_i T_0} - 1}{T_0 \lambda_i e^{\lambda_i T_s}}\right)^{-1},$$

Table 6.5a Final Stopping Boundaries $\alpha_K = \beta_K$

Δ	1	2	K 3	4	5
0	1.9599	1.9730	1.9902	2.0028	2.0143
0.1		1.9856	2.0074	2.0235	2.0373
0.2		2.0074	2.0361	2.0568	2.0717
0.3		2.0396	2.0821	2.1096	2.1303
0.4		2.0866	2.1521	2.1946	2.2256
0.5		2.1487	2.2532	2.3301	2.3737
0.6		2.2290	2.3898	2.5035	2.5896
0.7		2.3301	2.5678	2.7458	2.8871
0.8		2.4530	2.7929	3.0593	3.2798
0.9		2.6000	3.0685	3.4475	3.7759
1.0		2.7722	3.3947	3.9183	4.3823

Note: Equal info intervals, one-sided $\alpha = 0.025$.

ADAPTIVE GROUP SEQUENTIAL DESIGN

Table 6.5b Maximum Sample Size and Expected Sample Size Under H_o and H_a

Δ	1	2	K 3	4	5
0	3592	3636/2722/3142	3698/2558/2942	3744/2420/2826	3785/2346/2764
0.1		3680/2615/3050	3758/2449/2868	3818/2333/2760	3868/2260/2698
0.2		3755/2534/2974	3860/2342/2793	3937/2236/2692	3995/2167/2628
0.3		3868/2484/2918	4024/2251/2728	4128/2140/2628	4207/2073/2567
0.4		4037/2472/2893	4280/2193/2689	4442/2067/2587	4562/1994/2527
0.5		4265/2497/2897	4662/2181/2687	4931/2034/2584	5136/1950/2527
0.6		4573/2568/2937	5209/2226/2726	5675/2059/2630	6038/1959/2578
0.7		4984/2695/3017	5985/2348/2816	6775/2164/2724	7427/2047/2677
0.8		5525/2891/3143	7078/2580/2967	8402/2397/2879	9574/2272/2830
0.9		6238/3180/3327	8619/2972/3207	10805/2835/3131	12885/2736/3083
1.0		6238/3180/3327	10784/3591/3591	14358/3590/3590	17953/3591/3591

Note: Equal info intervals, one-sided $\alpha = 0.025$, $\delta = 0.1$, power $= 85\%$.

we obtain $\sigma_1^2 = 0.7622$, and $\sigma_2^2 = 1.303$. Note that

$$\delta = \frac{\lambda_2 - \lambda_1}{\sigma} = \frac{1 - 0.7}{\sqrt{0.7622 + 1.303}} = 0.20876.$$

The stopping boundaries ($\Delta = 0.1$) are given by $\alpha_3 = \beta_3 = 2.0074$ (Table 6.6). Thus, we have

$$\alpha_1 = 3.1152, \quad \alpha_2 = 2.3609;$$
$$\beta_1 = -0.79723, \quad \beta_2 = 0.91721.$$

Thus,

$$N_{\text{fixed}} = \frac{(z_{\alpha/2} + z_\beta)^2 \left(\sigma_1^2 + \sigma_2^2\right)}{(\lambda_2 - \lambda_1)^2}$$
$$= \frac{(1.96 + 1.0364)^2 (0.7622 + 1.303)}{(1 - 0.7)^2}$$
$$= 824.$$

The maximum sample size is given by

$$N_{\max} = 3758 \left(\frac{0.1}{0.20876}\right)^2 = 862.$$

The expected sample size under the null hypothesis is given by

$$\bar{N}_o = 2449 \left(\frac{0.1}{0.20876}\right)^2 = 562.$$

Table 6.6 Error Spending Functions

O'Brien-Fleming	$\alpha_1(s) = 2\{1 - \Phi(z_\alpha/\sqrt{s})\}$
Pocock	$\alpha_2(s) = \alpha \log[1 + (e-1)s]$
Lan-DeMets-Kim	$\alpha_3(s) = \alpha s^\theta, \theta > 0$
Hwang-Shih	$\alpha_4(s) = \alpha[(1 - e^{\zeta s})/(1 - e^{-\zeta})], \zeta \neq 0$

Source: Chow, Shao, and Wang (2003)

The expected sample size under the alternative hypothesis is given by

$$\bar{N}_a = 2868 \left(\frac{0.1}{0.20876} \right)^2 = 658.$$

6.4 Alpha Spending Function

Lan and DeMets (1983) proposed to distribute (or spend) the total probability of false positive risk as a continuous function of the information time in group sequential procedures for interim analyses. If the total information is scheduled to accumulate over the maximum duration T is known, the boundaries can be computed as a continuous function of the information time. This continuous function of the information time is referred to as the alpha spending function, denoted by $\alpha(s)$. The alpha spending function is an increasing function of information time. It is 0 when the information time is 0 and is equal to the overall significance level when information time is 1. In other words, $\alpha(0) = 0$ and $\alpha(1) = \alpha$. Let s_1 and s_2 be two information times, $0 < s_1 < s_2 \leq 1$. Also, denote $\alpha(s_1)$ and $\alpha(s_2)$ as their corresponding value of alpha spending function at s_1 and s_2. Then,

$$0 < \alpha(s_1) < \alpha(s_2) \leq \alpha.\alpha(s_1)$$

is the probability of type I error one wishes to spend at information time s_1. For a given alpha spending function $\alpha(s)$ and a series of standardized test statistic $Z_k, k = 1, \ldots, K$, the corresponding boundaries $c_k, k = 1, \ldots, K$ are chosen such that under the null hypothesis

$$P(Z_1 < c_1, \ldots, Z_{k-1} < c_{k-1}, Z_k \geq c_k)$$
$$= \alpha\left(\frac{k}{K}\right) - \alpha\left(\frac{k-1}{K}\right).$$

Some commonly used alpha spending functions are summarized in Table 6.6.

We now introduce the procedure for sample size calculation based on Lan-DeMets' alpha spending function, i.e.,

$$\alpha(s) = \alpha s^\theta, \quad \theta > 0.$$

Although alpha spending function does not require a fixed maximum number and equal spaced interim analyses, it is necessary to make those assumptions in order to calculate the sample size under the alternative hypothesis. The sample size calculation can be performed using computer simulations. As an example, in order to achieve a 90% power at the one-sided 2.5% level of significance, it is necessary to have $n_{\text{fixed}} = 84$ subjects per treatment group for classic design. The maximum sample size needed for achieving the desired power with 5 interim analyses using the Lan-DeMets type alpha spending function with $\delta = 2$ can be calculated as 92 subjects.

6.5 Group Sequential Design Based on Independent P-values

In this section, we discuss n-stage adaptive design based on individual p-values from each stage proposed by Chang (2005). In an adaptive group sequential design with K stages, a hypothesis test is performed at each stage, followed by certain actions according to the outcomes. Such actions could be early stopping for efficacy or futility, sample size re-estimation, modification of randomization, or other adaptations. At the kth stage, a typical set of hypotheses for the treatment difference is given by

$$H_{0k} : \eta_{k1} \geq \eta_{k2} \quad \text{vs.} \quad H_{ak} : \eta_{k1} < \eta_{k2}, \tag{6.6}$$

where η_{k1} and η_{k2} are the treatment response such as mean, proportion, or survival at the kth stage. We denote the test statistic for H_{0k} and the corresponding p-value by T_k and p_k, respectively.

The global test for the null hypothesis of no treatment effect can be written as an intersection of the individual hypotheses at different stages.

$$H_0 : H_{01} \cap \ldots \cap H_{0K} \tag{6.7}$$

Note that a one-sided test is assumed in this chapter. At the kth stage, the decision rules are given by

$$\begin{cases} \text{Stop for efficacy} & \text{if } T_k \leq \alpha_k, \\ \text{Stop for futility} & \text{if } T_k > \beta_k, \\ \text{Continue with adaptations} & \text{if } \alpha_k < T_k \leq \beta_k, \end{cases} \tag{6.8}$$

where $\alpha_k < \beta_k$ $(k = 1, \ldots, K-1)$, and $\alpha_K = \beta_K$. For convenience's sake, α_k and β_k are referred to as the efficacy and futility boundaries, respectively.

To reach the kth-stage, a trial has to pass all stages up to the $(k-1)^{th}$ stages, i.e.,

$$0 \leq \alpha_i < T_i \leq \beta_i \leq 1 (i = 1, \ldots, k-1).$$

Therefore, the cumulative distribution function of T_k is given by

$$\varphi_k(t) = \Pr(T_k < t, \alpha_1 < t_1 \leq \beta_1, \ldots, \alpha_{k-1} < t_{k-1} \leq \beta_{k-1})$$
$$= \int_{\alpha_1}^{\beta_1} \cdots \int_{\alpha_{k-1}}^{\beta_{k-1}} \int_0^t f_{T_1 \ldots T_k} \, dt_k \, dt_{k-1} \ldots dt_1, \qquad (6.9)$$

where $f_{T_1 \ldots T_k}$ is the joint probability density function of $T_1, \ldots,$ and T_k, and t_i is realization of T_i.

The joint probability density function $f_{T_1 \ldots T_k}$ in (6.5) can be any density function. However, it is desirable to choose T_i such that $f_{T_1 \ldots T_k}$ has a simple form. Note that when $\eta_{k1} = \eta_{k2}$, the p-value p_k from the sub-sample at the kth stage is uniformly distributed on $[0,1]$ under H_o and p_k $(k = 1, \ldots, K)$ are mutually independent. These two desirable properties can be used to construct test statistics for adaptive designs.

The simplest form of the test statistic at the kth stage is given by

$$T_k = p_k, \ k = 1, \ldots, K, \qquad (6.10)$$

due to independence of p_k, $f_{T_1 \ldots T_k} = 1$ under H_0 and

$$\varphi_k(t) = t \prod_{i=1}^{k-1} L_i, \qquad (6.11)$$

where $L_i = (\beta_i - \alpha_i)$. For convenience's sake, when the upper bound exceeds the lower bound, define $\prod_{i=1}^{K}(\cdot) = 1$. It is obvious that the error rate (α spent) at the kth stage is given by

$$\pi_k = \varphi_k(\alpha_k). \qquad (6.12)$$

When the efficacy is claimed at a certain stage, the trial is stopped. Therefore, the type I errors at different stages are mutually exclusive. Hence, the experiment-wise type I error rate can be written as

$$\alpha = \sum_{k=1}^{K} \pi_k. \qquad (6.13)$$

From (6.13), the experiment-wise type I error rate is given by

$$\alpha = \sum_{k=1}^{K} \alpha_k \prod_{i=1}^{k-1} L_i. \qquad (6.14)$$

ADAPTIVE GROUP SEQUENTIAL DESIGN

Note that (6.15) is the necessary and sufficient condition for determination of the stopping boundaries (α_i, β_i).

6.6 Calculation of Stopping Boundaries

Two-stage design

For a two-stage design, (6.14) becomes

$$\alpha = \alpha_1 + \alpha_2(\beta_1 - \alpha_1). \tag{6.15}$$

For convenience's sake, a table of stopping boundaries is constructed using (6.16) (Table 6.7). The adjusted p-value is given by

$$p(t, k) = \begin{cases} t & \text{if } k = 1, \\ \alpha_1 + (\beta_1 - \alpha_1)t & \text{if } k = 2. \end{cases} \tag{6.16}$$

K-stage design

For K-stage designs, it is convenient to define a function for L_i and α_i. Such functions could be of the form

$$L_k = b\left(\frac{1}{k} - \frac{1}{K}\right), \tag{6.17}$$

and

$$a_k = c\, k^\theta \alpha, \tag{6.18}$$

Table 6.7 Stopping Boundaries for Two-Stage Designs

	α_1	0.000	0.005	0.010	0.015	0.020
β_1						
0.15		0.1667	0.1379	0.1071	0.0741	0.0385
0.20		0.1250	0.1026	0.0789	0.0541	0.0278
0.25		0.1000	0.0816	0.0625	0.0426	0.0217
0.30		0.0833	0.0678	0.0517	0.0351	0.0179
0.35	α_2	0.0714	0.0580	0.0441	0.0299	0.0152
0.40		0.0625	0.0506	0.0385	0.026	0.0132
0.50		0.0500	0.0404	0.0306	0.0206	0.0104
0.80		0.0312	0.0252	0.0190	0.0127	0.0064
1.00		0.0250	0.0201	0.0152	0.0102	0.0051

Note: One-sided $\alpha = 0.025$.

where b, c, and θ are constants. Because of the equality $L_k = \beta_k - \alpha_k$, the futility boundaries become

$$\beta_k = b\left(\frac{1}{k} - \frac{1}{K}\right) + ck^\theta \alpha. \qquad (6.19)$$

Note that the coefficient b is used to determine how fast the continuation band shrinks when a trial proceeds from one stage to another. θ is used to determine the curvity of the stopping boundaries α_k and β_k. Substituting (6.18) and (6.19) into (6.16) and solving it for constant c, leads to

$$c = \left[\sum_{k=1}^{K}\left\{b^{k-1}k^\theta \prod_{i=1}^{k-1}\left(\frac{1}{i} - \frac{1}{K}\right)\right\}\right]^{-1} \qquad (6.20)$$

When K, b and θ are pre-determined, (6.20) can be used to obtain c. Then, (6.19) and (6.20) can be used to obtain the stopping boundaries α_k and β_k. For convenience, constant c is tabulated for different b, θ and K (Table 6.8).

Note that when $\theta < 0$, $\theta > 0$, and $\theta = 0$, the efficacy stopping boundaries are a monotonically decreasing function of k, an increasing function of k, and a constant, respectively. When the constant b increases, the continuation-band bound by the futility and efficacy stopping boundaries will shrink faster. It is suggested that b should be small enough such that all $\beta_k < 1$. Also, it should be noted that $L_K = 0$.

Trial Examples

To illustrate the group sequential methods described in the previous section, in what follows, two examples concerning clinical trials with group sequential designs are given. For illustration purposes, these two examples have been modified slightly from actual trials.

Example 6.1 Consider a two-arm comparative oncology trial comparing a test treatment with a control. Suppose that the primary efficacy endpoint of interest is time to disease progression (TTP). Based on data from previous studies, the median time for TTP is estimated to be 8 months (hazard rate = 0.08664) for the control group, and 10.5 months (hazard rate = 0.06601) for the test treatment group. Assume that there is a uniform enrollment with an accrual period of 9 months and the total study duration is expected to be 24 months. The logrank test will be used for the analysis. Sample size calculation will be performed under the assumption of an exponential survival distribution.

Assuming that the median time for TTP for the treatment group is 10.5 months, the classic design requires a sample size of 290 per treatment group in order to achieve an 80% power at the $\alpha = 0.025$ level

Table 6.8 Constant c in (6.18)

b	θ	2	3	K 4	5	6
0.25	−0.5	0.9188	0.8914	0.8776	0.8693	0.8638
	0.0	0.8889	0.8521	0.8337	0.8227	0.8154
	0.5	0.8498	0.8015	0.7776	0.7635	0.7540
	1.0	0.8000	0.7385	0.7087	0.6911	0.6795
0.50	−0.5	0.8498	0.7989	0.7733	0.7578	0.7475
	0.0	0.8000	0.7347	0.7023	0.6830	0.6702
	0.5	0.7388	0.6581	0.6190	0.5960	0.5808
	1.0	0.6667	0.5714	0.5267	0.5009	0.4840
0.75	−0.5	0.7904	0.7196	0.6840	0.6626	0.6483
	0.0	0.7273	0.6400	0.5972	0.5718	0.5549
	0.5	0.6535	0.5509	0.5022	0.4738	0.4553
	1.0	0.5714	0.4571	0.4052	0.3757	0.3567
1.00	−0.5	0.7388	0.6512	0.6074	0.5811	0.5635
	0.0	0.6667	0.5625	0.5120	0.4823	0.4627
	0.5	0.5858	0.4683	0.4138	0.3825	0.3622
	1.0	0.5000	0.3750	0.3200	0.2894	0.2699

of significance (based on a one-sided test). Suppose that an adaptive group sequential design is considered in order to improve efficiency and allow some flexibility of the trial. Under an adaptive group sequential design with an interim analysis, a sample size of 175 patients per treatment group is needed for controlling the overall type I error rate at 0.025 and for achieving the desired power of 80%. The interim analysis allows for early stopping for efficacy with stopping boundaries $\alpha_1 = 0.01$, $\beta_1 = 0.25$, and $\alpha_2 = 0.0625$ from Table 6.7. The maximum sample size allowed for adjustment is $n_{\max} = 350$. The simulation results are summarized in Table 6.8, where EESP and EFSP stand for early efficacy stopping probability and early futility stopping probability, respectively.

Note that power is the probability of rejecting the null hypothesis. Therefore, when the null hypothesis is true, the power is equal to the type I error rate α. From Table 6.9, it can be seen that the one-sided α is controlled at the 0.025 level as expected. The expected sample sizes under both hypothesis conditions are smaller than the sample size for

Table 6.9 Operating Characteristics of Adaptive Methods

Median Time				Expected	
Test	Control	EESP	EFSP	N	Power (%)
0	0	0.010	0.750	216	2.5
10.5	8	0.440	0.067	254	79

Note: 1,000,000 simulation runs.

the classic design (290/group). The power under the alternative hypothesis is 79%.

To demonstrate the calculation of the adjusted p-value, assume that (i) naive p-values from the logrank test (or other tests) are $p_1 = 0.1$ and $p_2 = 0.07$, and (ii) the trial stops at stage 2. Therefore, $t = p_2 = 0.07 > \alpha_2 = 0.0625$, and we fail to reject the null hypothesis of no treatment difference.

Example 6.2 Consider a phase III, randomized, placebo-controlled, parallel group study for evaluation of the effectiveness of a test treatment in adult asthmatics. Efficacy will be assessed based on the forced expiratory volume in one second (FEV1). The primary endpoint is the change in FEV1 from baseline. Based on data from phase II studies and other resources, the difference in FEV1 change from baseline between the test drug and the control is estimated to be $\delta = 8.18\%$ with a standard deviation σ of 18.26%. The classic design requires 87 subjects per group for achieving an 85% power at the significance level of $\alpha = 0.025$ (based on a one-sided test). Alternatively, a 4-stage adaptive group sequential design is considered for allowing comparisons at various stages. The details of the design and the corresponding operating characteristics are given in Table 6.10 and Table 6.11, respectively.

Note that the two sequential designs and the classic design have the same expected sample size under the alternative hypothesis condition. The two sequential designs have an increase in power as compared to the classic design.

6.7 Group Sequential Trial Monitoring

Data monitoring committee

As indicated in Offen (2003), the stopping rule can only serve as a guide for stopping a trial. For clinical trials with group sequential design, a Data Monitoring Committee (DMC) is usually formed. The DMC will

ADAPTIVE GROUP SEQUENTIAL DESIGN

Table 6.10 Four-Stage Adaptive Design Specifications

Design	Scenario	Stage k			
		1	2	3	4
GSD 1	α_i	0.01317	0.02634	0.03950	0.05267
	β_i	0.38817	0.15134	0.08117	0.05267
	N	60	120	170	220
GSD 2	α_i	0.00800	0.01600	0.02400	0.03200
	β_i	0.78200	0.28200	0.11533	0.03200
	N	50	95	135	180

Note: For design 1, $b = 0.5$, $\theta = 1$, and $c = 0.5267$.
For design 2, $b = 1.032$, $\theta = 1$, and $c = 0.32$.

usually evaluate all aspects of a clinical trial including integrity, quality, benefits, and the associated risks before a decision regarding the termination of the trial can be reached (Ellenberg, Fleming, and DeMets, 2002). In practice, it is recognized that although all aspects of the conduct of the clinical trial adhered exactly to the conditions stipulated during the design phase, the stopping rule chosen at the design phase may not be used directly because there are usually complicated factors that must be dealt with before such a decision can be made. In what follows, the rationales for closely monitoring a group sequential trial are briefly outlined.

DMC meetings are typically scheduled based on the availability of its members, which may be different from the schedules as specified

Table 6.11 Operating Characteristics of Various Designs

Design	Scenario	Expected N	Range of N	Power (%)
Classic	H_o	87	87–87	2.5
	H_a	87		85
GSD 1	H_o	85	60–220	2.5
	H_a	87		94
GSD 2	H_o	92	50–180	2.5
	H_a	87		89

Note: 500,000 and 100,000 simulation runs for each H_o and H_a scenarios, respectively.

at the design phase. In addition, the enrollment may be different from the assumption made at the design phase. The deviation of analysis schedule will affect the stopping boundaries. Therefore, the boundaries should be re-calculated based on the actual schedules.

In practice, the variability of the response variable is usually unknown. At interim analysis, an estimate of the variability can be obtained based on the actual data collected for the interim analysis. However, the estimate may be different from the initial guess of the variability at the design phase. The deviation of the variability will certainly affect the stopping boundaries. In this case, it is of interest to study the likelihood of success of the trial based on current available information such as conditional and predictive power and repeated confidence intervals. Similarly, the estimation of treatment difference in response could be different from the original expectation in the design phase. This could lead to the use of an adaptive design or sample size re-estimation (Jennison and Turnbull, 2000).

In general, efficacy is not the only factor that will affect DMC's recommendation regarding the stop or continuation of the trial. Safety factors are critical for DMC to make an appropriate recommendation to stop or continue the trial. The term benefit-risk ratio is probably the most commonly used composite criterion in assisting the decision making. In this respect, it is desirable to know the likelihood of success of the trial based on the conditional power or the predictive power.

In many clinical trials, the company may need to make critical decisions on its spending during the conduct of the trials due to some financial constraints. In this situation, the concept of benefit-risk ratio is also helpful when viewed from the financial perspective. In practice, the conditional and/or predictive powers are tools for the decision making. In group sequential trials, the simplest tool that is commonly used for determining whether or not to continue or terminate a trial is the use of sequential stopping boundaries. The original methodology for group sequential boundaries required that the number and timing of interim analyses be specified in advance in the study protocol. Whitehead (1983, 1994) introduced another type of stopping boundary method (the Whitehead triangle boundaries). This method permits unlimited analyses as the trial progresses. This method is referred to as a continuous monitoring procedure. In general, group sequential methods allow for symmetric or asymmetric boundaries. Symmetric boundaries would demand the same level of evidence to terminate the trial early and claim either lack of a beneficial effect or establishment of a harmful effect. Asymmetric boundaries might allow for less evidence for a negative harmful trend before an early termination is recommended. For example, the O'Brien-Fleming sequential boundary might be used for monitoring beneficial effects, while a Pocock-type sequential boundary could provide guidance for safety monitoring.

A practical and yet complicated method is to use the operating characteristics desired for the design, which typically include false positive error rate, the power curve, the sample size distribution or information levels, the estimates of treatment effect that would correspond to early stopping, the naive confidence interval, repeated confidence intervals, the curtailment (conditional power and predictive powers), and the futility index. Both the *conditional power* and the predictive power are the likelihood of rejecting the alternative hypothesis conditioning on the current data. The difference is that the *conditional power* is based on a frequentist approach and the *predictive power* is a Bayesian approach. *Futility index* is a measure of the likelihood of failure to reject H_o at k analysis given that H_a is true. The defining property of a $(1-\alpha)$-level sequence of repeated confidence interval (RCI) for θ is

$$\Pr\{\theta \in I_k \text{ for all } k = 1, \ldots, K\} = 1 - \alpha.$$

Here each I_k (k = 1, ..., K) is an interval computed from the information available at analysis k. The calculation of the RCI at analysis k is similar to the naive confidence interval but $z_{1-\alpha}$ is replaced with α_k, the stopping boundary on the standard z-statistic. For example, $CI = d \pm z_{1-\alpha}\sigma$; $RCI = d \pm \alpha_k \sigma$ (Jennison and Turnbull, 2000)

The conditional power method can be used to assess whether an early trend is sufficiently unfavorable that reversal to a significant positive trend is very unlikely or nearly impossible. The futility index can also be used to monitor a trial. Prematurely terminating a trial with a very small futility index might be inappropriate. It is the same for continuing a trial with very high futility index.

Principles for monitoring a sequential trial

Ellenberg, Fleming, and DeMets (2002) shared their experiences on DMC and provided the following six useful principles for monitoring a sequential trial.

Short-term versus long-term treatment effects When early data from the clinical trial appear to provide compelling evidence for short-term treatment effects, and yet the duration of patient follow-up is insufficient to assess long-term treatment efficacy and safety, early termination may not be warranted and perhaps could even raise ethical issues. The relative importance of short-term and long-term results depends on the clinical setting.

Early termination philosophies Three issues should be addressed. First, what magnitude of estimated treatment difference, and over what period of time, would be necessary before a beneficial trend would be sufficiently convincing to warrant early termination? Second, should the same level of evidence be required for a negative trend as for a positive trend before recommending early termination? Third, for a trial with no apparent trend, should the study continue to the scheduled termination?

Responding to early beneficial trends Determination of optimal length of follow-up can be difficult in a clinical trial having an early beneficial trend. Ideally, evaluating the duration of treatment benefit while continuing to assess possible side effects over a longer period of time would provide the maximum information for clinical use. However, for patients with life-threatening diseases such as heart failure, cancer, or advanced HIV/AIDS, strong evidence of substantial short-term therapeutic benefits may be compelling even if it is unknown whether these benefits are sustained over the long term. Under these circumstances, early termination might be justified to take advantage of this important short-term benefit, with some plan for continued follow-up implementation to identify any serious long-term toxicity.

Responding to early unfavorable trends When an unfavorable trend emerges, three criteria should be considered by a DMC as it wrestles with the question of whether trial modification or termination should be recommended: (i) Are the trends sufficiently unfavorable that there is very little chance of establishing a significant beneficial effect by the completion of the trial? (ii) Have the negative trends ruled out the smallest treatment effect of clinical interest? (iii) Are the negative trends sufficiently strong to conclude a harmful effect?

While the conditional power argument only allows a statement of failure to establish benefit, the symmetric or asymmetric boundary approach allows the researchers to rule out beneficial effects for a treatment or, with more extreme results, to establish harm. When early trends are unfavorable in a clinical trial that is properly powered, stochastic curtailment criteria would generally yield monitoring criteria for termination that would be similar to the symmetric lower boundary for lack of benefit. However, in underpowered trials having unfavorable trends, the stochastic curtailment criteria for early termination generally would be satisfied earlier than criteria based on the group sequential lower boundary for lack of benefit. Most trials comparing a new intervention to a standard of care or a control regimen do not set out to establish that the new intervention is inferior to the control. However, some circumstances may in fact lead to such a consideration.

Responding to unexpected safety concerns Statistical methods are least helpful when an unexpected and worrying toxicity profile begins to emerge. In this situation there can be no pre-specified statistical plan, since the outcome being assessed was unanticipated.

Responding when there are no apparent trends In some trials, no apparent trends of either beneficial or harmful effects emerge as the trial progresses to its planned conclusion. In such instances, a decision must be made as to whether the investment in participant, physician, and fiscal resources, as well as the burden of the trial to patients, remains viable and compelling.

6.8 Conditional Power

Conditional power at a given interim analysis in group sequential trials is defined as the power of rejecting the null hypothesis at the end of the trial conditional on the observed data accumulated up to the time point of the planned interim analysis. For many repeated significance tests such as Pocock's test, O'Brien and Fleming's test, and Wang and Tsiatis' test, the trial can only be terminated under the alternative hypothesis. In practice, this is usually true if the test treatment demonstrates substantial evidence of efficacy. However, it should be noted that if the trial indicates a strong evidence of futility (lack of efficacy) during the interim analysis, it is unethical to continue the trial. Hence, the trial may also be terminated under the null hypothesis. However, except for the inner wedge test, most repeated significance tests are designed for early stop under the alternative hypothesis. In such a situation, the analysis of conditional power (or equivalently futility analysis) can be used as a quantitative method for determining whether the trial should be terminated prematurely.

Comparing means

Let x_{ij} be the observation from the jth subject ($j = 1, \ldots, n_i$) in the ith treatment group ($i = 1, 2$). $x_{ij}, j = 1, \ldots, n_i$, are assumed to be independent and identically distributed normal random variables with mean μ_i and variance σ_i^2. At the time of interim analysis, it is assumed that the first m_i of n_i subjects in the ith treatment group have already been observed. The investigator may want to evaluate the power for rejection of the null hypothesis based on the observed data and appropriate assumption under the alternative hypothesis. More specifically, define

$$\bar{x}_{a,i} = \frac{1}{m_i} \sum_{j=1}^{m_i} x_{ij} \quad \text{and} \quad \bar{x}_{b,i} = \frac{1}{n_i - m_i} \sum_{j=m_i+1}^{n_i} x_{ij}.$$

At the end of the trial, the following Z test statistic is calculated:

$$Z = \frac{\bar{x}_1 - \bar{x}_2}{\sqrt{s_1^2/n_1 + s_2^2/n_2}}$$

$$\approx \frac{\bar{x}_1 - \bar{x}_2}{\sqrt{\sigma_1^2/n_1 + \sigma_2^2/n_2}}$$

$$= \frac{(m_1\bar{x}_{a,1} + (n_1 - m_1)\bar{x}_{b,1})/n_1 - (m_2\bar{x}_{a,2} + (n_2 - m_2)\bar{x}_{b,2})/n_2}{\sqrt{\sigma_1^2/n_1 + \sigma_2^2/n_2}}.$$

Under the alternative hypothesis, we assume $\mu_1 > \mu_2$. Hence, the power for rejecting the null hypothesis can be approximated by

$$1 - \beta = P(Z > z_{\alpha/2})$$

$$= P\left(\frac{\frac{(n_1-m_1)(\bar{x}_{b,1}-\mu_1)}{n_1} - \frac{(n_2-m_2)(\bar{x}_{b,2}-\mu_2)}{n_2}}{\sqrt{\frac{(n_1-m_1)\sigma_1^2}{n_1^2} + \frac{(n_2-m_2)\sigma_2^2}{n_2^2}}} > \tau\right)$$

$$= 1 - \Phi(\tau),$$

where

$$\tau = \left[z_{\alpha/2}\sqrt{\sigma_1^2/n_1 + \sigma_2^2/n_2} - (\mu_1 - \mu_2)\right.$$

$$\left. - \left(\frac{m_1}{n_1}(\bar{x}_{a,1} - \mu_1) - \frac{m_2}{n_2}(\bar{x}_{a,2} - \mu_2)\right)\right]$$

$$\left[\frac{(n_1 - m_1)\sigma_1^2}{n_1^2} + \frac{(n_2 - m_2)\sigma_2^2}{n_2^2}\right]^{-1/2}.$$

As it can be seen from the above, the conditional power depends not only upon the assumed alternative hypothesis (μ_1, μ_2) but also upon the observed values $(\bar{x}_{a,1}, \bar{x}_{a,2})$ and the amount of information that has been accumulated (m_i/n_i) at the time of interim analysis.

Comparing proportions

When the responses are binary, similar formulas can also be obtained. Let x_{ij} be the binary response observed from the jth subject ($j = 1, \ldots, n_i$) in the ith treatment group ($i = 1, 2$). Again, $x_{ij}, j = 1, \ldots, n_i$, are assumed to be independent and identically distributed binary variables with mean p_i. At the time of interim analysis, it is also assumed that the first m_i of n_i subjects in the ith treatment group have been observed. Define

$$\bar{x}_{a,i} = \frac{1}{m_i}\sum_{j=1}^{m_i} x_{ij} \quad \text{and} \quad \bar{x}_{b,i} = \frac{1}{n_i - m_i}\sum_{j=m_i+1}^{n_i} x_{ij}.$$

At the end of the trial, the following Z test statistic is calculated:

$$Z = \frac{\bar{x}_1 - \bar{x}_2}{\sqrt{\bar{x}_1(1-\bar{x}_1)/n_1 + \bar{x}_2(1-\bar{x}_2)/n_2}}$$

$$\approx \frac{\bar{x}_1 - \bar{x}_2}{\sqrt{p_1(1-p_1)/n_1 + p_2(1-p_2)/n_2}}$$

$$= \frac{(m_1\bar{x}_{a,1} + (n_1-m_1)\bar{x}_{b,1})/n_1 - (m_2\bar{x}_{a,2} + (n_2-m_2)\bar{x}_{b,2})/n_2}{\sqrt{p_1(1-p_1)/n_1 + p_2(1-p_2)/n_2}}.$$

Under the alternative hypothesis, we assume $p_1 > p_2$. Hence, the power for rejecting the null hypothesis can be approximated by

$$1 - \beta = P(Z > z_{\alpha/2})$$

$$= P\left(\frac{\frac{(n_1-m_1)(\bar{x}_{b,1}-\mu_1)}{n_1} - \frac{(n_2-m_2)(\bar{x}_{b,2}-\mu_2)}{n_2}}{\sqrt{\frac{(n_1-m_1)p_1(1-p_1)}{n_1^2} + \frac{(n_2-m_2)p_2(1-p_2)}{n_2^2}}} > \tau\right)$$

$$= 1 - \Phi(\tau),$$

where

$$\tau = \left[z_{\alpha/2}\sqrt{p_1(1-p_1)/n_1 + p_2(1-p_2)/n_2} - (\mu_1 - \mu_2) \right.$$
$$\left. - \left(\frac{m_1}{n_1}(\bar{x}_{a,1} - \mu_1) - \frac{m_2}{n_2}(\bar{x}_{a,2} - \mu_2)\right)\right]$$
$$\left[\frac{(n_1-m_1)p_1(1-p_1)}{n_1^2} + \frac{(n_2-m_2)p_2(1-p_2)}{n_2^2}\right]^{-1/2}.$$

Similarly, the conditional power depends not only upon the assumed alternative hypothesis (p_1, p_2) but also upon the observed values $(\bar{x}_{a,1}, \bar{x}_{a,2})$ and the amount of information that has been accumulated (m_i/n_i) at the time of interim analysis.

6.9 Practical Issues

The group sequential procedures for interim analyses are basically in the context of hypothesis testing, which is aimed at pragmatic study objectives, i.e., which treatment is better. However, most new treatments such as cancer drugs are very expensive or very toxic or both. As a result, only if the degree of the benefit provided by the new treatment exceeds some minimum clinically significant requirement, it will then be considered for the treatment of the intended medical conditions. Therefore, an adequate well-controlled trial should be able to provide not only the qualitative evidence whether the experimental treatment is effective but also the quantitative evidence from the unbiased estimation of the size of the effectiveness or safety over placebo given by the experimental therapy. For a fixed sample design without interim analyses for early termination, it is possible to achieve both qualitative and quantitative goals with respect to the treatment effect. However, with group sequential procedure, the size of benefit of the experimental treatment by the maximum likelihood method is usually overestimated because of the choice of stopping rule. Jennison and Turnbull (1990) pointed out that the sample mean might not be even contained in the final confidence interval. As a result, estimation of the size of treatment effect has received a lot of attention. Various estimation procedures have been proposed such as modified maximum likelihood estimator (MLE), median unbiased estimator (MUE), and the midpoint of the equal-tailed 90% confidence interval. For more details, see Cox (1952), Tsiatis et al. (1984), Kim and DeMets (1987), Kim (1989), Chang and O'Brien (1986), Chang et al. (1989), Chang (1989), Hughes and Pocock (1988), and Pocock and Hughes (1989).

The estimation procedures proposed in the above literature require extensive computation. On the other hand, simulation results (Kim, 1989; Hughes and Pocock, 1988) showed that the alpha spending function corresponding to the O'Brien-Fleming group sequential procedure is very concave and allocates only a very small amount of total nominal significance level to early stages of interim analyses, and hence, the bias, variance, and mean square error of the point estimator following O'Brien-Fleming procedure are also the smallest. Current researchers mainly focus upon the estimation of the size of the treatment effect for the primary clinical endpoints on which the group sequential procedure is based. However, there are many other secondary efficacy and safety endpoints to be evaluated in the same trial. The impact of early termination of the trial based on the results from primary clinical endpoints on the statistical inference for these secondary clinical endpoints is unclear. In addition, group sequential methods and their followed estimation procedures so far are only concentrated on the population average. On the other hand, inference of variability is sometimes also of vital importance for certain classes of drug products and diseases. Research on estimation of variability following early termination is still lacking. Other areas of interest for interim analyses include clinical trials with more than 2 treatments and bioequivalence assessment. For group sequential procedures for the trials with multiple treatments, see Hughes (1993) and Proschan et al. (1994). For group sequential bioequivalence testing procedure, see Gould (1995).

CHAPTER 7

Adaptive Sample Size Adjustment

In clinical trials, it is desirable to have a sufficient number of subjects in order to achieve a desired power for correctly detecting a clinically meaningful difference if such a difference truly exists. For this purpose, a pre-study power analysis is often conducted for sample size estimation under certain assumptions such as the variability associated with the observed response of the primary study endpoint (Chow, Shao, and Wang, 2003). If the true variability is much less than the initial guess of the variability, the study may be over-powered. On the other hand, if the variability is much larger than the initial guess of the variability, the study may not achieve the desired power. In other words, the results observed from the study may be due to chance alone and cannot be reproducible. Thus, it is of interest to adjust sample sizes adaptively based on accrued data at interim.

Adaptive sample size adjustment includes planned and unplanned (unexpected) sample size adjustment. Planned sample size adjustment is referred to as sample size re-estimation at interim analyses in a group sequential clinical trial design or an N-adjustable clinical trial design. Most unplanned sample size adjustments are due to changes made to on-going study protocols and/or unexpected administrative looks based on accrued data at interim. Chapter 2 provides an adjustment factor for sample size as the result of protocol amendments. In this chapter, we will focus on the case of planned sample size adjustment in a group sequential design.

In the next section, statistical procedures for sample size re-estimation without unblinding the treatment codes are introduced. Statistical methods such as Cui-Hung-Wang's idea, Proschan-Hunsberger's method, and Bauer and Köhne's approach for sample size re-estimation with unblinding data in group sequential trial designs are given in Sections 7.2, 7.3, and 7.4, respectively. Other methods such as the generalization of independent p-volume approaches and inverse-normal method are discussed in sections 7.5 and 7.6, respectively. Some concluding remarks are given in the last section of this chapter.

7.1 Sample Size Re-estimation without Unblinding Data

In clinical trials, the sample size is determined by a clinically meaningful difference and information on the variability of the primary endpoint. Since the natural history of the distribution is usually not known or the test treatment under investigation is a new class of drug, the estimate of variability for the primary endpoint for sample size estimation may not be adequate during the planning stage of the study. As a result, the planned sample size may need to be adjusted during the conduct of the trial if the observed variability of the accumulated response on the primary endpoint is very different from that used at the planning stage. To maintain the integrity of the trial, it is suggested that sample size re-estimation be performed without unblinding of the treatment codes if the study is to be conducted in a double-blind fashion. Procedures have been proposed for adjusting the sample size during the course of the trial without unblinding and altering the significance level (Gould, 1992, 1995; Gould and Shih, 1992). For simplicity, let us consider a randomized trial with two parallel groups comparing a test treatment and a placebo. Suppose that the distribution of the response of the primary endpoint is normally distributed. Then, the total sample size required for achieving a desired power of $1 - \beta$ for a two-sided alternative hypothesis can be obtained using the following formula (see, e.g., Chow, Shao, and Wang, 2003)

$$N = \frac{4\sigma^2(z_{\alpha/2} + z_\beta)}{\Delta^2},$$

where Δ is the difference of clinically importance. In general, σ^2 (the within-group variance) is unknown and needs to be estimated based on previous studies. Let σ^{*2} be the within-group variance specified for sample size determination at the planning stage of the trial. At the initiation of the trial, we expect the observed variability to be similar to σ^{*2} so that the trial will have sufficient power to detect the difference of clinically importance. However, if the variance turns out to be much larger than σ^{*2}, we will need to re-estimate the sample size without breaking the randomization codes. If the true within-group variance is in fact σ'^2, then the sample size to be adjusted to achieve the desired power of $1 - \beta$ at the α level of significance for a two-sided alternative is given by

$$N' = N\frac{\sigma'^2}{\sigma^{*2}},$$

where N is the planned sample size calculated based on σ^{*2}. However, σ'^2 is usually unknown and must be estimated from the accumulated data available from a total n of N patients. One simple approach to estimate σ'^2 is based on the sample variance calculated from the n responses, which is given by

$$s^2 = \frac{1}{n-1} \sum\sum (y_{ij} - \bar{y})^2,$$

where y_{ij} is the jth observation in group i and $\bar{y}$ is the overall sample mean, $j = 1, \ldots, n_i$, $i = 1$ (treatment), 2 (placebo), and $n = n_1 + n_2$. If n is large enough for the mean difference between groups to provide a reasonable approximation to Δ, then it follows that σ'^2 can be estimated by (Gould, 1995)

$$\sigma'^2 = \frac{n-1}{n-2}\left(s^2 - \frac{\Delta^2}{4}\right).$$

Note that the estimation of within-group variance σ'^2 does not require the knowledge of the treatment assignment, and hence the blindness of the treatment codes is maintained. However, one of the disadvantages of this approach is that it does depend upon the mean difference, which is not calculated and is unknown.

Alternatively, Gould and Shih (1992) and Gould (1995) proposed a procedure based on the concept of EM algorithm for estimating σ'^2 without a value for Δ. This procedure is briefly outlined below. Suppose that n observations, say, y_i, $i = 1, \ldots, n$ on a primary endpoint have been obtained from n patients. The treatment assignments for these patients are unknown. Gould and Shih (1992) and Gould (1995) considered randomly allocating these n observations to either of the two groups assuming that the treatment assignments are missing at random by defining the following π_i as the treatment indicator

$$\pi_i = \begin{cases} 1 & \text{if the treatment is the test drug} \\ 0 & \text{if the treatment is placebo.} \end{cases}$$

The E step is to obtain the provisional values of the expectation of π_i (i.e., the conditional probability that patient i is assigned to the test drug given y_i), which is given by

$$P(\pi_i = 1|y_i) = \left(1 + \exp\{(\mu_1 - \mu_2)(\mu_1 + \mu_2 - 2y_i)/2\sigma^2]\}\right)^{-1},$$

where μ_1 and μ_2 are the population mean of the test drug and the placebo, respectively. The M step involves the maximum likelihood estimates of μ_1, μ_2 and σ after updating π_i by their provisional values obtained from the E step in the log-likelihood function of the interim observations, which is given by

$$1 = n\log\sigma + \frac{\sum[\pi_i(y_i - \mu_1)^2 + (1-\pi_i)(y_i - \mu_2)^2]}{2\sigma^2}.$$

The E and M steps are iterated until the values converge. Gould and Shih (1992) and Gould (1995) indicated that this procedure can estimate within-group variance quite satisfactorily, but failed to provide a reliable estimate of $\mu_1 - \mu_2$. As a result, the sample size can be adjusted without knowledge of treatment codes. For sample size re-estimation procedure without unblinding treatment codes with respect to binary clinical endpoints, see Gould (1992, 1995). A review of the methods for sample size re-estimation can be found in Shih (2001).

7.2 Cui–Hung–Wang's Method

For a given group sequential trial, let N_k and T_k be the planned sample size and test statistic at stage k. Thus, we have

$$T_k = \frac{\sqrt{N_k}}{\sqrt{2}\sigma} \left(\frac{1}{N_k} \sum_{i=1}^{N_k} x_i - \frac{1}{N_k} \sum_{i=1}^{N_k} y_i \right).$$

Denote N_L and T_L by the planned cumulative sample size from stage 1 to stage L and the weighted test statistic from stage 1 to stage L. Thus, for a group sequential trial without sample size adjustment, the test statistic for mean difference between two groups at stage k can be expressed as weighted test statistics of the sub-samples from the previous stages as follows (see, e.g., Cui, Hung, and Wang, 1999)

$$T_{L+j} = T_L \left(\frac{N_L}{N_{L+j}} \right)^{1/2} + w_{L+j} \left[\frac{N_{L+j} - N_L}{N_{L+j}} \right]^{1/2}, \quad (7.1)$$

where

$$w_{L+j} = \frac{\sum_{i=N_L+1}^{N_L+j}(x_i - y_i)}{\sqrt{2(N_{L+j} - N_L)}}, \quad (7.2)$$

in which x_i and y_i are from treatment group 1 and 2, respectively, and M_L is the adjusted cumulative sample from stage 1 to stage L.

For group sequential trials with sample size adjustments, let M be the total sample size after adjustment and N be the original planned sample size. We may consider adjusting sample size with effect size as follows

$$M = \left(\frac{\delta}{\Delta_L} \right)^2 N, \quad (7.3)$$

where δ is the expected difference (effect size) given by

$$\frac{(\mu_2 - \mu_1)}{\sigma},$$

Table 7.1 Effects of Sample Adjustment Using Original Test Statistic and Stopping Boundaries

Time to N change, t_L	0.20	0.4	0.6	0.8	∞
Type-I error rate, α	0.038	0.035	0.037	0.033	0.025
Power	0.84	0.91	0.94	0.96	0.61

Note: $\delta = 0.03, \alpha = 0.025$, and power $= 0.9 \Rightarrow N = 250$/group.
True $\Delta = 0.21$. Sample size adjustment is based on equation 7.3.
Source: Cui, Hung, and Wang (1999).

and Δ_L is observed mean difference $\frac{\Delta \mu_L}{\sigma}$ at stage L. Based on the adjusted sample sizes, test statistic T_{L+j} becomes

$$U_{L+j} = T_L \left(\frac{N_L}{N_{L+j}}\right)^{1/2} + w^*_{L+j} \left[\frac{N_{L+j} - N_L}{N_{L+j}}\right]^{1/2}, \quad (7.4)$$

where

$$w^*_{L+j} = \frac{\sum_{i=N_L+1}^{M_{L+j}} (x_i - y_i)}{\sqrt{2(M_{L+j} - N_L)}}. \quad (7.5)$$

Cui, Hung, and Wang (1999) showed that using U_{L+j} and original boundary from the group sequential trial will not inflate the type I error rate, both mathematically and by means of computer simulation (see also Table 7.1 and Table 7.2).

Example 7.1
Cui, Hung, and Wang (1999) gave following example: A phase III two-arm trial for evaluating the effect of a new drug for prevention of myocardial infection in patients undergoing coronary artery bypass graft surgery has a sample size of 600 [300] patients per group to detect a 50% reduction in incidence from 22% to 11% with 95% power. However, at interim analysis based on data from 600 [300] patients, the test group has 16.5% incidence rate. If this incidence rate is the true rate, the power

Table 7.2 Effects of Sample Adjustment Using New Test Statistic and Original Stopping Boundaries

Time to N change, t_L	0.20	0.4	0.6	0.8	∞
Type-I error rate, α	0.025	0.025	0.025	0.025	0.025
Power	0.86	0.90	0.92	0.91	0.61

Note: $N = 250$/group, true, $\alpha = 0.025$. True $\Delta = 0.21$
Note: sample size adjustment is based on equation 7.3.
Source: Cui, Hung, and Wang (1999).

is about 40%. If using the Cui-Hung-Wang method to increase sample size to 1400 per group [unrealistically large], the power is 93% based on their simulation with 20,000 replications. (The calculations seem to be incorrect! All the sample sizes are twice as large as they should be.)

Remarks
Ciu-Hung-Wang's method has the following advantages. First, the adjustment of sample size is easy. Second, using the same stopping boundaries from the traditional group sequential trial is straightforward. The disadvantages include (i) their sample size adjustment is somewhat ad hoc, which does not aim a target power; and (ii) weighting outcomes differently for patients from different stages is difficult to explain clinically.

7.3 Proschan–Hunsberger's Method

For a given two-stage design, Proschan and Hunsberger (1995) and Proschan (2005) considered adjusting the sample size at the second stage based on the evaluation of conditional power given the data observed at the first stage. We will refer to their method as Proschan-Hunsberger's method. Let $P_c(n_2, z_\alpha | z_1, \delta)$ be the conditional probability that Z exceeds z_α, given that $Z_1 = z_1$ and $\delta = (\mu_x - \mu_y)/\sigma$ based on $n = n_1 + n_2$ observations. That is,

$$P_c(n_2, z_\alpha | z_1, \delta)$$
$$= \Pr\left(Z > z_\alpha | Z_1 = z_1, \delta\right)$$
$$= \Pr\left[\frac{n_1\left(\bar{Y}_1 - \bar{X}_1\right) + n_2\left(\bar{Y}_2 - \bar{X}_2\right)}{\sqrt{2\hat{\sigma}^2 n}} > z_\alpha | Z_1 = z_1, \delta\right]$$
$$= \Pr\left[\frac{n_2\left(\bar{Y}_2 - \bar{X}_2\right) - n_2\delta\sigma}{\sqrt{2n_2\hat{\sigma}^2}} > \frac{z_\alpha\sqrt{2\hat{\sigma}^2 n} - z_1\sqrt{2n_1\hat{\sigma}^2} - n_2\delta\sigma}{\sqrt{2n\hat{\sigma}^2}} | \delta\right].$$

If we treat $\hat{\sigma}$ as the true σ, we have

$$P_c(n_2, z_\alpha | z_1, \delta) = 1 - \Phi\left[\frac{z_\alpha\sqrt{2n} - z_1\sqrt{2n_1} - n_2\delta}{\sqrt{2n_2}}\right]. \qquad (7.6)$$

Since Z_1 is normally distributed, the type I error rate of this two-stage process without early stopping is given by

$$\int_{-\infty}^{\infty} P_c(n_2, z_\alpha | z_1, 0)\phi(z_1)dz_1 = \int_{-\infty}^{\infty} \left\{1 - \Phi\left[\frac{z_\alpha\sqrt{2n} - z_1\sqrt{2n_1}}{\sqrt{2n_2}}\right]\right\}\phi(z_1)dz_1.$$

Proschan and Hunsberger (1995) showed that without adjustment of reject regions, the type I error rate caused by sample size adjustment could be as high as

$$\alpha_{\max} = \alpha + 0.25 e^{-z_\alpha^2/2}.$$

In the interest of controlling the type I error rate at the nominal level, we may consider modifying the rejection region from z_α to z_c such that

$$\int_{-\infty}^{\infty} P_c(n_2, z_c|z_1, 0)\phi(z_1)dz_1 = \alpha, \tag{7.7}$$

where z_c is a function of z_1, n_1, and n_2. Since the integration is a constant α, we wish to find z_c such that $P_c(n_2, z_c|z_1, 0)$ depends only upon a function of z_1, say $A(z_1)$, i.e.,

$$P_c(n_2, z_c|z_1, 0) = A(z_1). \tag{7.8}$$

From (7.7) and (7.8), we can solve for z_c as follows

$$z_c = \frac{\sqrt{n_1}\,z_1 + \sqrt{n_2}\,z_A}{\sqrt{n_1 + n_2}}, \tag{7.9}$$

where $z_A = \Phi^{-1}(1 - A(z_1))$ and $A(z_1)$ is any increasing function with the range of [0, 1] satisfying

$$\int_{-\infty}^{\infty} A(z_1)\phi(z_1)dz_1 = \alpha. \tag{7.10}$$

To find the function of $A(z_1)$, it may be convenient to write $A(z_1)$ in the form of $A(z_1) = f(z_1)/\phi(z_1)$.(7.10) provides the critical value for rejecting the null hypothesis while protecting overall α. The next step is to choose the additional sample size n_2 at stage 2. At stage 1 we have the empirical estimate $\hat{\delta} = (\bar{y}_1 - \bar{x}_1)/\hat{\sigma}$ of the standard treatment difference. We may wish to power the trial to detect a value somewhere between the originally hypothesized difference and the empirical estimate. Whichever target difference δ we use, if we plug z_c from (7.9) into (7.6), we obtain the conditional power

$$P_c(n_2, z_c|z_1, \delta) = 1 - \Phi\left(z_A - \sqrt{n_2/2}\,\delta\right). \tag{7.11}$$

Supposing that the desired power is $1 - \beta_2$, we can immediately obtain the required sample size as follows

$$n_2 = \frac{2(z_A + z_{\beta_2})^2}{\delta^2}. \tag{7.12}$$

Plugging this into (7.9), we have

$$z_c = \frac{\delta\sqrt{\frac{n_1}{2}}\,z_1 + (z_A + z_{\beta_2})z_A}{\sqrt{\frac{n_1}{2}\delta^2 + (z_A + z_{\beta_2})^2}}. \tag{7.13}$$

Note that z_c is the reject region in n terms of $(\sqrt{n_1}z_1 + \sqrt{n_2}z_2)/\sqrt{n}$, usual z score on all $2n$ observations. If we use the empirical estimate $\hat{\delta}$, (7.12) and (7.13) become

$$n_2 = \frac{n_1(z_A + z_{\beta_2})^2}{z_1^2}, \quad (7.14)$$

and

$$z_c = \frac{z_1^2 + (z_A + z_{\beta_2})z_A}{\sqrt{z_1^2 + (z_A + z_{\beta_2})^2}}. \quad (7.15)$$

The fact that the value of β_2 can be changed after observing $Z_1 = z_1$ underscores the flexibility of the procedure. Note that (7.14) is the sample size formula to achieve power $1 - \beta$ in the fixed sample test at level $A(z_1)$. This interpretation allows us to see the benefit of extending our study relative to starting a new one. If $A(z_1) < \alpha$, we would be better off starting a new study than extending the old. We can extend the test procedure to two-stage with negative or positive early stopping with stopping rules in the first stage being

$$\begin{cases} \text{Stop not to reject } H_o, & z_1 < z_{cl}; \\ \text{Continue to stage 2,} & z_{cl} \le z_1 \le z_{cu}; \\ \text{Stop to reject } H_o, & z_1 > z_{cu}. \end{cases} \quad (7.16)$$

Then (7.7) should be modified as follows:

$$\alpha_1 + \int_{z_{cl}}^{z_{cu}} P_c(n_2, z_c|z_1, 0)\phi(z_1)dz_1 = \alpha \quad (7.17)$$

where $\phi(z_1)$ is the standard normal density function $\alpha_1 = \int_{z_{cu}}^{+\infty} \phi(z_1)dz_1$. Define

$$\tilde{P}_c(z_1; z_{c1}; \delta) = \begin{cases} 0 & z_1 < z_{cl}; \\ P_c(n_2, z_c|z_1, \delta) & z_{cl} \le z_1 \le z_{cu}; \\ 1 & z_1 > z_{cu}. \end{cases} \quad (7.18)$$

Note that

$$\alpha_1 = \int_{z_{cl}}^{z_{cu}} P_c(n_2, z_c|z_1, 0)\phi(z_1)dz_1.$$

Then (7.17) can be written

$$\alpha = \int_{-\infty}^{\infty} \tilde{P}_c(n_2, z_c|z_1, 0)\phi(z_1)dz_1, \quad (7.19)$$

ADAPTIVE SAMPLE SIZE ADJUSTMENT

Table 7.3 Corresponding Values z_{cu} for Different z_{cl}

α	.10	.15	$\alpha_0 = \Phi(1-z_{cl})$ .20	.25	.30	.35	.40	.45	.50
0.025	2.13	2.17	2.19	2.21	2.22	2.23	2.25	2.26	2.27
0.050	1.77	1.82	1.85	1.88	1.89	1.91	1.93	1.94	1.95

Source: Proschan and Hunsberger, 1995.

which in the same format as (7.7). Let $\tilde{P}_c(z_1; z_{c1}; \delta) = A(z_1)$, i.e.,

$$A(z_1) = \begin{cases} 0 & z_1 < z_{cl}; \\ P_c(n_2, z_c | z_1, \delta) & z_{cl} \leq z_1 \leq z_{cu}; \\ 1 & z_1 > z_{cu}. \end{cases} \quad (7.20)$$

Note that (7.10)–(7.18) are still valid when $A(z_1)$ is any increasing function with range [0, 1] satisfying the form of

$$A(z_1) = \begin{cases} 0 & z_1 < z_{cl}; \\ f(z_1)/\phi(z_1) & z_{cl} \leq z_1 \leq z_{cu}; \\ 1 & z_1 > z_{cu}. \end{cases} \quad (7.21)$$

Proschan (1995) and Hunsberger (2004) gave the following linear-error function:

$$A(z_1) = 1 - \Phi(\sqrt{2}z_\alpha - z_1).$$

Given observed treatment difference δ, we can use (7.12) or (7.14) re-estimate sample size and substitute (7.21) into (7.13) or (7.15) to determine reject region z_c. Note that this is a design without early stopping.

Example 7.2 Consider the following circular-function:

$$A(z_1) = \begin{cases} 0 & z_1 < z_{cl}; \\ 1 - \Phi(\sqrt{z_{cu}^2 - z_1^2}) & z_{cl} \leq z_1 \leq z_{cu}; \\ 1 & z_1 > z_{cu}. \end{cases} \quad (7.22)$$

For each z_{cl}, the corresponding z_{cu} can be calculated by substituting (7.21) into (7.11). and then calculated z_c from (7.12) or (7.14) with $A(z_1)$ of (7.21). For convenience's sake, we tabulate z_{cl}, z_{cu} and z_c in Table 7.3 for overall one-sided $\alpha = 0.025$ and 0.5.

7.4 Muller–Schafer Method

Muller and Schafer (2001) showed how one can make any data-dependent change in an on-going adaptive trial and still preserve the overall type I error. To achieve that, all one need do is preserve the conditional type I error of the remaining portion of the trial. Therefore, the Muller-Schafer method is a special conditional-error approach.

7.5 Bauer–Köhne Method

Two-stage design

Bauer-Köhne's method is based on the fact that under H_0 the p-value for the test of a particular null hypothesis, H_{0k}, in a stochastically independent sample, which is generally uniformly distributed on [0,1], where continuous test statistics are assumed (Bauer and Köhne, 1994, 1996). Usually, however, one obtains conservative combination tests when under H_0 the distribution of the p-values is stochastically larger than the uniform distribution.

Moreover, under H_0 the distribution of the resultant p-value is stochastically independent of previously measured random variables. Hence, provided H_0 is true, data-dependent planning (e.g., sample size change) does not change the convenient property of independently and uniformly distributed p-values, but some care is needed (Liu, Proschan, and Pledger, 2002). The modification considered here would imply that data are not allowed to be pooled over the whole trial. Data from the stages before and after that adaptive interim analysis have to be looked at separately. In the analysis, p-values from the partitioned sample have to be used. These are general measures of "deviation" from the respective null hypotheses. There are many ways to test the intersection H_o of two or more individual null hypotheses based on independently and uniformly distributed p-values for the individual test (Hedges and Olkin, 1985; Sonnesmann, 1991). Fisher's criterion using the product of the p-values has good properties. One obvious question is whether combination tests could be used that explicitly include a weighting of the p-values by the sample size. If the sample size itself is open to adaptation, then clearly the answer is no. To derive critical regions for test statistics explicitly containing random sample sizes, one would need to know or pre-specify the distribution. This, however, contradicts the intended flexibility of general approach.

Let P_1 and P_2 be the p-values for the sub-samples obtained from the first stage and second stage, respectively. Fisher's criterion leads to

Table 7.4 Stopping Boundaries α_0, α_1, and C_α

α	C_α	α_0	0.3	0.4	0.5	0.6	0.7	1.0
0.1	0.02045		0.0703	0.0618	0.0548	0.0486	0.0429	0.02045
0.05	0.00870	α_1	0.0299	0.0263	0.0233	0.0207	0.0183	0.00870
0.025	0.00380		0.0131	0.0115	0.0102	0.0090	0.0080	0.00380

Source: Table 1 of Bauer (1994).

rejection of H_0 at the end of trial if

$$P_1 P_2 \leq c_\alpha = e^{-\frac{1}{2}\chi^2_{4,1-\alpha}}, \tag{7.23}$$

where $\chi^2_{4,1-\alpha}$ is the $(1-\alpha)$-quantile of the central χ^2 distribution with 4 degrees of freedom (see Table 7.4). Decision rules at the first stage:

$$\begin{cases} P_1 \leq \alpha_1, & \text{Stop trial and reject } H_0 \\ P_1 > \alpha_0, & \text{Stop trial and accept } H_0 \\ \alpha_1 < P_1 \leq \alpha_0, & \text{Continue to the second stage.} \end{cases} \tag{7.24}$$

For determination of α_1 and α_0, the overall type I error rate is given by

$$\alpha_1 + \int_{\alpha_1}^{\alpha_0} \int_0^{\frac{c_\alpha}{P_1}} dP_2 dP_1 = \alpha_1 + c_\alpha \ln \frac{\alpha_0}{\alpha_1}. \tag{7.25}$$

Letting this error rate equal to α, and using the relationship

$$c_\alpha = e^{-\frac{1}{2}\chi^2_{4,1-\alpha}},$$

we have

$$\alpha_1 + \ln \frac{\alpha_0}{\alpha_1} e^{-\frac{1}{2}\chi^2_{4,1-\alpha}} = \alpha. \tag{7.26}$$

Decision rules at final stage are given by

$$\begin{cases} P_1 P_2 \leq e^{-\frac{1}{2}\chi^2_{4,1-\alpha}}, & \text{Reject } H_0 \\ \text{Otherwise,} & \text{Accept } H_0. \end{cases}$$

Assuming that z_i and n_i are the standardized mean and sample size for the sub-sample at stage i, under the condition that $n_1 = n_2$, the uniformly most powerful test is given by

$$\frac{z_1 + z_2}{\sqrt{2}} \geq z_{1-\alpha}.$$

Equivalently,

$$\Phi_o^{-1}(1 - P_1) + \Phi_o^{-1}(1 - P_2) \geq \sqrt{2}\Phi_o^{-1}(1 - \alpha).$$

Three-stage design

Let $p_i (i = 1, 2, 3)$ be the p-values for the hypothesis tests based on subsamples obtained at stage 1, 2, and 3, respectively.
Decision Rules:

Stage 1: $\begin{cases} \text{Stop with rejection of } H_0 \text{ if } p_1 \leq \alpha_1, \\ \text{Stop without rejection of } H_0 \text{ if } p_1 > \alpha_0, \\ \text{Otherwise continue to stage 2.} \end{cases}$

Stage 2: $\begin{cases} \text{Stop with rejection of } H_0 \text{ if } p_1 p_2 \leq c_{a_2} = e^{-\frac{1}{2}\chi_4^2(1-\alpha_2)}, \\ \text{Stop without rejection of } H_0 \text{ if } p_2 > \alpha_0, \\ \text{Otherwise continue.} \end{cases}$

Stage 3: $\begin{cases} \text{Stop with rejection of } H_0 \text{ if } p_1 p_2 p_3 \leq d_a = e^{-\frac{1}{2}\chi_6^2(1-\alpha)}, \\ \text{Otherwise stop without rejection of } H_0. \end{cases}$

To avoid qualitative interaction between stages and treatments, choose

$$c_{a_2} = d_\alpha / \alpha_0.$$

Then, no values of $p_3 \geq \alpha_0$ can lead to the rejection of H_0 because the procedure would have stopped beforehand. On the other hand, if

$$\alpha_1 \geq c_{\alpha_2}/\alpha_0,$$

then no $p_2 \geq \alpha_0$ can lead to the rejection of H_0. Note that

$$\alpha_1 + \int_{\alpha_1}^{\alpha_0} \int_0^{d_\alpha/(\alpha_0 p_1)} dp_1 dp_2 + \int_{\alpha_1}^{\alpha_0} \int_{d_\alpha/(\alpha_0 p_1)}^{\alpha_0} \int_0^{d_\alpha/(p_1 p_2)} dp_1 dp_2 dp_3$$

$$= \alpha_1 + \frac{d_\alpha}{\alpha_0}(\ln \alpha_0 - \ln \alpha_1) + d_\alpha(2\ln \alpha_0 - \ln d_\alpha)(\ln \alpha_0 - \ln \alpha_1)$$

$$+ \frac{d_\alpha}{2}(\ln^2 \alpha_0 - \ln^2 \alpha_1).$$

Now, let it be equal to α. We can then solve for α_1 given α and α_0. For $\alpha_0 = 0.025$, $d_\alpha = 0.000728$.

7.6 Generalization of Independent p-Value Approaches

General Approach

Consider a clinical trial with K stages and at each stage a hypothesis test is performed, followed by some actions that are dependent on the analysis results. Such actions could be an early futility or efficacy stopping, sample size re-estimation, modification of randomization, or

Table 7.5 Stopping Boundaries

α_0	α_1	α_2
.4	.0265	.0294
.6	.0205	.0209
.8	.0137	.0163

Source: Bauer and Köhne (1995)

other adaptations. The objective of the trial (e.g., testing the efficacy of the experimental drug) can be formulated using a global hypothesis test, which is the intersection of the individual hypothesis tests from the interim analyses.

$$H_0 : H_{01} \cap \ldots \cap H_{0K}, \qquad (7.27)$$

where H_{0k} ($k = 1, \ldots, K$) is the null hypothesis test at the kth interim analysis. Note that the H_{0k} have some restrictions, that is, rejection of any H_{0k} ($k = 1, \ldots, K$) will lead to the same clinical implication (e.g., drug is efficacious). Otherwise the global hypothesis cannot be interpreted. In the rest of the paper, H_{0k} will be based on sub-samples from each stage with the corresponding test statistic denoted by T_k and p-value denoted by p_k. The stopping rules are given by

$$\begin{cases} \text{Stop for efficacy} & \text{if } T_k \leq \alpha_k, \\ \text{Stop for futility} & \text{if } T_k > \beta_k, \\ \text{Continue with adaptations} & \text{if } \alpha_k < T_k \leq \beta_k, \end{cases} \qquad (7.28)$$

where $\alpha_k < \beta_k$ ($k = 1, \ldots, K-1$), and $\alpha_K = \beta_K$. For convenience, α_k and β_k are called the efficacy and futility boundaries, respectively.

To reach the kth stage, a trial has to pass the 1st to $(k-1)$th stages, therefore the CDF of T_k is given by

$$\varphi_k(t) = \Pr(T_k < t, \alpha_1 < t_1 \leq \beta_1, \ldots, \alpha_{k-1} < t_{k-1} \leq \beta_{k-1})$$
$$= \int_{\alpha_1}^{\beta_1} \ldots \int_{\alpha_{k-1}}^{\beta_{k-1}} \int_0^t f_{T_1 \ldots T_k} \, dt_k \, dt_{k-1} \ldots dt_1, \qquad (7.29)$$

where $f_{T_1 \ldots T_k}$ is the joint PDF of $T_1, \ldots,$ and T_k. The error rate (α spent) at the kth stage is given by $\Pr(T_k < \alpha_k)$, that is,

$$\pi_k = \varphi_k(\alpha_k). \qquad (7.30)$$

When the efficacy is claimed at a certain stage, the trial is stopped. Therefore, the type I errors at different stages are mutually exclusive. Hence the experiment-wise type I error rate can be written as

$$\alpha = \sum_{k=1}^{K} \pi_k. \quad (7.31)$$

(7.33) is the key to determining the stopping boundaries as illustrated in the next four sections with two-stage adaptive designs.

There are different p-values that can be calculated: unadjusted p-value and adjusted p-value. Both are measures of the statistical strength for treatment effect. The unadjusted p-value (p_u) associates with π_k when the trial stops at the kth stage, while the adjusted p-value associates with the overall α. The unadjusted p-value corresponding with an observed t when the trial stops at the kth stage is given by

$$p_u(t;k) = \varphi_k(t), \quad (7.32)$$

where $\varphi_k(t)$ is obtained from (7.31). The adjusted p-value corresponding to an observed test statistic $T_k = t$ at the kth stage is given by

$$p(t;k) = \sum_{i=1}^{k-1} \pi_i + p_u(t;k), \ k = 1, \ldots K. \quad (7.33)$$

Note that the adjusted p-value is a measure of statistical strength for rejecting H_0. The later the H_0 is rejected, the larger the adjusted p-value is and the weaker the statistical evidence is.

Selection of Test Statistic

Without losing generality, assume H_{0k} is a test for the efficacy of the experimental drug, which can be written as

$$H_{0k}: \eta_{k1} \geq \eta_{k2} \text{ vs. } H_{ak}: \eta_{k1} < \eta_{k2}, \quad (7.34)$$

where η_{k1} and η_{k2} are the treatment response (mean, proportion, or survival) in the two comparison groups at the kth stage. The joint PDF $f_{T_1\ldots T_k}$ in (7.31) can be any density function; however, it is desirable to chose T_k such that $f_{T_1\ldots T_k}$ has a simple form. Note that when $\eta_{k1} = \eta_{k2}$, the p-value p_k from the sub-sample at the kth stage is uniformly distributed on [0,1] under H_0. This desirable property can be used to construct test statistics for adaptive designs.

In what follows, two different combinations of the p-values will be studied: (i) linear combination of p-values (Chang, 2005), and (ii) product of p-values. The linear combination is given by

$$T_k = \Sigma_{i=1}^{k} w_{ki} p_i, \ k = 1, \ldots, K, \quad (7.35)$$

where $w_{ki} > 0$, and K is the number of analyses planned in the trial. There are two interesting cases of (7.37) that will be studied. They are the test based on the individual p-value for the sub-sample obtained at each stage and the test based on the sum of the p-values from the sub-samples.

The test statistic using the product of p-values is given by

$$T_k = \Pi_{i=1}^k p_i, \quad k = 1, \ldots, K. \tag{7.36}$$

This form has been proposed by Bauer and Köhne (1994) using Fisher's criterion. Here, it will be generalized without using Fisher's criterion so that the selection of stopping boundaries is more flexible. Note that p_k in (7.37) and (7.38) is the p-value from the sub-sample at the kth stage, while $p_u(t;k)$ and $p(t;k)$ in the previous section are unadjusted and adjusted p-values, respectively, calculated from the test statistic, which are based on the cumulative sample up to the kth stage where the trial stops.

Test Based on Individual P-values

The test statistic in this method is based on individual p-values from different stages. The method is referred to as method of individual p-values (MIP). By defining the weighting function as $w_{ki} = 1$ if $i = k$, and $w_{ki} = 0$ otherwise, (7.37) becomes

$$T_k = p_k. \tag{7.37}$$

Due to the independence of p_k, $f_{T_1 \ldots T_k} = 1$ under H_0 and

$$\varphi_k(t) = t \prod_{i=1}^{k-1} L_i, \tag{7.38}$$

where $L_i = (\beta_i - \alpha_i)$ and for convenience, when the upper bound exceeds the lower bound, define $\prod_{i=1}^0 (\cdot) = 1$. The family experiment-wise type I error rate is given by

$$\alpha = \sum_{k=1}^K \alpha_k \prod_{i=1}^{k-1} L_i. \tag{7.39}$$

(7.41) is the necessary and sufficient condition for determining the stopping boundaries, (α_i, β_i).

For a two-stage design, (7.41) becomes

$$\alpha = \alpha_1 + \alpha_2(\beta_1 - \alpha_1) \tag{7.40}$$

Table 7.6 Stopping Boundaries with MIP

	α_1	0.000	0.005	0.010	0.015	0.020
β_1						
0.15		0.1667	0.1379	0.1071	0.0741	0.0385
0.20		0.1250	0.1026	0.0789	0.0541	0.0278
0.25		0.1000	0.0816	0.0625	0.0426	0.0217
0.30		0.0833	0.0678	0.0517	0.0351	0.0179
0.35	α_2	0.0714	0.0580	0.0441	0.0299	0.0152
0.40		0.0625	0.0506	0.0385	0.026	0.0132
0.50		0.0500	0.0404	0.0306	0.0206	0.0104
0.80		0.0312	0.0252	0.0190	0.0127	0.0064
1.00		0.0250	0.0201	0.0152	0.0102	0.0051

Note: One-sided $\alpha = 0.025$.

For convenience, a table of stopping boundaries has been constructed using (7.42) (Table 7.6). The adjusted p-value is given by

$$p(t,k) = \begin{cases} t & \text{if } k=1, \\ \alpha_1 + (\beta_1 - \alpha_1)t & \text{if } k=2. \end{cases} \quad (7.41)$$

Test Based on Sum of P-values

This method is referred to as the method of sum of p-values (MSP). The test statistic in this method is based on the sum of the p-values from the sub-samples. Defining the weights as $w_{ki} = 1$, (7.37) becomes

$$T_k = \sum_{i=1}^{k} p_i, \quad k=1, \ldots, K. \quad (7.42)$$

For two-stage designs, the α spent at stage 1 and stage 2 are given by

$$\Pr(T_1 < \alpha_1) = \int_0^{\alpha_1} dt_1 = \alpha_1, \quad (7.43)$$

and

$$\Pr(T_2 < \alpha_2, \alpha_1 < T_1 \leq \beta_1) = \begin{cases} \int_{\alpha_1}^{\beta_1} \int_{t_1}^{\alpha_2} dt_2 dt_1, & \text{for } \beta_1 \leq \alpha_2, \\ \int_{\alpha_1}^{\alpha_2} \int_{t_1}^{\alpha_2} dt_2 dt_1, & \text{for } \beta_1 > \alpha_2, \end{cases} \quad (7.44)$$

respectively. Carrying out the integrations in (7.46) and substituting the results into (7.33), it is immediately obtained that

$$\alpha = \begin{cases} \alpha_1 + \alpha_2(\beta_1 - \alpha_1) - \frac{1}{2}(\beta_1^2 - \alpha_1^2), & \text{for } \beta_1 < \alpha_2, \\ \alpha_1 + \frac{1}{2}(\alpha_2 - \alpha_1)^2, & \text{for } \beta_1 \geq \alpha_2. \end{cases} \quad (7.45)$$

Table 7.7 Stopping Boundaries with MSP

	α_1	0.000	0.005	0.010	0.015	0.020
β_1						
0.05		0.5250	0.4719	0.4050	0.3182	0.2017
0.10		0.3000	0.2630	0.2217	0.1751	0.1225
0.15	α_2	0.2417	0.215 4	0.187 1	0.1566	0.1200
0.20		0.2250	0.2051	0.1832	0.1564	0.1200
>0.25		0.2236	0.2050	0.1832	0.1564	0.1200

Note: One-sided $\alpha = 0.025$.

Various stopping boundaries can be chosen from (7.47). See Table 7.7 for examples of the stopping boundaries.

The adjusted p-value can be obtained by replacing α_1 with t in (7.45) if the trial stops at stage 1 and by replacing α_2 with t in (7.47) if the trial stops at stage 2.

$$p(t;k) = \begin{cases} t, & k=1, \\ \alpha_1 + t(\beta_1 - \alpha_1) - \frac{1}{2}(\beta_1^2 - \alpha_1^2), & k=2 \text{ and } t \leq \alpha_2, \\ \alpha_1 + \frac{1}{2}(t - \alpha_1)^2, & k=2 \text{ and } t > \alpha_2, \end{cases} \quad (7.46)$$

where $t = p_1$ if the trial stops at stage 1 ($k = 1$) and $t = p_1 + p_2$ if the trial stops at stage 2 ($k = 2$).

Test Based on Product of P-values

This method is known as the method of products of p-values (MPP). The test statistic in this method is based on the product of the p-values from the sub-samples. For two-stage designs, (7.37) becomes

$$T_k = \Pi_{i=1}^{k} p_i, \quad k = 1, 2. \quad (7.47)$$

The α spent in the two stages are given by

$$\Pr(T_1 < \alpha_1) = \int_0^{\alpha_1} dt_1 = \alpha_1 \quad (7.48)$$

and

$$\Pr(T_2 < \alpha_2, \alpha_1 < T_1 \leq \beta_1) = \int_{\alpha_1}^{\beta_1} \int_0^{\alpha_2} \frac{1}{t_1} dt_2 dt_1. \quad (7.49)$$

Table 7.8 Stopping Boundaries with MPP

	α_1	0.005	0.010	0.015	0.020
β_1					
0.15		0.0059	0.0055	0.0043	0.0025
0.20		0.0054	0.0050	0.0039	0.0022
0.25		0.0051	0.0047	0.0036	0.0020
0.30		0.0049	0.0044	0.0033	0.0018
0.35	α_2	0.0047	0.0042	0.0032	0.0017
0.40		0.0046	0.0041	0.0030	0.0017
0.50		0.0043	0.0038	0.0029	0.0016
0.80		0.0039	0.0034	0.0025	0.0014
1.00		0.0038	0.0033	0.0024	0.0013

Note: One-sided $\alpha = 0.025$.

(7.51) can also be written as

$$\Pr(T_2 < \alpha_2, \alpha_1 < T_1 \leq \beta_1)$$
$$= \left\{ \int_{\alpha_1}^{\beta_1} \int_0^{\alpha_2} \frac{1}{t_1} dt_2 dt_1, \quad \text{for } \beta_1 \leq \alpha_2. \right. \tag{7.50}$$

Carrying out the integrations in (7.52) and substituting the results into (7.33), it is immediately obtained that

$$\alpha = \left\{ \alpha_1 + \alpha_2 \ln \frac{\beta_1}{\alpha_1}, \quad \text{for } \beta_1 \leq \alpha_2. \right. \tag{7.51}$$

Note that the stopping boundaries based on Fisher's criterion are special cases of (7.53), where

$$\beta_1 < \alpha_2$$

and

$$\alpha_2 = \exp\left[-\frac{1}{2}\chi_4^2(1-\alpha)\right], \tag{7.52}$$

that is, $\alpha_2 = 0.0380$ for $\alpha = 0.025$. Examples of the stopping boundaries using (7.49) are provided in Table 7.8.

The adjusted p-value can be obtained by replacing α_1 with t in (7.50) if the trial stops at stage 1 and replacing α_2 with t in (7.53) if the trial stops at stage 2.

$$p(t;k) = \begin{cases} t, & k=1, \\ \alpha_1 + t \ln \frac{\beta_1}{\alpha_1}, & k=2 \text{ and } t \leq \alpha_2, \end{cases} \tag{7.53}$$

ADAPTIVE SAMPLE SIZE ADJUSTMENT

where $t = p_1$ if the trial stops at stage 1 ($k = 1$) and $t = p_1 + p_2$ if the trial stops at stage 2 ($k = 2$).

Rules for Sample Size Adjustment The primary rule for adjustment is based on the ratio of the initial estimate of effect size (E_0) to the observed effect size (E), specifically,

$$N = \left|\frac{E_0}{E}\right|^a N_0, \qquad (7.54)$$

where N is the newly estimated sample size, N_0 is the initial sample size which can be estimated from a classic design, and a is a constant,

$$E = \frac{\hat{\eta}_{i2} - \hat{\eta}_{i1}}{\hat{\sigma}_i}. \qquad (7.55)$$

With large sample size assumption, the common variance for the two treatment groups is given by

$$\hat{\sigma}_i^2 = \begin{cases} \hat{\sigma}_i^2, & \text{for normal endpoint,} \\ \bar{\eta}_i(1 - \bar{\eta}_i), & \text{for binary endpoint,} \\ \bar{\eta}_i^2 \left[1 - \frac{e^{\bar{\eta}_i T_0} - 1}{T_0 \bar{\eta}_i e^{\bar{\eta}_i T_s}}\right]^{-1}, & \text{for survival endpoint,} \end{cases} \qquad (7.56)$$

where

$$\bar{\eta}_i = \frac{\hat{\eta}_{i1} + \hat{\eta}_{i1}}{2}.$$

$\bar{\eta}_i = \frac{\hat{\eta}_{i1} + \hat{\eta}_{i2}}{2}$ and the logrank test is assumed to be used for the survival analysis. Note that the standard deviations for proportion and survival have several versions. There are usually slight differences in sample size or power among the different versions.

The sample size adjustment in (7.56) should have the following additional constraints: (i) It should be smaller than $N_{\max}$ (due to financial and or other constraints) and greater than or equal to $N_{\min}$ (the sample size for the interim analysis), and (ii) If E and E_0 have different signs, no adjustment will be made.

Operating characteristics

The operating characteristics are studied using the following example, which is modified slightly from an oncology trial.

Example 7.3 In a two-arm comparative oncology trial, the primary efficacy endpoint is time to progression (TTP). The median TTP is estimated to be 8 months (hazard rate = 0.08664) for the control group, and 10.5 months (hazard rate = 0.06601) for the test group. Assume a uniform enrollment with an accrual period of 9 months and a total study duration of 24 months. The log-rank test will be used for the analysis.

Table 7.9 Operating Characteristics of Adaptive Methods

Median time				Expected	Power (%)
Test	Control	EESP	EFSP	N	MIP/MSP/MPP
0	0	0.010	0.750	216	2.5/2.5/2.5
9.5	8	0.174	0.238	273	42.5/44.3/45.7
10.5	8	0.440	0.067	254	78.6/80.5/82.7
11.5	8	0.703	0.015	219	94.6/95.5/96.7

Note: 1,000,000 simulation runs.

An exponential survival distribution is assumed for the purpose of sample size calculation.

When there is a 10.5 month median time for the test group, the classic design requires a sample size of 290 per group with 80% power at a level of significance (one-sided) α of 0.025. To increase efficiency, an adaptive design with an interim sample size of 175 patients per group is used. The interim analysis allows for early efficacy stopping with stopping boundaries (from Tables 7.6, 7.7, and 7.8) $\alpha_1 = 0.01$, $b_1 = 0.25$ and $\alpha_2 = 0.0625$ (MIP), 0.1832 (MSP), 0.00466 (MPP). The sample size adjustment is based on the rules described in the appendix where $a = 2$. The maximum sample size allowed for adjustment is $N_{\max} = 350$. The simulation results are presented in Table 7.9, where the abbreviations EESP and EFSP stand for early efficacy stopping probability and early futility stopping probability, respectively.

Note that power is the probability of rejecting the null hypothesis. Therefore when the null hypothesis is true, the power is the type I error rate α. From Table 7.9, it can be seen that the one-sided α is controlled at a 0.025 level as expected for all three methods. The expected sample sizes under all four scenarios are smaller than the sample size for the classic design (290/group). In terms of power, MPP has 1% more power than MSP, and MSP has about 1% more power than MIP. If the stopping boundaries are changed to $\alpha_1 = 0.005$ and $\beta_1 = 0.2$, then the power (median TTP = 10.5 months for the test group) will be 76, 79, and 82 for MIP, MSP and MPP, respectively. The detailed results are not presented.

To demonstrate how to calculate the adjusted p-value (e.g., using MSP), assume that naive p-values from logrank test (or other test) are $p_1 = 0.1$, $p_2 = 0.07$, and the trial stops at stage 2. Therefore, $t = p_1 + p_2 = 0.17 < \alpha_2$, and the null hypothesis of no treatment difference is rejected. In fact, the adjusted p-value is 0.0228 (< 0.025) which is obtained from Eq. 7.46 using $t = 0.17$ and $\alpha_1 = 0.01$.

Remarks

With respect to the accuracy of proposed methods, a larger portion of the stopping boundaries in Tables 7.6 through 7.8 is validated using computer simulations with 10,000,000 runs for each set of boundaries $(\alpha_1, \beta_1, \alpha_2)$. To conduct an adaptive design using the methods proposed, follow the steps below:

Step 1: If MIP is used for the design, use (7.42) or Table 7.6 to determine the stopping boundaries $(\alpha_1, \beta_1, \alpha_2)$, and use (7.43) to calculate the adjusted p-value when the trial is finished.

Step 2: If MSP is used for the design, use (7.45) or Table 7.7 to determine the stopping boundaries, and use (7.48) to calculate the adjusted p-value.

Step 3: If MPP is used for the design, use (7.53) or Table 7.8 to determine the stopping boundaries, and (7.54) to calculate the adjusted p-value.

To study the operating characteristics before selecting an optimal design, simulations must be conducted with various scenarios. A SAS program for the simulations can be obtained from the author. The program has fewer than 50 lines of executable code and is very user-friendly.

7.7 Inverse-Normal Method

Lehmacher and Wassmer (1999) proposed normal-inverse method. The test statistic that results from the inverse normal method of combining independent p values (Hedges and Olkin, 1985) is given by

$$\frac{1}{\sqrt{k}} \sum_{i=1}^{k} \Phi^{-1}(1 - p_i) \qquad (7.57)$$

where $\Phi^{-1}(\cdot)$ denotes the inverse cumulative standard normal distribution function. The proposed approach involves using the classical group sequential boundaries for the statistics (7.59). Since the

$$\Phi^{-1}(1 - p_i)'s, k = 1, 2, \ldots, K,$$

are independent and standard normally distributed, the proposed approach maintains α exactly for any (adaptive) choice of sample size.

Example 7.4 Lehmacher and Wassmer gave the following example to demonstrate their method. In a randomized, placebo-controlled, double-blind study involving patients with acne papulopustulosa, Plewig's grade Il-Ill, the effect of treatment under a combination of 1% chloramphenicol (CAS 56-75-7) and 0.5% pale sulfonated shale oil versus the alcoholic vehicle (placebo) was investigated (Fluhr et al., 1998). After 6 weeks of treatment, reduction of bacteria from baseline, examined on agar plates (log CFU/cm^2; CFU, colony forming units), of the active group as compared to the placebo group were assessed. The available data were from 24 and 26 patients in the combination drug and the placebo groups, respectively. The combination therapy resulted in a highly significant reduction in bacteria as compared to placebo using a two-sided t-test for the changes (p = 0.0008).

They further illustrated the method. Suppose that it was intended to perform a three-stage adaptive Pocock's design with $\alpha = 0.01$, and after 2×12 patients the first interim analysis was planned. The two-sided critical bounds for this method are $\alpha_1 = \alpha_2 = \alpha_3 = 2.873$ (Pocock, 1977). After ni = 12 patients per group, the test statistic of the t-test is 2.672 with one-sided p-value $p_1 = 0.0070$, resulting from an observed effect size $\bar{x}_{ii} - \bar{x}_{21} = 1.549$ and an observed standard deviation $s_i = 1.316$. The study should be continued since

$$\Phi^{-1}(i - P_1) = 2.460 < \alpha_1.$$

The observed effect is fairly near to significance. We therefore plan the second interim analysis to be conducted after observing the next 2×6 patients, i.e., the second interim analysis will be performed after fewer patients than the first. The t-test statistic of the second stage is equal to 1.853 with one-sided p value $P_2 = 0.0468$ ($\bar{x}_{12} - \bar{x}_{22} = 1.580$, standard deviation of the second stage $s_2 = 1.472$). The test statistic becomes

$$\sqrt{2}(\Phi^{-1}(1 - p_1) + \Phi^{-1}(1 - p_2)) = 2.925,$$

yielding a significant result after the second stage of the trial. Corresponding approximate 99% RCIs are (0.12, 3.21) and (0.21, 2.92) for the first and the second stages, respectively.

7.8 Concluding Remarks

One of the purposes for adaptive sample size adjustment based on accrued data at interim in clinical trials is not only to achieve statistical significance with a desired power for detecting a clinically significant difference, but also to have the option for stopping the trial early for safety or futility/benefits. To maintain the integrity of the trial, it is strongly recommended that an independent data monitoring committee (DMC) should be established to perform (safety) data monitoring and interim analyses for efficacy/benefits regardless of whether the review or analysis is blinded or unblinded. Based on sample size re-assessment, the DMC can then recommend one of the following: (i) continue the trial with no changes; (ii) decrease/increase the sample size for achieving statistical significance with a desired power; (iii) stop the trial early for safety, futility or benefits; and (iv) modifications to the study protocol. In a recent review article by Montori et al. (2005), it is indicated that there is a significant increasing trend in the percentage of randomized clinical trials that are stopped early for benefits in the past decade. Pocock (2005), however, criticized that the majority of the trials stopped early for benefits do not have correct infrastructure/system in place, and hence the decisions/recommendations for stopping early may not be appropriate. Chow (2005) suggested that so-called reproducibility probability be carefully evaluated if a trial is to be stopped early for benefits, in addition to an observed small p-value.

It should be noted that current methods for adaptive sample size adjustment are mostly developed in the interest of controlling an overall type I error rate at the nominal level. These methods, however, are conditional and may not be feasible to reflect current best medical practice. As indicated in Chapter 2, the use of adaptive design methods in clinical trials could result in a moving target patient population after protocol amendments. As a result, sample size required in order to have an accurate and reliable statistical inference on the moving target patient population is necessarily adjusted unconditionally. In practice, it is then suggested that current statistical methods for group sequential designs should be modified to incorporate the randomness of the target patient population over time. In other words, sample sizes should be adjusted adaptively to account for random boundaries at different stages.

CHAPTER 8

Adaptive Seamless Phase II/III Designs

A seamless phase II/III trial design is a program that addresses within a single trial the objectives that are normally achieved through separate trials in phases IIb and III (Gallo et al., 2006; Chang et al., 2006). An adaptive seamless phase II/III design is a combination of phase II and phase III, which aims at achieving the primary objectives normally achieved through the conduct of separate phase II and phases III trials, and would use data from patients enrolled before and after the adaptation in the final analysis (Maca et al., 2006). In a seamless design, there is usually a so-called learning phase that serves the same purpose as a traditional phase II trial, and a confirmatory phase that serves the same objective as a traditional phase III study. Compared to traditional designs, a seamless design can not only reduce sample size but also shorten the time to bring a positive drug candidate to the marketplace. In this chapter, for illustration purposes, we will discuss different seamless designs and their utilities, through real examples. We will also discuss the issues that are commonly encountered followed by some recommendations for assuring the validity and integrity of a clinical trial with seamless design.

In the next section, the efficiency of an adaptive seamless design is discussed. Section 8.2 introduces step-wise tests with respect to some adaptive procedures employed in a seamless trial design. Statistical methods based on the concepts of contrast test and naïve p-value are described in Section 8.3. Section 8.4 compares several seamless designs. Drop-the-loses adaptive designs are discussed in Section 8.5. A brief summary is given in the last section of this chapter.

8.1 Why a Seamless Design Is Efficient

The use of a seamless design enjoys the following advantages. There are opportunities for savings when (i) a drug is not working through early stopping for futility and when (ii) a drug has a dramatic effect by early stopping for efficacy. A seamless design is efficient because there is no lead time between the learning and confirmatory phases. In addition, the data collected at the learning phase are combined with those data obtained at the confirmatory phase for final analysis.

The most notable difference between an adaptive seamless phase II/III design and the traditional approach that has separate phase II and phase III trials is the control of the overall type I error rate (alpha) and the corresponding power for correctly detecting a clinically meaningful difference. In the traditional approach, the actual α is equal to $\alpha_{II}\alpha_{III}$, where α_{II} and α_{III} are the type I error rates controlled at phase II and phase III, respectively. If two phase III trials are required, then

$$\alpha = \alpha_{II}\alpha_{III}\alpha_{III}.$$

In a seamless adaptive phase II/III design, actual $\alpha = \alpha_{III}$. If two phase III studies are required, then $\alpha = \alpha_{III}\alpha_{III}$. Thus, the α for a seamless design is actually $1/\alpha_{II}$ times larger than the traditional design. Similarly, we can steal power (permissible) by using a seamless design. Here *power* refers to the probability of correctly detecting a *true* but not *hypothetical* treatment difference. In a classic design, the actual power is given by

$$power = power_{II} * power_{III},$$

while in a seamless adaptive phase II/III design, actual power is

$$power = power_{III},$$

which is $1/power_{II}$ times larger than the traditional design.

In practice, it is not necessary to gain much power by combining the data from different phases. Table 7.9 provides a summary of the results (power) using individual p-values from the sub-sample of each stage (MIP), sum of the p-values from different stages (MSP), and Fisher's combination of the p-values from sub-samples from each stage (MPP) under a two-group parallel design. Power differences between methods are small.

8.2 Step-Wise Test and Adaptive Procedures

Consider a clinical trial with K stages. At each stage, a hypotheses testing is performed followed by some actions that are dependent on the analysis results. In practice, three possible actions are often considered. They are (i) an early futility stopping, (ii) an early stopping due to efficacy, or (iii) dropping the losers (i.e., inferior arms including pre-determined sub-populations are dropped after the review of analysis results at each stage). In practice, the objective of the trial (e.g., testing for efficacy of the experimental drug) can be formulated as a global hypotheses testing problem. In other words, the null hypothesis is the intersection of individual null hypotheses at each stage, that is

$$H_0 : H_{01} \cap \ldots \cap H_{0K}, \qquad (8.1)$$

where H_{0k} ($k = 1, \ldots, K$) is the null hypothesis at the kth stage. Note that the H_{0k} have some restrictions, that is, the rejection of any H_{0k} ($k = 1, \ldots, K$) will lead to the common clinical implication of the efficacy of the study medication. Otherwise, the global hypothesis cannot be interpreted. The following step-wise test procedure is often employed. Let T_k be the test statistic associated with H_{0k}. Note that for convenience's sake, we will only consider one-sided tests throughout this chapter.

Stopping Rules

To test (8.1), first, we need specify stopping rules at each stage. The stopping rules considered here are given by

$$\begin{cases} \text{Stop for efficacy} & \text{if } T_k \leq \alpha_k, \\ \text{Stop for futility} & \text{if } T_k > \beta_k, \\ \text{Drop losers and continue} & \text{if } \alpha_k < T_k \leq \beta_k, \end{cases} \qquad (8.2)$$

where $\alpha_k < \beta_k$ ($k = 1, \ldots, K - 1$), and $\alpha_K = \beta_K$. For convenience's sake, we denote α_k and β_k as the efficacy and futility boundaries, respectively. The test statistic is defined as

$$T_k = \prod_{i=1}^{k} p_i, \ k = 1, \ldots, K, \qquad (8.3)$$

where p_i is the naive p-value for testing H_{0k} based on sub-samples collected at the kth stage. It is assumed that p_k is uniformly distributed under the null hypothesis H_{0k}.

8.3 Contrast Test and Naive p-Value

In clinical trials with M arms, the following general one-sided contrast hypotheses testing is often considered:

$$H_0 : L(\mathbf{u}) \leq 0; \text{ vs. } H_a : L(\mathbf{u}) = \varepsilon > 0, \qquad (8.4)$$

where

$$L(\mathbf{u}) = \sum_{i=1}^{M} c_i u_i$$

is a linear combination of u_i, $i = 1, \ldots, M$, in which c_i are the contrast coefficients satisfying

$$\sum_{i=1}^{M} c_i = 0,$$

and ε is a pre-specified constant. In practice, u_i can be the mean, proportion, or hazard rate for the ith group depending on the study endpoint. Under the null hypothesis of (8.4), a contrast test can be obtained as follows:

$$Z = \frac{L(\hat{\mathbf{u}}; H)}{\sqrt{var L(\hat{\mathbf{u}})}}, \qquad (8.5)$$

where $\hat{\mathbf{u}}$ is an unbiased estimator of $\mathbf{u}$, where $\mathbf{u} = (u_i)$ and

$$\hat{u}_i = \sum_{j=1}^{n_{ij}} \frac{x_{ij}}{n_{ij}}.$$

Let

$$\varepsilon = E(L(\hat{\mathbf{u}})), \quad v^2 = var(L(\hat{\mathbf{u}})), \qquad (8.6)$$

where homogeneous variance assumption under H_0 and H_a is assumed. It is also assumed that u_i, $i = 1, \ldots, M$ are mutually independent. Without loss of generality, assume that $c_i u_i > 0$ as an indication of efficacy. Then, for a superiority design, if the null hypothesis H_0 given in (8.4) is rejected for some c_i satisfying $\sum_{i=1}^{M} c_i = 0$, then there is a difference among u_i, $i = 1, \ldots, M$.

Let $\hat{\mathbf{u}}$ be the mean for a normal endpoint (proportion for a binary endpoint, or MLE of the hazard rate for a survival endpoint). Then, by the *Central Limit Theorem*, the asymptotic distribution of the test statistic and the pivotal statistic can be obtained as follows:

$$Z = \frac{L(\hat{\mathbf{u}}|H_0)}{v} \sim N(0, 1), \qquad (8.7)$$

and

$$Z = \frac{L(\hat{\mathbf{u}}|H_a)}{v} \sim N(\frac{\varepsilon}{v}, 1), \qquad (8.8)$$

where

$$v^2 = \sum_{i=1}^{M} c_i^2 var(\hat{u}_i) = \sigma^2 \sum_{i=1}^{M} \frac{c_i^2}{n_i} = \frac{\theta^2}{n}, \qquad (8.9)$$

and

$$\theta^2 = \sigma^2 \sum_{i=1}^{M} \frac{c_i^2}{f_i}, \qquad (8.10)$$

in which n_i is the sample size for the ith arm, $f_i = \frac{n_i}{n}$ is the size fraction, $n = \sum_{i=0}^{k} n_i$, and σ^2 is the variance of the response under H_0. Thus, the power is given by

$$\text{power} = \Phi_0\left(\frac{\varepsilon\sqrt{n} - \theta z_{1-\alpha}}{\theta}\right), \tag{8.11}$$

where Φ_0 is cumulative distribution function of $N(0, 1)$. Thus, the sample size required for achieving a desired power can be obtained as

$$n = \frac{(z_{1-\alpha} + z_{1-\beta})^2 \theta^2}{\varepsilon^2}. \tag{8.12}$$

It can be seen from above that (8.11) and (8.12) include the commonly employed one-arm or two-arm superiority design and non-inferiority designs as special cases. For example, for a one-arm design, $c_1 = 1$, and for a two-arm design, $c_1 = -1$ and $c_2 = 1$. Note that a minimal sample size is required when the response and the contrasts have the same shape under a balanced design. If, however, an inappropriate set of contrasts is used, the sample size could be several times larger than the optimal design.

When the shape of the c_i is similar to the shape of u_{ik}, the test statistic is a most powerful test. However, u_i is usually unknown. In this case, we may consider the adaptive contrasts $c_{ik} = \hat{u}_{ik-1}$ at the kth stage, where $\hat{u}_{ik-1}$ is the observed response at the previous stage, i.e., the $(k-1)^{th}$ stage. Thus, we have

$$Z_k = \sum_{i=1}^{m} (\hat{u}_{ik-1} - \bar{u}_{k-1})\hat{u}_{ik}, \tag{8.13}$$

which are conditionally, given data at the $(k-1)^{th}$ stage, normally distributed. It can be shown that the correlation between z_{k-1} and z_k is zero since p_k (=α) is independent of $c_m = u_m$, $m = 1, \ldots, M$ and p_k is independent of Z_{k-1} or p_{k-1}. It follows that Z_1 and Z_2 are independent.

8.4 Comparison of Seamless Designs

There are many possible seamless adaptive designs. It is helpful to classify these designs into the following four categories according to the design features and adaptations: (i) fixed number of regimens, which includes stopping early for futility, biomarker-informed stopping early for futility, and stopping early for futility/efficacy with sample size re-estimation; (ii) flexible number of regimens, which includes a flexible number of regimens, adaptive hypotheses, and response-adaptive randomization; (iii) population adaptation, where the number of patient groups can be changed from the learning phase to the confirmatory phase; and (iv) combinations of (ii) and (iii). For seamless adaptive designs in category (iii), patient groups are often correlated, such as the entire patient population and sub-population with certain genomic markers. When all patient groups are mutually independent, categories (iii) and (iv) are statistically equivalent. Chang (2005) discussed various designs in category (i) and proposed the use of a Bayesian biomarker-adaptive design in a phase II/III clinical program.

In this section, we will focus on seamless adaptive designs with a flexible number of regimens. We will compare four different seamless adaptive designs with normal endpoints. Each design has five treatment groups including a control group in the learning phase. Since there are multiple arms, contract tests are considered for detecting treatment difference under the null hypothesis of

$$H_0 : \sum_{i=1}^{5} c_i u_i > 0,$$

where c_i is the contrast for the ith group that has an expected response of u_i. The test statistic is $T = \Sigma_{i=1}^{5} c_i \hat{u}_i$. The four seamless designs considered here include (i) a five-arm group sequential design; (ii) an adaptive hypotheses design, where contracts c_i change dynamically according to the shape of the response (u_i) for achieving the most power; (iii) a drop-the-losers design, where inferior groups (losers) will be dropped, but two groups and the control will be kept in the confirmatory phase; and (iv) a keep-the-winner design, where we keep the best group and the control at the confirmatory phase. Since the maximum power is achieved for a balanced design when the shape of the contrasts is consistent with the shape of the response (Stewart and Ruberg, 2000; Chang and Chow, 2006; Chang, Chow, and Pong, 2006), in the adaptive hypotheses approach, the contrasts in the confirmatory phase are re-shaped based on the observed responses in the learning phase. Three different response and contrast shapes are presented (see Table 8.1). The powers of the adaptive designs are summarized in Table 8.2, where the generalized Fisher combination method (Chang, 2005) with efficacy and futility stopping boundaries of $\alpha_1 = 0.01, \beta_1 = 1, \alpha_2 = 0.0033$ are used.

Table 8.1 Response and Contrast Shapes

Shape	u_1	u_2	u_3	u_4	u_5	c_1	c_2	c_3	c_4	c_5
Monotonic	1.0	2.0	3.5	4.0	4.5	−1.9	−0.9	0.1	1.1	1.6
Convex	1.0	1.0	4.0	1.0	3.0	−1.0	−1.0	2.0	−1.0	1.0
Step	1.0	3.4	3.4	3.4	3.4	−1.92	0.48	0.48	0.48	0.48

Table 8.2 Power (%) of Contrast Test

Response	Design	Monotonic	Contrast Wave	Step
Monotonic	Sequential	96.5	27.1	71.0
	Adaptive	83.4	50.0	70.0
	Drop-losers	94.6	72.7	87.9
	Keep-winner	97.0	84.9	94.2
Wave	Sequential	26.5	95.8	23.3
	Adaptive	49.5	82.1	48.0
	Drop-losers	56.1	85.6	54.6
	Keep-winner	67.7	88.7	66.6
Step	Sequential	42.6	14.6	72.4
	Adaptive	41.0	26.4	54.6
	Drop-losers	64.9	49.6	78.9
	Keep-winner	77.5	64.6	87.9

Note: $\sigma = 10$, one-sided $\alpha = 0.025$, interim n = 64/group.
Expected total n = 640 under the alternative hypothesis for all the designs. For simplicity, assume the best arm is correctly predetermined at interim analysis for the drop-losers and keep-winner designs.

It can be seen that the keep-the-winner design is very robust for different response and contrast shapes.

It can be seen from Table 8.1 and Table 8.2, when the contrast shape is consistent with the response shape, it gives the most power regardless the type of design. When the response shape is unknown, adaptive design (may be drop-the-losers) is the most powerful design. Note that the examples provided here controlled the type I error under the global null hypothesis.

8.5 Drop-the-Loser Adaptive Design

In pharmaceutical research and development, it is desirable to shorten the time of the conduct of clinical trials, data analysis, submission, and regulatory review and approval process in order to bring the drug product to the marketplace as early as possible. Thus, any designs which can help to achieve the goals are very attractive. As a result, various strategies are proposed. For example, Gould (1992) and Zucker et al. (1999) considered using blinded data from the pilot phase to design a clinical trial and then combine the data for final analysis. Proschan and Hunsberger (1995) proposed a strategy which allows re-adjustment of the sample size based upon unblinded data so that a clinical trial is properly powered. Other designs have been proposed to combine studies conducted at different phases of traditional clinical development into a single study. For example, Bauer and Kieser (1999) proposed a two-stage design which enables investigators to terminate the trial entirely or drop a subset of the regimens for lack of efficacy at the end of the first stage. Their procedure is highly flexible, and the distributional assumptions are kept to a minimum. Bauer and Kieser's method has the advantage of allowing hypothesis testing at the end of the confirmation stage. However, it is difficult to construct confidence intervals. Brannath, Koening, and Bauer (2003) examined adjusted and repeated confidence intervals in group sequential designs, where the responses are normally distributed. Such confidence intervals are important for interpreting the clinical significance of the results.

In practice, drop-the-losers adaptive designs are useful in combining phase II and phase III clinical trials into a single trial. In this section, we will introduce the application of the drop-the-losers adaptive designs under the assumption of normal distributions. The concept, however, can be similarly applied to other distributions. The drop-the-losers adaptive design consists of two stages with a simple data-based decision made at the interim. In the early phase of the trial, the investigators may administer K experimental treatments (say $\tau_1, \ldots, \tau_K$) to n subjects per treatment. A control treatment, τ_0, is also administered during this phase. Unblinded data on patient responses are collected at end of the first stage. The best treatment group (based on observed mean) and the control group are retained and other treatment groups are dropped at the second stage.

Cohen and Sackrowitz (1989) provided an unbiased estimate using data from both stages. Cohen and Sackrowitz considered using a conditional distribution on a specific event to construct conditionally unbiased estimators. Following a similar idea, the test statistic and confidence intervals can be derived. The specific conditional distribution used in the final analysis depends on the outcomes from the first stage. Provided the set of possible events from the first stage on which one condition is a partition of the sample space, the *conditional corrections* also hold *unconditionally*. In our setting, conditional level α tests are unconditional level α tests. In other words, if all of the null hypotheses are true for all of the treatments, the probability of rejecting a null hypothesis is never greater than α, regardless of which treatment is selected (Sampson and Sill, 2005).

Sampson and Sill assume the following ordered outcome after the first stage,

$$Q = \{X : \bar{X}_1 > \bar{X}_2 > \cdots > \bar{X}_k\}$$

so that τ_1 continues into the second stage (other outcomes would be equivalently handled by relabeling). Typically, at the end of the trial, we want to make inferences on the mean μ_1 of treatment τ_1, and compare it with the control (e.g., test $H_0 : \mu_1 - \mu_0 \leq \Delta_{10}$ or construct a confidence interval about $\mu_1 - \mu_0$). Therefore, we can construct uniformly most powerful (UMP) unbiased tests for hypotheses concerning Δ_1 based upon the conditional distribution of W given (X^*, T). To see this, note that the test is based on the conditional event Q. Lehmann (1983) gives a general proof for this family, which shows that conditioning on sufficient statistics associated with nuisance parameters causes them to drop from the distribution. In addition, the theorem states that the use of this conditional distribution to draw inferences about a parameter of interest yields hypothesis testing procedures which are uniformly most powerful unbiased unconditionally (i.e., UMPU before conditioning on the sufficient statistics). The test statistic is

$$W = \frac{n_0 (n_A + n_B)}{(n_0 + n_A + n_B) \sigma^2} (\bar{Z} - \bar{Y}_0),$$

which has the distribution of

$$W \sim f_a (W|\Delta_1, X^*, T) = C_N \exp\left\{-\frac{1}{2G} (W - G\Delta_1)^2\right\} D$$

where

$$\bar{Z} = \frac{(n_A \bar{X}_M + n_B \bar{Y})}{n_A + n_B},$$

$\bar{X}_M = \max(\bar{X}_1, \ldots, \bar{X}_k) =$ maximum mean observed mean at first stage,

$$G = \frac{n_0 (n_A + n_B)}{(n_0 + n_A + n_B) \sigma^2},$$

$$T = \frac{n_0 \bar{Y}_0 + (n_A + n_B) \bar{Z}}{n_0 + n_A + n_B},$$

$$D = \Phi\left[\frac{\sqrt{n_A (n_A - n_B)} \left(\sigma^2 W + (n_A + n_B) (T - \bar{X}_2)\right)}{\sqrt{n_A (n_A + n_B)} \sigma}\right],$$

and C_N is the normalization constant, which involves integrating W over real line.

In order to test

$$H_0 : \mu_1 - \mu_0 \leq \Delta_{10} \text{ versus } H_a : \mu_1 - \mu_0 > \Delta_{10},$$

we consider the following function

$$F_Q (W|\Delta_{10}, X^*, T) = \int_{-\infty}^{W} f_Q (t |\Delta_{10}, X^*, T) \, dt.$$

We can use the function to obtain a critical value, W_u, through $F_Q(W_u|\Delta_{10}, X^*, T) = 1 - \alpha$. Note that $100(1-\alpha)\%$ confidence intervals, $[\Delta_L, \Delta_U]$, can be constructed from

$$F_Q(W_{obs}|\Delta_L, X^*, T) = 1 - \alpha/2,$$

and

$$F_Q(W|\Delta_{10}, X^*, T) = \alpha/2$$

because $W|X^*, T$ is monotonic likelihood ratio in T. Computer programs are available at

$$http://www.gog.org/sdcstaff/mikesill$$

or

$$http://sphhp.buffalo.edu/biostat/.$$

To illustrate the calculation, Sampson and Sill (2005) simulated a data set from a design, where $k = 7$, $\mu_1 = \cdots = \mu_7 = 0$, $n_A = n_B 1 = 100$, $n_0 = 200$, and $\sigma = 10$. The experimental data have been relabeled in decreasing order. Suppose we want to test

$$H_0: \mu_1 - \mu_0 \leq 0 \text{ versus } H_1: \mu_1 - \mu_0 > 0.$$

The simulated data are given as follows:

$$\bar{X}_1 = 1.8881,$$
$$\bar{X}_2 = 0.9216,$$
$$\bar{X}_3 = 0.0691,$$
$$\bar{X}_4 = -0.3793,$$
$$\bar{X}_5 = -0.3918,$$
$$\bar{X}_6 = -0.8945,$$
$$\bar{X}_7 = -0.9276,$$
$$\bar{Y} = 0.7888,$$
$$\bar{Y}_0 = -0.4956.$$

Based on these data, $W_{obs} = 1.83$. Thus, the rejection region is given by $(2.13, \infty)$. Hence, we fail to reject H_0. The 95% confidence interval is given by $(-0.742, 3.611)$.

8.6 Summary

The motivation behind the use of an adaptive seamless design is probably the possibility of shortening the time of development of a new medication. As indicated earlier, an adaptive seamless phase II/III design is not only flexible but also efficient as compared to separate phase II and phase III studies. However, benefits and drawbacks for implementing an adaptive seamless phase II/III design must be carefully weighed against each other. In practice, not all clinical developments may be candidates for such a design. Maca et al. (2006) proposed a list of criteria for determining the feasibility of the use of an adaptive seamless design in clinical development plan. These criteria include endpoints and enrollment, clinical development time, and logistical considerations, which are briefly outlined below.

One of the most important feasibility considerations for an adaptive seamless design is the amount of time that a patient needs in order to reach the endpoint, which will be used for dose escalation. If the endpoint duration is too long, the design could result in unacceptable inefficiencies. In this case, a surrogate marker with much shorter duration might be used. Thus, Maca et al. (2006) suggested that well-established and understood endpoints (or surrogate markers) be considered when implementing an adaptive seamless design in clinical development. It, however, should be noted that if the goal of a phase II program is to learn about the primary endpoint to be carried forward into phase III, an adaptive seamless design would not be feasible. As the use of an adaptive seamless design is to shorten the time of development, whether the adaptive seamless design would achieve the study objectives within a reduced time frame would be another important factor for feasibility consideration, especially when the adaptive seamless trial is the only pivotal trial required for regulatory submission. In the case where there are two pivotal trials, whether the second seamless trial can shorten the overall development time should be taken into feasibility consideration as well. Logistical considerations are drug supply and drug packaging. It is suggested that development programs which do not have costly or complicated drug regimens would be better suited to adaptive seamless designs.

Although adaptive seamless phase II/III designs are efficient and flexible as compared to the traditional separate phase II and phase III studies, potential impact on statistical inference and p-value after adaptations are made should be carefully evaluated. It should be noted that although more adaptations allow higher flexibility, this could result in a much more complicated statistical analysis at the end of trial.

CHAPTER 9

Adaptive Treatment Switching

For evaluation of the efficacy of a test treatment for progressive disease such as cancer or HIV, a parallel-group active control randomized clinical trial is often conducted. Under the study design, qualified patients are randomly assigned to receive either an active control (a standard therapy or a treatment currently available in the marketplace) or the test treatment under investigation. Patients are allowed to switch from one treatment to another due to ethical consideration such as lack of response or evidence of disease progression. In practice, it is not uncommon that up to 80% of patients may switch from one treatment to another. This certainly has an impact on the evaluation of the efficacy of the test treatment. Despite allowing a switch between two treatments, many clinical studies are to compare the test treatment with the active control agent as if no patients had ever switched. Sommer and Zeger (1991) referred to the treatment effect among patients who complied with treatment as *biological efficacy*. In practice, the survival time of a patient who switched from the active control to the test treatment might be on the average longer than his/her survival time that would have been if he/she had adhered to the original treatment (either the active control or the test treatment), if switching is based on prognosis to optimally assign patients' treatments over time. We refer to the difference caused by treatment switch as *switching effect*. The purpose of this chapter is to discuss some models for treatment switch with switching effect and methods for statistical inference under these models.

The remainder of this chapter is organized as follows. In the next section, the latent event times model under the parametric setting is described. In Section 9.2, the concept of latent hazard rate is considered by incorporating the switching effect in the latent hazard functions. Statistical inferences are also derived using Cox's regression with some additional covariates and parameters in this section. A simulation study is carried out in Section 9.3 to examine the performance of the method as compared to two other methods, where the one ignoring the switching data and the other one including the switching data but ignoring the switching effect. A mixed exponential model is considered to assess the total survival time in Section 9.4. Some concluding remarks are given in the last section of this chapter.

9.1 Latent Event Times

Suppose that patients are randomly assigned to two treatment groups: a test treatment and an active control. Consider the case where there is no treatment switch and the study objective is to compare the efficacy of the two treatments. Let $T_1, \ldots, T_n$ be independent non-negative survival times and $C_1 \ldots, C_n$ be independent non-negative censoring times that are independent of survival times. Thus, the observations are $Y_i = min(T_i, C_i)$, $i = 1$ if $T_i \leq C_i$, and $i = 0$ if $T_i > C_i$. Assume that the test treatment acts multiplicatively on a patient's survival time, i.e., an accelerated failure time model applies. Denote the magnitude of this multiplicative effect by $e^{-\beta}$, where β is an unknown parameter. Assume further that the survival time distribution under the active control has a parametric form $F_\theta(t)$, where θ is an unknown parameter vector and $F_\theta(t)$ is a known distribution when θ is known. Let k_i be the treatment indicator for the ith patient, i.e., $k_i = 1$ for the test treatment and $k_i = 0$ for the active control. Then, the distribution of the survival time is given by

$$P(T_i \leq t) = F_\theta(e^{\beta k_i} t), \quad t > 0. \tag{9.1}$$

If F_θ has a density f_θ, then the density of T_i is given by $e^{\beta k_i}$, $t > 0$.

Consider the situation where patients may switch their treatments and the study objective is to compare the biological efficacy. Let $S_i > 0$ denote the ith patient's switching time. Branson and Whitehead (2002) introduced the concept of *latent event time* in the simple case where only patients in the control group may switch. We define the latent event time in the general case as follows. For a patient with no treatment switch, the latent event time is the same as his/her survival time. For patient i who switches at time S_i, the latent event time $\tilde{T}_i$ is an abstract quantity defined to be the patient's survival time that would have been if this patient had not switched the treatment. For patients who switch from the active control group to the test treatment group, Branson and Whitehead (2002) suggested the following model conditional on S_i:

$$\tilde{T}_i \stackrel{d}{=} S_i + e^\beta (T_i - S_i), \tag{9.2}$$

where d denotes equality in distribution. That is, the survival time for a patient who switched from the active control to the test treatment could be back-transformed to the survival time that would have been if the patient had not switched. For the case where patients may switch from either group, the model (9.2) can be modified as follows:

$$\tilde{T}_i \stackrel{d}{=} S_i + e^{\beta(1-2k_i)}(T_i - S_i), \tag{9.3}$$

where k_i is the indicator for the original treatment assignment, not for the treatment after switching.

Model (9.2) or (9.3), however, does not take into account the fact that treatment switch is typically based on prognosis and/or investigator's judgment. For example, a patient in one group may switch to another because he/she does not respond to the original assigned treatment. This may result in a somewhat optimal treatment assignment for the patient and a survival time longer than those patients who did not switch. Ignoring such a switching effect will lead to a biased assessment of the treatment effect Shao, Chang and Chow (2005) consider the following model conditional on S_i:

$$\tilde{T}_i \stackrel{d}{=} S_i + e^{\beta(1-2k_i)} w_{k,\eta}(S_i)(T_i - S_i), \tag{9.4}$$

where η is an unknown parameter vector and $w_{k,\eta}(S)$ are known functions of the switching time S when η and k are given. Typically, $w_{k,\eta}(S)$ should be close to 1 when S is near 0, i.e., the switching effect is negligible if switching occurs too early. Note that

$$\lim_{S \downarrow 0} w_{k,\eta}(S) = 1.$$

An example is

$$w_{k,\eta}(S) = exp\left(\eta_{k,0}S + \eta_{k,1}S^2\right),$$

where $\eta_{k,l}$ are unknown parameters.

Under model (9.1) and model (9.4), the distributions of the survival times for patients who switched treatments are given by (conditional on S_i)

$$\begin{aligned} P(T_i \leq t) &= P(\tilde{T}_i \leq S_i + e^{\beta(1-2k_i)} w_{k,\eta}(S_i)(t - S_i)) \\ &= F_\theta(e^{\beta k_i}[S_i + e^{\beta(1-2k_i)} w_{k,\eta}(S_i)(t - S_i)]) \\ &= F_\theta(e^{\beta k_i} S_i + e^{\beta(1-k_i)} w_{k,\eta}(S_i)(t - S_i)) \end{aligned}$$

for $k_i = 0, 1$. The distributions for patients who never switch are

$$F_\theta(e^{\beta k_i} t), k_i = 0, 1.$$

Assume that F has a density f_θ. For convenience's sake, we denote $S_i = \infty$ for patient i who never switch. Then, the conditional likelihood function given S_i is

$$L(\theta, \beta, \eta)$$
$$= \prod_{i:S_i=\infty} [e^{\beta k_i} f_\theta(e^{\beta k_i} Y_i)]^{\delta_i} [1 - F_\theta(e^{\beta k_i} Y_i)]^{1-\delta_i}$$
$$\times \prod_{i:S_i<\infty} [e^{\beta(1-k_i)} w_{k_i}(s_i) f_\theta(e^{\beta k_i} S_i + e^{\beta(1-k_i)} w_{k_i}(S_i)(Y_i - S_i))]^{\delta_i}$$
$$\times [1 - F_\theta(e^{\beta k_i} S_i + e^{\beta(1-k_i)} w_{k_i}(S_i)(Y_i - S_i))]^{\delta_i}.$$

Let $\gamma = (\theta, \beta, \eta)$. The parameter vector can be estimated by solving the following likelihood equation

$$\frac{\partial \log L(\gamma)}{\partial \gamma} = 0. \tag{9.5}$$

Under some regularity conditions, the estimate of γ is asymptotically normal with mean vector $\mathbf{0}$ and covariance matrix

$$\left[E \frac{\partial^2 \log L(\gamma)}{\partial \gamma \partial \gamma'}\right]^{-1} Var\left[E \frac{\partial \log L(\gamma)}{\partial \gamma}\right] \left[E \frac{\partial^2 \log L(\gamma)}{\partial \gamma \partial \gamma'}\right]^{-1}, \tag{9.6}$$

which can be estimated by substituting with its estimate. Statistical inference can then be obtained based on the asymptotic results.

Branson and Whitehead (2002) proposed an iterative parameter estimation (IPE) method for statistical analysis of data with treatment switch. The idea of the method is to relate the distributions of the survival times of the two treatments under a parametric model. Thus, under model (9.2), IPE can be described as follows. First, an initial estimate $\hat{\beta}$ of β is obtained. Then, latent event times are estimated as

$$\hat{T}_i = S_i + b^{\hat{\beta}}(T_i - S_i)$$

for patients who switched their treatments. Next, a new estimate of β is obtained by using the estimated latent event times as if they were the observed data. Finally, the previously described procedure is iterated until the estimate of β converges.

Note that although a similar IPE method can be applied under model (9.4), it is not recommended for the following reason. If initial estimates of model parameters are obtained by solving the likelihood equation given in (9.5), then iteration does not increase the efficiency of estimates and hence adds unnecessary complexity for computation. On the other hand, if initial estimates are not solutions of the likelihood equation given in (9.5), then they are typically not efficient and the estimates obtained by IPE (if they converge) may not be as efficient as the solutions of the likelihood equation (9.5). Thus, directly solving the likelihood equation (9.5) produces estimates that are either more efficient or computationally simpler than the IPE estimates.

9.2 Proportional Hazard Model with Latent Hazard Rate

The above parametric approach for latent event times is useful. However, statistical analysis under such a parametric model may not be robust against model mis-specifications. For survival data in clinical trials, alternatively, we may consider the following Cox's proportional hazard model, which is a semi-parametric model.

Let $F(t)$ be the distribution of the survival time and $f(t)$ be its corresponding density. Then, the hazard rate at time t is defined as

$$\lambda(t) = f(t)/[1 - F(t)].$$

The Cox's proportional hazard model is then given by

$$\lambda_{k_i}(t) = \lambda_0(t) e^{\beta k_i}, \tag{9.7}$$

where k_i is the treatment indicator and $\lambda_0(t)$ is left unspecified. In a more general setting, we can replace k_i in (9.7) by a covariate vector associated with the ith patient and β by a parameter vector. Under model (9.7), if there is no treatment switch, an estimator of β can be obtained by maximizing the following partial likelihood function

$$L(\beta) = \prod_i \left(\frac{e^{\beta k_i}}{\sum_{j \in R_i} e^{\beta k_j}} \right)^{\delta_i}, \tag{9.8}$$

where R_i is the set of patients who are alive and observed just before time T_i. When there is treatment switch but the switching effect is ignored (i.e., patients switch treatments at random), model (9.7) can be modified by replacing k_i by the time-dependent covariate $k_i(t)$ as follows:

$$k_i(t) = \begin{cases} 1 - k_i, & t \geq S_i \\ k_i & t < S_i, \end{cases}$$

where S_i is the switching time for the ith patient and $0 \leq t < \infty$. Note that by definition, $S_i = \infty$ if the ith patient never switched. This reduces to a special case of the proportional hazard model with time-dependent covariates (see, e.g., Kalb and Prentice, 1980; Cox and Oakes, 1984).

Consider the case where the switching effect $w_{k,\eta}(S_i)$ may depend on prognosis and/or investigator's assessment, which is an unknown parameter vector. Instead of including the switching effect in the model as latent event times (9.4), we include it in the proportional hazard

model as follows:
$$\lambda_{k_i}(t) = \lambda_0(t) e^{\beta k_i(t)} w_{k,\eta}(t, S_i), \qquad (9.9)$$
where
$$w_{k,\eta}(t, S_i) = \begin{cases} w_{k,\eta}(S_i), & t \geq S_i \\ 1, & t < S_i \end{cases}.$$

We refer to this model as the latent hazard rate model since $\lambda_{ki}(t)$ in (9.9) corresponds to a latent event time and hence can be treated as a latent hazard rate. Under the latent hazard rate model (9.9), the partial likelihood is given by

$$L(\beta, \eta) = \prod_{i:S_i = \infty} \left[e^{\beta k_i} w_{k,\eta}(T_i, S_i) \left(\sum_{j \in R_i} e^{\beta k_j} w_{k,\eta}(T_i, S_i) \right)^{-1} \right]^{\delta_i}. \qquad (9.10)$$

Estimators of β and η can be obtained by solving

$$\frac{\partial \log L(\gamma)}{\partial \gamma} = 0,$$

where $\gamma = (\beta, \eta)$. Under some regularity conditions, these estimators are asymptotically normal with mean vector $\mathbf{0}$ and covariance matrix as given in (9.6). Based on the asymptotic results, statistical inference can be obtained.

If $\log w_{k,\eta}(s)$ is linear in η such as

$$w_{k,\eta}(s) = e^{\eta_{k,0} S + \eta_{k,1} S^2},$$

then model (9.9) is another special case of the proportional hazard model with time-dependent covariates since the switching effect term can be written as

$$w_{k,\eta}(t, S_i) = e^{\eta_{k_i,0} S_i(t) + \eta_{k_i,1} S_i^2(t)}, \qquad (9.11)$$

where

$$S_i(t) = \begin{cases} S_i, & t \geq S_i \\ 0, & t < S_i \end{cases},$$

which can be treated as another time-dependent covariate. That is, model (9.9) is the proportional hazard model with time-dependent covariates $k_i(t)$ and $S_i(t)$, where $S_i(t)$ is additional time-independent covariate. Thus, the parameter vector is given by

$$\gamma = (\beta, \eta_{0,0}, \eta_{0,1}, \eta_{1,0}, \eta_{1,1})$$

and it can be estimated by solving

$$\sum_i \delta_i \left(z_{ii} - \frac{\sum_{j \in R_i} Z_{ij} e^{\gamma' Z_{ij}}}{\sum_{j \in R_i} e^{\gamma' Z_{ij}}} \right) = 0,$$

where

$$Z_{ij} = \left(k_j(T_i), (1-k_j) S_j(T_i), (1-k_j) S_j^2(T_i), k_j S_j(T_i), k_j S_j^2(T_i) \right).$$

The resulting estimator, denoted by $\hat{\gamma}$, is asymptotically normal with mean $\mathbf{0}$ and a covariance matrix that can be estimated by

$$\hat{B}^{-1} \hat{A} \hat{B}^{-1},$$

where

$$\hat{A} = \sum_i \delta_i \left(z_{ii} - \frac{\sum_{j \in R_i} Z_{ij} e^{\hat{\gamma}' Z_{ij}}}{\sum_{j \in R_i} e^{\hat{\gamma}' Z_{ij}}} \right) \left(z_{ii} - \frac{\sum_{j \in R_i} Z_{ij} e^{\hat{\gamma}' Z_{ij}}}{\sum_{j \in R_i} e^{\hat{\gamma}' Z_{ij}}} \right)',$$

and

$$\hat{B} = \sum_i \delta_i \left(\frac{\sum_{j \in R_i} Z_{ij} e^{\hat{\gamma}' Z_{ij}}}{\sum_{j \in R_i} e^{\hat{\gamma}' Z_{ij}}} \right) \left(\frac{\sum_{j \in R_i} Z_{ij} e^{\hat{\gamma}' Z_{ij}}}{\sum_{j \in R_i} e^{\hat{\gamma}' Z_{ij}}} \right)'$$

$$- \sum_i \delta_i \frac{\sum_{j \in R_i} Z_{ij} Z_{ij}' e^{\hat{\gamma}' Z_{ij}}}{\sum_{j \in R_i} e^{\hat{\gamma}' Z_{ij}}}.$$

The above results can be easily extended to the case where there are some other time-independent and/or time-dependent covariates in model (9.9). The latent event times approach described in the previous section coincides with the latent hazard rate model when the survival time distribution is exponential, i.e.,

$$F(t) = 1 - e^{-t/\theta}$$

with an unknown parameter $\theta > 0$. However, for other types of survival time distributions, the two approaches are different. If we apply the latent event times model (9.4) under the semi-parametric approach in which Cox's proportional hazard model is used for data without treatment switch, then the resultant latent hazard model for $\log \lambda_{k_i}(t)/\lambda_0(t)$ depends on t is rather complicated. Statistical inference under such models could be very difficult.

9.2.1 Simulation results

In this section, we studied the finite sample performance of the Cox's proportional hazard model with switching effect through simulation. Consider a clinical trial comparing a test treatment with an active control agent. Suppose 300 patients per treatment group is planned. The survival time was generated according to the exponential distribution with hazard rate 0.0693 for the active control group (mean = 14.43 months) and 0.0462 for the treatment group (mean = 21.65 months). For both treatment groups, the random censoring time was generated according to the uniform distribution over the range of 15–20 months. This results in the censoring percentage of 24.6% for the active control group and 34.6% for the treatment group. On the other hand, the patient treatment switch time was generated according to the exponential distribution with a mean of 7.22 months for the active control group and a mean of 10.82 months for the treatment group. The switching rate is about 67% for both the active control group and the treatment group. This choice of switching rate is within the range of 60–80% practical experience of patients who switch from one treatment to another.

For each combination of parameters (β and $\eta_{k,j}$), 1000 simulation runs were done. The results are summarized in Table 9.1. As it can be seen from Table 9.1, the estimators based on the method of latent hazard rate perform well. The relative bias is within 3% in all cases. The performance of the estimator of β (the treatment effect) is generally better than that of the estimators of η's (switching effects) in terms of both relative bias and the coefficient of variation. We note that the estimated standard deviation has very little bias. Furthermore, the coverage probability of the asymptotic confidence interval is close to the nominal level of 95%.

In the simulation, two other methods were also considered for the purpose of comparison. One method is to estimate β under model (9.7) with $w_{k,\eta}(t; S_i) \equiv 1$, (i.e., ignoring the switching effect), which is clearly biased. The other method is to estimate β under model (9.7) based on data from patients who adhered to their original randomized treatments (i.e., ignoring data from patients who switched). Simulation results indicated

Table 9.1 Simulation Results Based on 1000 Simulation Runs

Parameter	Proposed Method					Other*	Other†
	β	$\eta_{0,0}$	$\eta_{0,1}$	$\eta_{1,0}$	$\eta_{1,1}$	β	β
True value	−0.406	0.100	0.009	0.080	0.010	−0.406	−0.406
Mean of estimates	−0.396	0.098	0.009	0.082	0.010	−0.393	0.033
SD of estimates	0.128	0.052	0.004	0.049	0.004	0.147	0.094
Mean of estimated SD	0.129	0.053	0.004	0.049	0.004	0.148	0.093
Coverage probability	0.951	0.951	0.949	0.952	0.956	0.951	0.003

*The method that ignores data from patients who switched.
†The method that ignores switching effect, i.e., uses model with $w_{k_i,\eta}(t; S_i) \equiv 1$.

that this method has little bias in estimating β. However, the estimator from this method has larger standard deviation (less efficiency). The efficiency gain in using data from patients who switched is about 15% under the switching rate of 67%. This gain is not as large as what is hoped for, because of the fact that the proposed method estimates four additional parameters $\eta_{k,j}$. However, a 15% gain in efficiency in terms of standard deviation amounts to approximately a 32% of reduction in sample size. For example, suppose that a sample size 100 is required in the case of no switching. If the switching rate is 67% and we ignore data from patients who switched, then we need a sample size of approximately 300 in order to retain the efficiency. On the other hand, with the same switching rate and the proposed method, the sample size required to retain the same efficiency is 228.

9.3 Mixed Exponential Model

As indicated earlier, treatment switch is a common and flexible medical practice in cancer trials due to ethical considerations. Treatment switch is in fact a response-adaptive switch. Due to the treatment switch, however, the treatment effect can only be partially observed, and the effects of different treatments are difficult to separate from each other. In this case, the commonly used exponential models with a single parameter may not be appropriate. Alternatively, a mixed exponential model (MEM) with multiple parameters is more flexible and hence suitable for a wide range of applications (see, e.g., Mendenhal and Hader, 1985; Susarda and Pathala, 1965; Johnson et al., 1994).

In clinical trials, the target patient population often consists of two or more subgroups based on heterogeneous baseline characteristics (e.g., the patients could be a mixture of the second-line and the third-line oncology patients). The median survival time of the third-line patients is usually shorter than that of the second-line patients. If the survival times of the two subgroup populations are modeled by exponential distributions with hazard rates λ_1 and λ_2, respectively, then the survival distribution of the total population in the trial is a mixed exponential distribution with a probability density function of

$$P_1 \lambda_1 e^{-\lambda_1 t} + P_2 \lambda_2 e^{-\lambda_2 t} (t > 0),$$

where t is the survival time and P_1 and P_2 (fixed or random) are the proportions of the two sub-populations. Following the similar idea of Mendenhal and Hader (1958), the maximum likelihood estimates of the parameters λ_i and P_i can be obtained. In clinical trials, a patient's treatment is switched in the middle of the study often because there is a biomarker, such as disease progression, indicating the failure of the initial treatment regimen. If the test drug is more effective than the control, then the majority of patients in the control group will switch to the test drug. In this case, the response or survival difference between the two treatment groups will be dramatically reduced in comparison to the case without treatment switching. Moreover, if the test drug is much more effective in treating a patient after disease progression than before disease progression, it could lead to an erroneous conclusion that the test drug is inferior to the control without considering the switching effect, but in fact it is not. This biomarker-based treatment switch is obviously not a random switch but a response-adaptive treatment switch. In what follows, we will focus on the application of mixed exponential model to a clinical trial with biomarker response-adaptive treatment switching (Chang, 2005).

9.3.1 Biomarker-based survival model

In cancer trials, there are often some signs/symptoms (or more generally biomarkers) that indicate the state of the disease and the ineffectiveness or failure of a treatment. A cancer patient often experiences several episodes of progressed diseases before death. Therefore, it is natural to construct a survival model based on the disease mechanism. In what follows, we consider a mixed exponential model, which is derived from the more general mixed Gamma model. Let τ_i be the time from the $(i-1)^{th}$ disease progression to the ith disease progression, where $i = 1,..,n$. τ_i is assumed to be mutually independent with probability density function of $f_i(\tau_i)$. The survival time t for a subject can be written as follows:

$$t = \sum_{i=1}^{n} \tau_i. \tag{9.13}$$

Note that the nth disease progression is death. The following lemma regarding the distribution of linear combination of two random variables is useful.

Lemma Given $x \sim f_x(x)$ and $y \sim f_y(y)$. Define $z = ax + by$. Then, the probability density function of z is given by

$$f_z(z) = \frac{1}{a} \int_{-\infty}^{\infty} f\left(\frac{z-by}{a}, y\right) dy \tag{9.14}$$

Proof.

$$F_z(z) = P(Z \leq z) = \iint_{ax+by \leq z} f(x,y) dx dy = \int_{-\infty}^{\infty} \int_{-\infty}^{\frac{z-by}{a}} f(x,y) dx dy \tag{9.15}$$

Take the derivative with respect to z and exchange the order of the two limit processes, (9.14) is immediately obtained. □

Corollary When x and y are independent, then

$$f_z(z) = \frac{1}{a}\int_{-\infty}^{\infty} f_X\left(\frac{z-by}{a}\right) f_Y(y) dy. \qquad (9.16)$$

Theorem If n independent random variables τ_i, $i = 1, \ldots, n$ are exponentially distributed with parameter λ_i, i.e.,

$$\tau_i \sim f_i(\tau_i) = \lambda_i e^{-\lambda_i \tau_i}, \quad (\tau_i \geq 0),$$

then the probability density function of random variable $t = \sum_{i=1}^{n} \tau_i$ is given by

$$f(t;n) = \sum_{i=1}^{n} \frac{\lambda_i e^{-\lambda_i t}}{\prod_{\substack{k=1 \\ k \neq i}}^{n}\left(1 - \frac{\lambda_i}{\lambda_k}\right)}, \quad t > 0, \qquad (9.17)$$

where $\lambda_i \neq \lambda_k$ if $k \neq i$ for $i, k \in m_0 \leq n$ and m_i is the number of replicates for λ_i with the same value.

Proof. By mathematical induction, when $n = 2$, Lamma (9.14) gives ($\lambda_i \neq \lambda_k$ if $i \neq k$)

$$f(t;2) = \lambda_1 \lambda_2 \int_0^t \exp(-\lambda_1 t - (\lambda_2 - \lambda_1)\tau_2) d\tau_2 = \frac{\lambda_1 e^{-\lambda_1 t}}{1 - \frac{\lambda_1}{\lambda_2}} + \frac{\lambda_2 e^{-\lambda_2 t}}{1 - \frac{\lambda_2}{\lambda_1}}.$$

Therefore, (9.17) is proved for $n = 2$.

Now assume (9.17) holds for any $n \geq 2$, and it will be proven that (9.17) also holds for $n+1$. From (9.17) and corollary (9.16), we have

$$f(t;n+1) = \int_0^t f(t - \tau_{n+1}; n) f_{n+1}(\tau_{n+1}) d\tau_{n+1}$$

$$= \int_0^t \sum_{i=1}^{n} \frac{\lambda_i e^{-\lambda_i(t-\tau_{n-1})}}{\prod_{\substack{k=1 \\ k \neq i}}^{n}\left(1 - \frac{\lambda_i}{\lambda_k}\right)} \lambda_{n+1} e^{-\lambda_{n+1}\tau_{n+1}} d\tau_{n+1}$$

$$= \sum_{i=1}^{n} \frac{1}{\prod_{\substack{k=1 \\ k \neq i}}^{n}\left(1 - \frac{\lambda_i}{\lambda_k}\right)} \left[\frac{\lambda_i e^{-\lambda_i t}}{1 - \frac{\lambda_i}{\lambda_{n+1}}} + \frac{\lambda_{n+1} e^{-\lambda_{n+1} t}}{1 - \frac{\lambda_{n+1}}{\lambda_i}}\right]$$

$$= \sum_{i=1}^{n+1} \frac{\lambda_i e^{-\lambda_i t}}{\prod_{\substack{k=1 \\ k \neq i}}^{n+1}\left(1 - \frac{\lambda_i}{\lambda_k}\right)}.$$

This completes the proof. □

For the exponential distribution $f_i(\tau_i) = \lambda_i e^{-\lambda_i \tau}$, by the above theorem, the probability density function of t, which is a mixed Gamma distribution, is given by

$$f(t;n) = \left\{ \sum_{i=1}^{n} w_i \lambda_i e^{-\lambda_i t}, t > 0; \lambda_i \neq \lambda_k \quad \text{if } k \neq i, \right. \tag{9.18}$$

where $\lambda_i \neq \lambda_k$ if $k \neq i$ for $i, k \leq m_0 \leq n$, m_i is the number of replicates for λ_i with the same value, and

$$\prod_{\substack{k=1 \\ k \neq i}}^{1} \left(1 - \frac{\lambda_i}{\lambda_k}\right) = 1.$$

For disease progression, it is usually true that $\lambda_i > \lambda_k$ for $i > k$. Note that $f(t;n)$ does not depend on the order of λ_i in the sequence, and

$$f(t;n)_{\lambda_n \to +\infty} = f(t;n-1).$$

The survival function $S(t)$ can be easily obtained from (9.18) by integration and the survival function is given by

$$S(t;n) = \sum_{i=1}^{n} w_i e^{-\lambda_i t}; \quad t > 0, \quad n \geq 1, \tag{9.19}$$

where the weight is given by

$$w_i = \left[\prod_{k=1, k \neq i}^{n} \left(1 - \frac{\lambda_i}{\lambda_k}\right) \right]^{-1}. \tag{9.20}$$

The mean survival time and its variance are given by

$$\mu = \sum_{i=1}^{n} \frac{w_i}{\lambda_i} \quad \text{and} \quad \sigma^2 = \sum_{i=1}^{n} \frac{w_i}{\lambda_i^2}, \tag{9.21}$$

respectively. When $n = 1$, $w_1 = 1$, (9.19) reduces to the exponential distribution. It can be shown that the weights have the properties of $\sum_{i=1}^{n} w_i = 1$ and $\sum_{i=1}^{n} w_i \lambda_i = 0$.

9.3.2 Effect of patient enrollment rate

In this section, we will examine the effect of the accrual duration on the survival distribution. Let N be the number of patients enrolled and let $(0, t_0)$ be the patient enrollment period defined as the time elapsed from the first patient enrolled to the last patient enrolled. Also, let t denote the time elapsed from the beginning of the trial. Denote $f_d(t)$ and $f_e(\tau_e)$, where $\tau_e \in [0, T_0]$, the probability density function of failure (death) and the patient enrollment rate, respectively. The failure function (or the probability of death before time t) can be expressed as

$$F(t) = \int_0^t f_d(\tau) d\tau = \int_0^t \int_0^{\min(\tau, t_0)} f(\tau - \tau_e) f_e(\tau_e) d\tau_e d\tau. \quad (9.22)$$

For a uniform enrollment rate,

$$f_e(\tau_e) = \begin{cases} \frac{N}{t_0}, & \tau_e \in [0, t_0] \\ 0, & \text{otherwise} \end{cases}$$

and probability density function (9.18), (9.22) becomes

$$F(t) = \int_0^t \int_0^{\min(\tau, t_0)} \sum_{i=1}^n w_i \frac{\lambda_i e^{-\lambda_i(\tau - \tau_e)}}{t_0} d\tau_e d\tau.$$

After the integration, we have

$$F(t) = \begin{cases} \frac{1}{t_0} \{ t + \sum_{i=1}^n \frac{w_i}{\lambda_i} \left[e^{-\lambda_i t} - 1 \right] \}, & t \le t_0 \\ \frac{1}{t_0} \{ t_0 + \sum_{i=1}^n \frac{w_i}{\lambda_i} \left[e^{-\lambda_i t} - e^{-\lambda_i(t-t_0)} \right] \}, & t > t_0 \end{cases}. \quad (9.23)$$

Differentiating it with respect to t, it can be obtained that

$$f(t) = \begin{cases} \frac{1}{t_0} \left(1 - \sum_{i=1}^n w_i e^{-\lambda_i t} \right), & t \le t_0 \\ \frac{1}{t_0} \sum_{i=1}^n w_i \left[e^{-\lambda_i(t-t_0)} - e^{-\lambda_i t} \right], & t > t_0 \end{cases}. \quad (9.24)$$

The survival function is then given by

$$S(t) = 1 - F(t), \quad (9.25)$$

and the number of deaths among N patients can be written as

$$D(t) = NF(t). \quad (9.26)$$

Note that (9.23) is useful for sample size calculation with a non-parametric method. For $n = 1$, (9.26) reduces to the number of deaths with the exponential survival distribution, i.e.,

$$D = \begin{cases} R(t - \frac{1}{\lambda} e^{-\lambda t}), & t \le t_0 \\ R \left[t_0 - \frac{1}{\lambda}(e^{\lambda t_0} - 1) e^{-\lambda t} \right], & t > t_0 \end{cases},$$

where the uniform enrollment rate $R = \frac{N}{t_0}$.

Parameter estimate

It is convenient to use the paired variable $(\hat{t}_j, \delta_j)$ defined as $(\hat{t}_j, 1)$ for a failure time $\hat{t}_j$ and $(\hat{t}_j, 0)$ for a censored time $\hat{t}_j$. The likelihood then can be expressed as

$$L = \prod_{j=1}^N \left[f(\hat{t}_j) \right]^{\delta_j} \left[S(\hat{t}_j) \right]^{1-\delta_j}, \quad (9.27)$$

where the probability density function $f(t)$ and survival function $S(t)$ are given by (9.18) and (9.19), respectively, for instantaneous enrollment, but (9.24) and (9.25) otherwise. Note that for an individual whose survival time is censored at $\hat{t}_j$, the contribution to the likelihood is given by the probability of surviving beyond that point in time, i.e., $S(\hat{t}_j)$. To reduce the number of parameters in the model, we can assume that the hazard rates take the form of a geometric sequence, i.e., $\lambda_i = a\lambda_{i-1}$ or $\lambda_i = a^i \lambda_0$; $i = 1, 2, \ldots, n$. This leads to a two-parameter model regardless of n, the number of progressions. The maximum likelihood estimates of λ and a can be easily obtained through numerical iterations.

Example 9.1 To illustrate the mixed exponential model for obtaining the maximum likelihood estimates with two parameters of λ_1 and λ_2, independent x_{1j} and x_{2j}, $j = 1, \ldots, N$ from two exponential distributions with λ_1 and λ_2, respectively were generated. Let $\tau_j = x_{1j} + x_{2j}$. Then τ_j has a mixed exponential distribution with parameters λ_1 and λ_2. Let $\hat{t}_j = \min(\tau_j, T_s)$, where T_s is the duration of the study. Now, we have the paired variables $(\hat{t}_j, \delta_j)$, $j = 1, \ldots, N$, which were used to obtain the maximum likelihood estimators $\hat{\lambda}_1$ and $\hat{\lambda}_2$. Using (9.21) and the invariance principle of maximum likelihood estimators, the maximum likelihood estimate of mean survival time, $\hat{\mu}$, can be obtained as

$$\hat{\mu} = \sum_{j=1}^{2} \frac{\hat{w}_j}{\hat{\lambda}_j} = \frac{1}{\hat{\lambda}_1} + \frac{1}{\hat{\lambda}_2}. \qquad (9.28)$$

For each of the three scenarios (i.e., $\lambda_1 = 1, \lambda_2 = 1.5$; $\lambda_1 = 1, \lambda_2 = 2$; $\lambda_1 = 1, \lambda_2 = 5$), 5000 simulation runs were done. The results of the means and coefficients of variation of the estimated parameters are summarized in Table 9.2. As it can be seen from Table 9.2, the mixed exponential model performs well, which gives an excellent estimate of mean survival time for all three cases with virtually no bias and a less than 10% coefficient of variation. The maximum likelihood estimate of λ_1 is reasonably good with a bias less than 6%. However, there are about 5% to 15% over-estimates for λ_2 with large coefficients of variation ranging from 30% to 40%. The bias increases as the percent of the censored observations increases. Thus, it is suggested that the maximum likelihood estimate of mean survival time rather than the maximum likelihood estimate of the hazard rate be used to assess the effect of a test treatment.

Table 9.2 Simulation Results with Mixed Exponential Model

	λ_1	λ_2	μ	λ_1	λ_2	μ	λ_1	λ_2	μ
True	1.00	1.50	1.67	1.00	2.00	1.50	1.00	5.00	1.20
Mean*	1.00	1.70	1.67	1.06	2.14	1.51	1.06	5.28	1.20
CV*	0.18	0.30	0.08	0.20	0.37	0.08	0.18	0.44	0.09
PDs (%)		93			96			96	
Censors (%)		12			8			5	

Note: Study duration $T = 3.2$ with quick enrollment. Number of subjects $N = 100$.
*Mean and coefficient of variation of the estimates from 5000 runs for each scenario

9.3.3 Hypothesis test and power analysis

In a two-arm clinical trial comparing treatment difference in survival, the hypotheses can be written as

$$H_0 : \mu_1 \geq \mu_2 \tag{9.29}$$

$$H_a : \mu_1 < \mu_2.$$

Note that hazard rates for the two treatment groups may change over time. In practice, the proportional hazard rates do not generally hold for a mixed exponential model. In what follows, we will introduce two different approaches for hypotheses testing: nonparametric and simulation methods.

Nonparametric method

In most clinical trials, there are some censored observations. In this case, the parametric method is no longer valid. Alternatively, nonparametric methods such as the logrank test (Marubini and Valsecchi, 1995) are useful. Note that procedure for sample size calculation using the logrank test under the assumption of an exponential distribution is available in the literature (see, e.g., Marubini and Valsecchi, 1995; Chang and Chow, 2005). In what follows, we will derive a formula for sample size calculation under the mixed exponential distribution based on logrank statistic. The total number of deaths required for a one-sided logrank test for the treatment difference between two equal-sized independent groups is given by

$$D = \left[z_{1-\alpha} + 2z_{1-\beta} \frac{\sqrt{\theta}}{1+\theta} \right]^2 \left(\frac{1+\theta}{1-\theta} \right)^2, \tag{9.30}$$

where the hazard ratio is

$$\theta = \frac{\ln F_1(T_s)}{\ln F_2(T_s)}, \qquad (9.31)$$

T_s is trial duration, and $F_k(T_s)$ is the proportion of patients with the event in the kth group. The relationship between $F_k(T_s)$ and t_0 and T_s and hazard rates is given by (9.23). From (9.23) and (9.26), the total number patients required for the case where the enrollment is uniformly distributed can be obtained as follows:

$$N = \frac{\left[z_{1-\alpha} + 2z_{1-\beta}\frac{\sqrt{\theta}}{1+\theta}\right]^2 \left(\frac{1+\theta}{1-\theta}\right)^2}{F_1 + F_2}, \qquad (9.32)$$

where t_0 is the duration of enrollment.

Example 9.2 Assume a uniform enrollment with a duration of $t_0 = 10$ months and trial duration $T_s = 14$ months. At the end of the study, the proportions of failures are $F_1 = 0.8$ and $F_2 = 0.75$ for the control (group 1) and the active drug (group 2), respectively. Choose a power of 90% and one-sided $\alpha = 0.025$. The hazard ratio is calculated using (9.31) as $\theta = 1.29$. From (9.32), the total number of patients required is $N = 714$. If hazard rates are given instead of the proportions of failures, we may use (9.23) to calculate the proportion of failures first.

Simulation method

The computer simulation is a very useful tool, which can be directly applied to almost all hypotheses testing problems and power analysis for sample size calculations. It can be used with or without censoring. It can also be easily applied to a trial with treatment switching. The following is the simulation algorithm:

Step 1: Generate simulation data under H_0

Generate x_i and y_i independently from a mixed exponential distribution with parameters λ_{11} and λ_{12}, the hazard rates under the null hypothesis H_o, using the method as described in the previous section.

Step 2: Find the distribution of test statistic T under H_0

For each set of data, calculate the test statistic T as defined (e.g., the maximum likelihood estimate of mean difference). By repeating step 1 M times, M values of the test statistic T, and its distribution can be obtained. The precision of the distribution will increase as the number of replications, M, increases.

Step 3: Calculate p-value

Sort the Ts obtained from step 2, and calculate the test statistic $\hat{T}$ based on the observed value from the trial. The p-value is the proportion of the simulated Ts whose values are larger (less) than $\hat{T}$.

Step 4: Calculate test statistic under H_a

For the power calculation, data under H_a must be generated (i.e., generate x_i ($i = 1, \ldots, N$) from a mixed exponential distribution with parameters λ_{11} and λ_{12}, and y_i ($i = 1, \ldots, N$) from another mixed exponential distribution with parameters λ_{21} and λ_{22}, as described in section 4). Calculate the test statistic as in step 2.

Step 5: Calculate the power of test

Repeat step 4 M times to form the distribution of the test statistic under H_a. The power of the test with N subjects per group is the proportion of the simulated test statistic T with its value exceeding the critical value T_c.

Note that steps 4 and 5 are for power analysis for sample size calculations. For hypotheses testing, only the distribution of the test statistic under H_0 is required. However, for power and sample size calculation, distributions under both H_0 and H_a are required. This simulation approach is useful in dealing with adaptive treatment switching.

9.3.4 Application to trials with treatment switch

As indicated earlier, it is not uncommon to switch a treatment when there is evidence of lack of efficacy or disease progression. Due to the natural course of the disease, most patients will have disease progression during the trial. When this happens, the clinician often gives an alternative treatment. Patients who were initially treated with the standard therapy are often switched to the test drug, but patients who were initially treated with the test drug are not necessarily switched to the standard therapy; rather, they could be switched to a different drug that has a similar effect as the control.

For a typical patient in the Kth group who experiences disease progression and dies, the time to disease progression is assumed to be an exponential distribution with a hazard rate of λ_{k1}, and the time from the progression to death is another exponential distribution with a hazard rate of λ_{k2}. Due to treatment switching, a patient in treatment 1 will have a hazard rate of $\lambda_{12}^* = \lambda_{22}$ after switching to treatment 2, and a patient in treatment 2 will have a hazard rate of $\lambda^*_{22} = \lambda_{12}$ after switching to treatment 1. Further, assume all patients eventually have progressive disease and will switch treatment if the trial lasts long enough. Under these conditions, the probability density function and survival function for the kth group are given by

$$f^*_k = w^*_{k1}\lambda_{k1}e^{-\lambda_{k1}t} + w^*_{k2}\lambda^*_{k2}e^{-\lambda^*_{k2}t} \tag{9.33}$$

and

$$S^*_k = w^*_{k1}e^{-\lambda_{k1}t} + w^*_{k2}e^{-\lambda_{k2}t}, \tag{9.34}$$

respectively, where

$$w^*_{k1} = \left[1 - \frac{\lambda_{k1}}{\lambda^*_{k2}}\right]^{-1},$$

and

$$w^*_{k2} = \left[1 - \frac{\lambda^*_{k2}}{\lambda_{k1}}\right]^{-1}.$$

The likelihood for kth group is similar to (9.27), i.e.,

$$L^*_k = \prod_{j=1}^{N} \left[f^*_k(\hat{t}_j)\right]^{\delta_j} \left[S^*_k(\hat{t}_j)\right]^{1-\delta_j}. \tag{9.35}$$

The likelihood for the two groups combined is given by

$$L^* = L^*_1 L^*_2.$$

Under the assumption that all patients will eventually switch treatment, maximizing L^* is equivalent to maximizing both L^*_1 and L^*_2. After obtaining the maximum likelihood estimates of $\hat{\lambda}_{11}$, $\hat{\lambda}_{22}$, $\hat{\lambda}_{21}$, and $\hat{\lambda}_{12}$ using (9.35), one can calculate the mean survival times $\hat{\mu}_1$ and $\hat{\mu}_2$ for the two groups using

$$\hat{\mu}_k = \left(\frac{1}{\hat{\lambda}_{k1}} + \frac{1}{\hat{\lambda}_{k2}}\right). \tag{9.36}$$

$\hat{\mu}_k$ is called the estimator of latent survival time μ_k. The latent survival time can be interpreted as (i) the survival time that would have been observed if the patient had not switched the treatment, or (ii) overall survival benefit of the drug in treating patients with different baseline severities (e.g., 2nd-line and 3rd-line oncology patients). In the first interpretation, it is assumed that the drug has that magnitude of re-treatment effect, which implies that the investigator should not switch treatment at all. The second interpretation is appropriate regardless of the re-treatment effect of the drug. For the hypotheses testing

$$H_o : \mu_1 \geq \mu_2 \text{ versus } H_a : \mu_1 < \mu_2,$$

the test statistic is defined as

$$T = \hat{\mu}_2 - \hat{\mu}_1.$$

Example 9.3 Suppose that a clinical trial comparing two parallel treatment groups was conducted to demonstrate that the test drug (group 2) is better than the control (group 1) in survival. The study duration was 3.2 years and the enrollment was quick (i.e., $t_0 = 0$). The trial protocol allowed the investigator to switch a patient's treatment if his/her disease progression was observed. Suppose that $\lambda_{11} = 1$, $\lambda_{12} = 5$, $\lambda_{21} = 0.7$, and $\lambda_{22} = 1.5$. The latent mean survival times for the two groups calculated using (9.21) are $\mu_1 = 1.2$ and $\mu_2 = 2.095$ for the control and test groups, respectively. The latent survival times indicate that the test drug is better than the control in survival. However, if the treatment switch is not taken into account, the mean survival will be calculated as follows:

$$\mu_1 = \frac{1}{\lambda_{11}} + \frac{1}{\lambda_{22}} = 1.667$$

and

$$\mu_2 = \frac{1}{\lambda_{21}} + \frac{1}{\lambda_{12}} = 1.629,$$

which could lead to a wrong conclusion that the control is better than the test drug. Therefore, it is critical to consider the switching effect in the statistical analysis.

Note that the nonparametric method may not be appropriate for trials with treatment switching. In this case, it is suggested that the method of computer simulation be used. Table 9.3 presents results of computer simulation. The results indicate that under H_0, the critical point T_c for rejecting the null hypothesis is 0.443 for the test statistic (the observed mean survival difference). Using $T_c = 0.443$ to run the simulation under H_a with $N = 250$ patients per group shows that the trial has 86% power for detecting the difference. The distributions of the test statistic under H_0 and H_a are plotted in Figure 9.1. Under H_a, there is about a 3% overestimate of μ_1 and a 3% under-estimate of μ_2. There is about a 13% under-estimate in mean difference $\mu_2 - \mu_1$ with a standard deviation of 0.34. The expected standard deviation for mean survival difference

$$\sigma = \sqrt{\sigma_1^2 + \sigma_2^2} = 1.88,$$

where σ_1^2 and σ_2^2 are calculated from (9.21). We can see that the method of computer simulation improves the precision at the cost of accuracy.

Remarks For patients who are never switched regardless of treatment failure or other reasons, the probability density function and survival

Table 9.3 Simulation Results with Treatment Switching

	Under H_0 Condition						
	λ_{11}	λ_{12}	μ_1	λ_{21}	λ_{22}	μ_2	$\mu_2-\mu_1$
True	1	5	1.2	1	5	1.2	0.00
Mean*	1.03	5.17	1.20	1.02	5.13	1.20	0.004
SD*	0.11	1.63	.12	0.11	1.60	.12	0.22
PDs (%)	96			96			
Censors (%)	5			5			
	Under H_a Condition						
	λ_{11}	λ_{12}	μ_1	λ_{21}	λ_{22}	μ_2	$\mu_2-\mu_1$
True	1	5	1.2	0.7	1.5	2.10	0.90
Mean*	1.00	5.25	1.24	0.71	1.64	2.06	0.82
SD*	0.14	1.81	0.17	0.07	0.42	0.20	0.34
PDs (%)	96			89			
Censors (%)	11			12			

*Mean and standard deviation of the estimates (5000 runs).

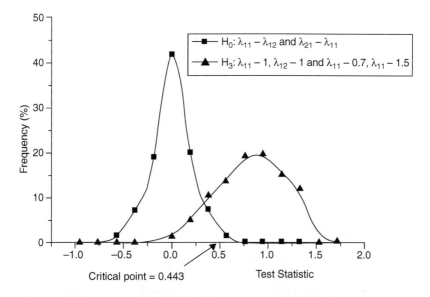

Figure 9.1 Distribution of test statistic with $n = 250$ (5000 runs).

function are given by (9.18) and (9.19), respectively. Denote P_s the proportion of patients who are willing to switch. Then, the distribution of survival time for a typical patient in the trial is given by

$$\tilde{f}_k(t) = P_s f_k^* + (1 - P_s) f_k,$$

which is the unconditional distribution. For patients who already switched and for patients who did not switch at a certain time, the conditional distributions will be different. This case will not be studied here. It is assumed that re-treatment of a patient with the same drug after disease progression is not an option, and all patients will eventually develop progressed disease and switch their treatments at the time of disease progression if the trial lasts long enough. In the simulation, the sample size N has been adjusted several times in order to meet the power requirement. Note that every time N changes, the critical point also changes due to the nature of the test statistic.

9.4 Concluding Remarks

Branson and Whitehead's method considered the use of latent event times to model a patient's observed survival time after switching and the survival time that would have been observed if this patient had not switched treatment. Their model does not take into account the fact that a treatment switch is often based on the observed effect of the current treatment. For example, the survival time of a patient who switches from the active control to the test treatment might be longer than his survival time if he had adhered to the original treatment. Therefore, Branson and Whitehead's model is a model for random treatment switching with a constant latent hazard rate over time. In fact, even in the case of random switching, the hazard rate increases after the switch, and the later the switch occurs, the bigger the hazard rate after the switch. Shao, Chang, and Chow's method considered a generalized time-dependent Cox's proportional hazard model and provided maximum likelihood estimates (MLE) of the parameters. However, the method for hypothesis testing was not provided.

On the other hand, the biomarker-based mixed exponential model provides a great flexibility for modeling. The maximum likelihood estimate does not require the collection of biomarker data in the trial. Instead, the time to biomarker response can be estimated using one of the hazard rates in the mixed exponential model. One can use the data to improve the maximum likelihood estimates of the parameters if the biomarker response data are available.

CHAPTER 10

Bayesian Approach

As pointed out by Woodcock (2005), Bayesian approaches to clinical trials are of great interest in the medical product development community because they offer a way to gain valid information in a manner that is potentially more parsimonious of time, resources, and investigational subjects than our current methods. The need to streamline the product development process without sacrificing important information has become increasingly apparent. Temple (2005) also indicated that the FDA's reviewers have already used some of the thinking processes that involve Bayesian approaches, although the Bayesian approaches are not implemented. In Bayesian paradigm, initial beliefs concerning a parameter of interest (discrete or continuous) are expressed by a prior distribution. Evidence from further data is then modeled by a likelihood function for the parameter. The normalized product of the prior and the likelihood forms so-called posterior distribution. Based on the posterior distribution, conclusions regarding the parameter of interest can then be drawn. The possible use of Bayesian methods in clinical trials has been studied extensively in the literature in recent years. See, for example, Brophy and Joseph (1995), Lilford and Braunholtz (1996), Berry and Stangl (1996), Gelman, Carlin, and Rubin (2003), Spiegelhalter, Abrams, and Myles (2004), Goodman (1999, 2005), Louis (2005), and Berry (2005).

Bayesian approaches for dose-escalation trials have been discussed in Chapter 4. In this chapter, our focus will be placed on the use of different utilities of Bayesian approaches in clinical trials. In the next section, some basic concepts of Bayesian approach such as Bayes rule and Bayesian power are given. Section 10.2 discusses the determination of prior distribution. In Section 10.3, Bayesian approaches to multiple-stage design for a single-arm trial are discussed. Section 10.4 introduces the use of Bayesian optimal adaptive designs in clinical trials. Some concluding remarks are given in the last section of this chapter.

10.1 Basic Concepts of Bayesian Approach

In this section, basic concepts of a Bayesian approach such as Bayes rule and Bayesian power are briefly described.

10.1.1 Bayes rule

Let θ be the parameter of interest. Denote the prior distribution of θ as $\pi(\theta)$. Also let $f(x|\theta)$ be the sampling distribution of X given θ. Basically, a Bayesian approach involves the following four elements:

- The joint distribution of (θ, X), which is given by

$$\varphi(\theta, x) = f(x|\theta)\pi(\theta); \qquad (10.1)$$

- The marginal distribution of X, which can be obtained as

$$m(x) = \int \varphi(\theta, x)\, d\theta = \int f(x|\theta)\pi(\theta)\, d\theta; \qquad (10.2)$$

- The posterior distribution of θ, which can be obtained by Bayes' formula

$$\pi(\theta|x) = \frac{f(x|\theta)\pi(\theta)}{m(x)}; \qquad (10.3)$$

- The predictive probability distribution, which is given by

$$P(y|x) = \int P(x|y, \theta)\pi(\theta|x)\, d\theta. \qquad (10.4)$$

To illustrate the use of a Bayesian approach, the following examples are useful. We first consider the case where the study endpoint is discrete.

Example 10.1 Assume that x follows a binomial distribution with the probability of success p, i.e., $X \sim B(n, p)$. Also, assume that the parameter of interest p follows a beta distribution with parameters α and β, i.e., $p \sim Beta(\alpha, \beta)$. Thus, the prior distribution is given by

$$\pi(p) = \frac{1}{B(\alpha, \beta)} p^{\alpha-1}(1-p)^{\beta-1}, \quad 0 \le p \le 1, \qquad (10.5)$$

where

$$B(\alpha, \beta) = \frac{\Gamma(\alpha)\Gamma(\beta)}{\Gamma(\alpha+\beta)}.$$

Furthermore, the sampling distribution of X given p is given by

$$f(x|p) = \binom{n}{x} p^x (1-p)^{n-x}, \quad x = 0, 1, \ldots, n. \qquad (10.6)$$

BAYESIAN APPROACH

Thus, the joint distribution of (p, X) is given by

$$\varphi(p, x) = \frac{\binom{n}{x}}{B(\alpha, \beta)} p^{\alpha+x-1} (1-p)^{n-x\beta-1}. \tag{10.7}$$

and the marginal distribution of X is given by

$$m(x) = \frac{\binom{n}{x}}{B(\alpha, \beta)} B(\alpha + x, n - x + \beta). \tag{10.8}$$

As a result, the posterior distribution of p given X can be obtained as

$$\pi(p|x) = \frac{p^{\alpha+x-1}(1-p)^{n-x\beta-1}}{B(\alpha+x, \beta+n-x)} = Beta(\alpha+x, \beta+n-x). \tag{10.9}$$

For another example, consider the case where the study endpoint is a continuous variable.

Example 10.2 Assume that x follows a normal distribution with mean θ and variance σ^2/n, i.e., $X \sim N(\theta, \sigma^2/n)$. Also, assume that the parameter of interest θ follows a normal distribution with mean μ and variance σ^2/n_0, i.e., $\theta \sim N(\mu, \sigma^2/n_0)$. Thus, we have

$$\pi(\theta|X) \propto f(X|\theta)\pi(\theta).$$

As a result, the posterior distribution of θ given X can be obtained as

$$\pi(\theta|X) = Ce^{-\frac{(X-\theta)^2 n}{2\sigma^2}} e^{-\frac{(\theta-\mu)^2 n_0}{2\sigma^2}}, \tag{10.10}$$

where C is a constant with θ. It can be verified that (10.10) is a normal distribution with mean $\theta \frac{n_0\mu + nx}{n_0+n}$ and variance $\frac{\sigma^2}{n_0+n}$, i.e.,

$$\theta|X \sim N\left(\theta\frac{n_0\mu + nX}{n_0+n}, \frac{\sigma^2}{n_0+n}\right).$$

Now, based on (10.10), we can make predictions concerning future values of x by taking into account for the uncertainty about its mean θ. For this purpose, we rewrite $X = (X - \theta) + \theta$ so that X is the sum of two independent quantities, i.e., $(X - \theta) \sim N(0, \sigma^2/n)$ and $\theta \sim N(\mu, \sigma^2/n_0)$. As a result, the predictive probability distribution can be obtained as (see, e.g., Spiegelhalter, Abrams, and Rubin, 2004)

$$X \sim N\left(\mu, \sigma^2\left(\frac{1}{n} + \frac{1}{n_0}\right)\right). \tag{10.11}$$

Note that if we observe the first n_1 observations (i.e., the mean of the first n_1 observations, x_{n_1} is known), then the predictive probability distribution is given by

$$X|x_{n_1} \sim N\left(\frac{n_0\mu + n_1 x_{n_1}}{n_0 + n_1}, \sigma^2\left(\frac{1}{n_0+n_1} + \frac{1}{n}\right)\right). \quad (10.12)$$

The above basic Bayesian concepts can be easily applied to some classical designs in clinical trials. However, it may affect the power and consequently sample size calculation. For illustration purposes, we consider the following example.

Example 10.3 Consider a two-arm parallel-group design comparing a test treatment and a standard therapy or an active control agent. Under the two-arm trial, it can be verified that the power is a function of effect size of ε (see, e.g., Chow, Shao, and Wang, 2003). That is,

$$\text{power}(\varepsilon) = \Phi_0\left(\frac{\sqrt{n}\varepsilon}{2} - z_{1-\alpha}\right), \quad (10.13)$$

where Φ_0 is cumulative distribution function of the standard normal distribution. Suppose the prior distribution of the uncertainty ε is $\pi(\varepsilon)$. Then the expected power is given by

$$P_{\exp} = \int \Phi_0\left(\frac{\sqrt{n}\varepsilon}{2} - z_{1-\alpha}\right) \pi(\varepsilon) d\varepsilon. \quad (10.14)$$

In practice, a numerical integration is usually employed for evaluation of (10.14). To illustrate the implication of (10.14), we assume a one-sided $\alpha = 0.025$ (i.e., $z_{1-\alpha} = 1.96$) and the following prior for ε

$$\pi(\varepsilon) = \begin{cases} 1/3, & \varepsilon = 0.1, 0.25, 0.4 \\ 0, & \text{otherwise.} \end{cases} \quad (10.15)$$

Conventionally, we use the mean (median) of the effect size $\bar{\varepsilon} = 0.25$ to design the trial and perform sample size calculation assuming that $\bar{\varepsilon} = 0.25$ is the true effect size. For the two-arm balanced design with $\beta = 0.2$ or $power = 80\%$, the classical approach gives the following sample size:

$$n = \frac{4(z_{1-\alpha} + z_{1-\beta})^2}{\varepsilon^2} = \frac{4(1.96 + 0.842)^2}{0.25^2} = 502. \quad (10.16)$$

BAYESIAN APPROACH

On the other hand, the Bayesian approach based on the expected power from (10.14) yields

$$
\begin{aligned}
P_{\exp} &= \frac{1}{3}\left[\Phi_0\left(\frac{0.1\sqrt{n}}{2} - z_{1-\alpha}\right) + \Phi_0\left(\frac{0.25\sqrt{n}}{2} - z_{1-\alpha}\right)\right.\\
&\quad \left.+ \Phi_0\left(\frac{0.4\sqrt{n}}{2} - z_{1-\alpha}\right)\right] (10.1)\\
&= \frac{1}{3}\left[\Phi_0\left(\frac{0.1\sqrt{502}}{2} - 1.96\right) + \Phi_0\left(\frac{0.25\sqrt{502}}{2} - 1.96\right)\right.\\
&\quad \left.+ \Phi_0\left(\frac{0.4\sqrt{502}}{2} - 1.96\right)\right]\\
&= \frac{1}{3}\left[\Phi_0\left(-0.839\,73\right) + \Phi_0\left(0.840\,67\right) + \Phi_0\left(2.\,521\,1\right)\right]\\
&= \frac{1}{3}\left(0.2005 + 0.7997 + 0.9942\right) = 0.664\,8 = 66\%. \quad (10.17)
\end{aligned}
$$

As it can be seen from the above, the expected power is only 66%, which is lower than the desired power of 80%. As a result, in order to reach the same power, the sample size is necessarily increased.

If $\pi(\varepsilon)$ follows a normal distribution as $N(\mu, \sigma^2/n_0)$, then the expected power can be obtained using the predictive distribution by evaluating the chance that the critical event occurs, i.e.,

$$P\left(X > \frac{1}{\sqrt{n}}z_{1-\alpha}\sigma\right).$$

This gives

$$P_{\exp} = \Phi\left(\sqrt{\frac{n_0}{n_0+n}}\left(\frac{\mu\sqrt{n}}{\sigma} - z_{1-\alpha}\right)\right). \quad (10.18)$$

As indicated earlier, the total sample size required for achieving the desired power is a function of the effect size ε, i.e.,

$$n(\varepsilon) = \frac{4(z_{1-\alpha} + z_{1-\beta})^2}{\varepsilon^2}. \quad (10.19)$$

Thus, the expected total sample size can be obtained as

$$n_{\exp} = \int \frac{4(z_{1-\alpha} + z_{1-\beta})^2}{\varepsilon^2} \pi(\varepsilon)\,d\varepsilon. \quad (10.20)$$

For a given flat prior, i.e., $\pi(\varepsilon) \sim \frac{1}{b-a}$, where $a \leq \varepsilon \leq b$, we have

$$n_{\exp} = \int_a^b \frac{4(z_{1-\alpha}+z_{1-\beta})^2}{\varepsilon^2} \frac{1}{b-a} d\varepsilon$$

$$= \frac{4}{ab}(z_{1-\alpha}+z_{1-\beta})^2. \tag{10.21}$$

This gives the following sample size ratio

$$R_n = \frac{n_{\exp}}{n} = \frac{\varepsilon^2}{ab}.$$

As it can be seen from the above, if $\varepsilon = 0.25$, $\alpha = 0.025$, $\beta = 0.8$, $n = 502$, $a = 0.1$, $b = 0.4$ (note that $(a+b)/2 = \varepsilon$), then

$$R_n = \frac{0.25^2}{(0.1)(0.4)} = 1.56.$$

This indicates that the frequentist approach could substantially underestimate the sample size required for achieving the desired power.

10.1.2 Bayesian power

For testing the null hypothesis that $H_0 : \theta \leq 0$ against an alternative hypothesis that $H_a : \theta > 0$, we defined the Bayesian significance as

$$P_B = P(\theta < 0 \mid data) < \alpha_B.$$

Note that the Bayesian significance can be easily found based on the posterior distribution. For the case where the data and the prior both follow a normal distribution, the posterior distribution is given by

$$\pi(\theta|x) = N\left(\frac{n_0 \mu + nx}{n_0 + n}, \frac{\sigma^2}{n_0 + n}\right). \tag{10.22}$$

Thus, Bayesian significance can be calculated if the parameter estimate X satisfies

$$X > \frac{\sqrt{n_0 + n} z_{1-\alpha} \sigma - n_0 \mu}{n}. \tag{10.23}$$

Note that the Bayesian power is then given by

$$P_B(n) = \Phi\left(\frac{\mu\sqrt{n_0+n}\sqrt{n_0}}{\sigma\sqrt{n}} - \sqrt{\frac{n_0}{n}} z_{1-\alpha}\right). \tag{10.24}$$

Example 10.4 For illustration purposes, consider a phase II hypotension study comparing a test treatment with an active control agent. Suppose the primary endpoint is the reduction in systolic blood pressure (SBP). Assume that the estimated treatment effect is normally distributed, i.e.,

$$\theta \sim N\left(\mu, \frac{2\sigma^2}{n_0}\right).$$

The design is targeted to achieve the Bayesian power at $(1-\beta_B)$ at the Bayesian significance level of $\alpha_B = 0.2$. For the sample size, the sample mean difference

$$\hat{\theta} \sim N\left(\theta, \frac{2\sigma^2}{n}\right),$$

where n is the sample size per group. For a large sample size, we can assume that σ is known. In this case, the sample size n is the solution of the following equation:

$$\Phi\left(\frac{\mu\sqrt{n_0} + n\sqrt{n_0}}{\sigma\sqrt{2n}} - \sqrt{\frac{n_0}{n}}z_{1-\alpha_B}\right) = 1 - \beta_B. \qquad (10.25)$$

This leads to

$$\frac{\mu\sqrt{n_0} + n\sqrt{n_0}}{\sqrt{2n}} - \sqrt{\frac{n_0}{n}}z_{1-\alpha_B} = z_{1-\beta_B}. \qquad (10.26)$$

The above can be rewritten as follows:

$$An + B\sqrt{n} + C = 0, \qquad (10.27)$$

where

$$\begin{cases} A = z_{1-\beta_B}^2 - \mu^2 n_0, \\ B = 2z_{1-\beta_B}z_{1-\alpha}\sqrt{2n_0}, \\ C = 2z_{1-\alpha}^2 n_0 - \mu^2 n_0^2. \end{cases} \qquad (10.28)$$

As a result, we can solve (10.27) for n, which is given by

$$n = \left(\frac{-B + \sqrt{B^2 - 4AC}}{2A}\right)^2 \qquad (10.29)$$

10.2 Multiple-Stage Design for Single-Arm Trial

As indicated in Chapter 6, in phase II cancer trials, it is undesirable to stop a study early when the test drug is promising, and it is desirable to terminate the study as early as possible when the test treatment is not effective due to ethical consideration. For this purpose, a multiple-stage design single-arm trial is often employed to determine whether the test treatment is promising for further testing. For a multiple-stage single-arm trial, the classical method and the Bayesian approach are commonly employed. In this section, these two methods are briefly described.

10.2.1 Classical approach for two-stage design

The most commonly used two-stage design in phase II cancer trials is probably Simon's optimal two-stage design (Simon, 1989). The concept of Simon's optimal two-stage design is to permit early stopping when a moderately long sequence of initial failure occurs. Thus, under a two-stage trial design, the hypotheses of interest are given below:

$$H_0 : p \leq p_0 \text{ versus } H_a : p \geq p_1,$$

where p_0 is the undesirable response rate and p_1 is the desirable response rate ($p_1 > p_0$). If the response rate of a test treatment is at the undesirable level, one may reject it as an ineffective treatment with a high probability, and if its response rate is at the desirable level, one may not reject it as a promising compound with a high probability. Note that under the above hypotheses, the usual type I error is the false positive in accepting an ineffective drug and the type II error is the false negative in rejecting a promising compound.

Let n_1 and n_2 be the number of subjects in the first and second stage, respectively. Under a two-stage design, n_1 patients are treated at the first stage. If there are fewer than r_1 responses, then stop the trial. Otherwise, additional n_2 patients are recruited and tested at the second stage. A decision regarding whether the test treatment is promising is then made based on the response rate of the $n = n_1 + n_2$ subjects. Note that the rejection of H_0 (or H_a) means that further (or not further) study of the test treatment should be carried out. Simon (1989) proposed to select the optimal two-stage design that achieves the minimum expected sample size under the null hypothesis. Let n_{exp} and P_{et} be the expected sample size and the probability of early termination after the first stage. Thus, we have

$$n_{\text{exp}} = n_1 + (1 - P_{et})n_2.$$

At the end of the first stage, we would terminate the trial early and reject the null hypothesis if r_1 or fewer responses are observed. As a result, P_{et} is given by

$$P_{et} = B_c(r_1; n_1, p),$$

where $B_c(r_1; n_1, p)$ denotes the cumulative binomial distribution that $X \leq r_1$. Thus, we reject the test treatment at the end of the second stage if r or fewer responses are observed. The probability of rejecting the test treatment with success probability p is then given by

$$B_c(r_1; n_1, p) + \sum_{x=r_1+1}^{\min(n_1,r)} B(x; n_1, p) B_c(r - x; n_2, p),$$

where $B(x; n_1, p)$ denotes the binomial probability density function. For specific values of p_0, p_1, α, and β, Simon's optimal two-stage design can be obtained as the two-stage design that satisfies the error constraints and minimizes the expected sample size when the response rate is p_0.

Example 10.5 Assume the undesirable and desirable response rates under the null hypothesis and the alternative hypothesis are given by 0.05 and 0.25, respectively. For a given one-sided $\alpha = 0.05$ with a desired power of 80%, we obtain the sample size and the operating characteristics as follows. The sample size required at stage 1 is $n_1 = 9$. The cumulative sample size at stage 2 is $n = 17$. The actual overall α and the actual power are given by 0.047 and 0.812, respectively. The stopping rules are specified as follows. At stage 1, stop and accept the null hypothesis if the response rate is less than or equal to 0/9. Otherwise, continue to stage 2. The probability of stopping for futility is 0.63 when H_0 is true and 0.075 when H_a is true. At stage 2, stop and accept the null hypothesis if the response rate is less than or equal to 2/17. Otherwise, stop and reject the null hypothesis.

10.2.2 Bayesian approach

Assume that $X \sim B(n, p)$ and $p \sim Beta(a, b)$. At the first stage with n_1 subjects, the posterior distribution of p given X is given by

$$\pi_1(p|x) = Beta(a + x, b + n_1 - x). \tag{10.30}$$

Similarly, at the end of the second stage with n subjects, the posterior distribution of p given X is

$$\pi(p|x) = Beta(a + x, b + n - x). \tag{10.31}$$

As a result, the cutoff point for stopping the trial is chosen in a way such that the Bayesian power at the first stage is $(1 - \beta_1)$ at Bayesian significance level of α_{B1}. Similarly, the n is chosen such that the Bayesian power at the second stage is $(1 - \beta)$ at Bayesian significance level α_B. Based on (10.30) and (10.31), conditional power and predictive power can be derived. Given X out of n_1 patients who respond at the first stage, the probability (or conditional power) of having at least y additional responses out of the n_2 additional patients at the second stage is given by

$$P(y|x, n_1, n_2) = \sum_{i=y}^{n_2} \binom{n_2}{i} \left(\frac{x}{n_1}\right)^i \left(1 - \frac{x}{n_1}\right)^{n_2 - i}. \tag{10.32}$$

However, Bayesian approach provides a different look. Assume that the prior follows a binomial prior distribution $p \in [0, 1]$. Thus, the sampling distribution of X given p is given by

$$P(X = x|p) = \binom{n_1}{x} p^x (1-p)^{n_1-x}.$$

Since

$$P(a < p < b \cap X = x) = \int_a^b \binom{n_1}{x} p^x (1-p)^{n_1-x} dp,$$

and

$$P(X = x) = \int_0^1 \binom{n_1}{x} p^x (1-p)^{n_1-x} dp,$$

the posterior distribution of p given X can be obtained as

$$P(a < p < b \mid X = x) = \frac{\int_a^b \binom{n_1}{x} p^x (1-p)^{n_1-x} dp}{\int_0^1 \binom{n_1}{x} p^x (1-p)^{n_1-x} dp}$$

$$= \frac{\int_a^b p^x (1-p)^{n_1-x} dp}{B(x+1, n_1-x+1)},$$

where

$$B(x+1, n_1-x+1) = \frac{\Gamma(x+1)\Gamma(n_1-x+1)}{\Gamma(n_1+2)}.$$

Thus, the posterior distribution of p conditionally on $X = x$ responses out of n_1 is a *Beta* distribution, i.e.,

$$\pi(p|x) = \frac{p^x (1-p)^{n_1-x}}{B(x+1, n_1-x+1)}. \tag{10.33}$$

As a result, the predictive power (which is different from the frequentist's conditional power) or the predictive probability of having at least y responders out of additional m patients, given the observed response rate of x/n_1 at the first stage, is given by

$$P(y|x, n_1, n_2) = \int_0^1 P(X \geq k|p, n_2) \pi(p|x) dp$$

$$= \int_0^1 \sum_{i=y}^{n_2} \binom{n_2}{i} p^i (1-p)^{n_2-i} \frac{p^x (1-p)^{n_1-x}}{B(x+1, n_1-x+1)} dp. \tag{10.34}$$

Carrying out the integration, we have

$$P(y|x, n_1, n_2) = \sum_{i=y}^{n_2} \binom{n_2}{i} \frac{B(x+i+1, n_2+n_1-x-i+1)}{B(x+1, n_1-x+1)}.$$

Note that the above results follow directly from the fact that

$$\int_0^1 p^a (1-p)^b \, dp = B(a+1, b+1). \tag{10.35}$$

As a result, the conditional and/or predictive power can be used to design the sequential or other adaptive designs.

10.3 Bayesian Optimal Adaptive Designs

In practice, different adaptations and choices of priors with many possible probabilistic outcomes (good or bad) could lead to different types of adaptive designs. How to select an efficient adaptive design among these designs has become an interesting question to the investigators. In this section, we propose to evaluate so-called utility index for choosing a Bayesian optimal adaptive design. The utility index is an indicator of patients' health outcomes. Bayesian optimal design is a design that has maximum expected utility under financial, time, and other constraints.

For illustration purposes, we apply the approach for choosing a Bayesian optimal design among the three commonly considered two-arm designs in pharmaceutical research and development. The three commonly considered two-arm trial designs include a classical approach of two separate two-arm designs (i.e., a two-arm phase II design followed by a two-arm phase III design) and two different seamless phase II/III designs, which are group sequential designs with O'Brien-Fleming boundary and Pocock boundary, respectively. For each design, we calculate the utility index and weighted by its prior probability to obtain the expected utility for the design. For a given design, the Bayesian optimal design is the one with maximum utility. For convenience's sake, we consider three scenarios of prior knowledge, which are given in Table 10.1.

Assume that there is no dose selection issue (i.e., the dose has been determined by the toxicity and biomaker response in early studies). For the classical approach of two separate two-arm designs, we consider a phase IIb and a phase III (assuming that one phase III study is sufficient for regulatory approval). For the phase II study, we assume $\delta = 0.2$, one-sided $\alpha = 0.1$ and power $= 0.8$. Thus, the total sample size required is

Table 10.1 Prior Knowledge

Scenario	Effect Size	Prior Prob.
1	0	0.2
2	0.1	0.2
3	0.2	0.6

Table 10.2 Characteristics of Classic Phase II and III Designs

Scenario, i	Effect Size	Prior Prob. π	Prob. of Continue to Phase III, P_c	Phase III Power, P_3
1	0	0.2	0.1	0.025
2	0.1	0.2	0.4	0.639
3	0.2	0.6	0.9	0.996

$n_1 = 450$. For the phase III trial, we assume

$$\delta = 0.2(0) + 0.2(0.1) + 0.6(0.2)$$
$$= 0.14,$$

which was calculated from Table 10.1. Furthermore, assuming that $\alpha = 0.025$ (one-sided) and power $= 0.9$, the total sample size required is $n = 2144$. If the phase II study didn't show any statistical significance, we will not conduct the phase III trial. Note that the rule is not always followed in practice. The probability that continues to phase III is the weighted continual probability given in Table 10.2, i.e.,

$$P_c = \sum_{i=1}^{3} P_c(i) \pi(i)$$
$$= 0.2(0.1) + 0.2(0.4) + 0.6(0.9)$$
$$= 0.64.$$

Thus, the expected sample size for phase II and phase III trials as a whole is given by

$$\bar{N} = (1 - P_c) n_1 + P_c n$$
$$= (1 - 0.64)(450) + 0.64(2144)$$
$$= 1500.$$

The overall expected power is then given by

$$\bar{P} = \sum_{i=1}^{3} P_c(i) \pi(i) P_3(i)$$
$$= (0.2)(0.1)(0.025) + (0.2)(0.4)(0.639) + (0.6)(0.9)(0.996)$$
$$= 0.59$$

In conclusion, the classical approach for separate phase II and phase III designs (i.e., a phase II design followed by a phase III design) has an overall power of 59% with expected total (combined) sample size of 1500. On the other hand, for seamless phase II/III designs, we assume

BAYESIAN APPROACH

Table 10.3 Characteristics of Seamless Phase II/III Design with OB Boundary

Scenario, i	Effect Size	Prior Prob. π	$N_{\exp}$	Power
1	0	0.2	1600	0.025
2	0.1	0.2	1712	0.46
3	0.2	0.6	1186	0.98

(i) $\delta = 0.14$, (ii) one-sided $\alpha = 0.025$, (iii) power $= 0.90$, (iv) O'Brien-Fleming efficacy stopping boundary, and (v) symmetrical futility stopping boundary. Suppose there is one planned interim analysis when 50% of patients are enrolled. Thus, this design has one interim analysis and one final analysis. Thus, we have:

- The sample sizes for the two analyses are 1,085, and 2,171, respectively.
- The sample size ratio between the two groups is 1.
- The maximum sample size for the design is 2,171.
- Under the null hypothesis, the expected sample size is 1,625.
- Under the alternative hypothesis, the expected sample size is 1,818.

The decision rules are specified as follows. At stage 1, accept the null hypothesis if $z_1 < 0$. We would reject the null hypothesis if $z_1 \geq 2.79$; Otherwise, continue. At stage 2, accept the null hypothesis if $z < 1.974$ and reject the null hypothesis if $z \geq 1.97$. The stopping probabilities at the first stage are given by

- Stopping for H_0 when H_0 is true is 0.5000,
- Stopping for H_a when H_0 is true is 0.0026,
- Stopping for H_0 when H_a is true is 0.0105,
- Stopping for H_a when H_a is true is 0.3142.

The operating characteristics are summarized in Table 10.3. Furthermore, the average total expected sample size can be obtained as

$$\sum \pi(i) N_{\exp}(i) = 0.2(1600) + 0.2(1712) + 0.6(1186)$$
$$= 1374.$$

Table 10.4 Characteristics of Seamless Phase II/III Design with Pocock Boundary

Scenario, i	Effect Size	Prior Prob. π	N_{exp}	Power
1	0	0.2	1492	0.025
2	0.1	0.2	1856	0.64
3	0.2	0.6	1368	0.996

and the average power is given by

$$\sum \pi(i) N_{\text{exp}}(i) \, Power(i) = 0.2(0.025) + 0.2(0.46) + 0.6(0.98)$$
$$= 0.69.$$

Now, consider another type of adaptive seamless phase II/III trial design using Pocock's efficacy stopping boundary and the symmetric futility stopping boundary. Based on the same parameter specifications, i.e., $\alpha = 0.025$, power $= 0.9$, mean difference $= 0.14$, and standard deviation $= 1$, we have:

- The sample sizes for the two analyses are 1,274, and 2,549, respectively.
- The sample size ratio between the two groups is 1.
- The maximum sample size for the design is 2,549.
- Under the null hypothesis, the expected sample size is 1,492.
- Under the alternative hypothesis, the expected sample size is 1,669.

The decision rules are specified as follows. At stage 1, accept the null hypothesis if the p-value > 0.1867 (i.e., $z_1 < 0.89$). We would reject the null hypothesis if p-value ≤ 0.0158 (i.e., $z_1 \geq 2.149$); otherwise, continue. At stage 2, accept the null hypothesis if the p-value > 0.0158 (i.e., $z = 2.149$) and reject the null hypothesis if the p-value ≤ 0.0158. The stopping probabilities at the first stage are given by

- Stopping for H_0 when H_0 is true is 0.8133,
- Stopping for H_a when H_0 is true is 0.0158,
- Stopping for H_0 when H_a is true is 0.0538,
- Stopping for H_a when H_a is true is 0.6370.

Other operating characteristics are summarized in Table 10.4.

Table 10.5 Comparison of Classic and Seamless Designs

Design	N_{max}	Average N_{exp}	Average Power	Expected utility
Classic		1500	0.59	$0.515B
OB		1374	0.69	$0.621B
Pocock		1490	0.73	$0.656B

Furthermore, the average total expected sample size can be obtained as

$$\sum \pi(i) N_{exp}(i) = 0.2(1492) + 0.2(1856) + 0.6(1368)$$
$$= 1490,$$

and the average power is given by

$$\sum \pi(i) N_{exp}(i) \, Power(i) = 0.2(0.025) + 0.2(0.64) + 0.6(0.996)$$
$$= 0.73.$$

In addition, we may compare these designs from the financial perspective. Assume that the pre-patient cost of the trial is about $50K and the value of regulatory approval before deducting the cost of the trial is $1B. For simplicity, potential time savings are not included in the calculation. We consider the following expected utility

Expected utility = (average power)($80M$) − (average N_{exp})($50K$).

Table 10.5 summarizes the comparison of the classical separate phase II and phase III design and the two seamless phase II/III designs using O'Brien-Fleming boundary and Pocock boundary.

As it can be seen from Table 10.5, Pocock's design is the best among the three designs based on power or the expected utility.

10.4 Concluding Remarks

The Bayesian approach has several advantages in pharmaceutical development. First, it provides the opportunity to continue updating the information/knowledge regarding the test treatment under study. Second, Bayesian approach is a decision-making process that specifically ties to a particular trial, a clinical development program, and a company's portfolio for pharmaceutical development. In practice, regulatory agencies require the type I error rate be controlled with many externally mandated restrictions when implementing a Bayesian design, which might decrease the application of Bayesian methods in clinical trials. In essence, once Bayesian methods become more familiar to clinical scientists, they will face fewer externally mandated restrictions.

In the past several decades, the process of pharamaceutical development has been criticized for not being able to bring promising and safe compounds to the marketplace in a timely fashion. As a result, there is increasing demand from political bodies and consumer groups to make drug development more efficient, safer, and yet faster. However, it is a concern that we may abandon fundamental scientific principles for pharmaceutical (clinical) research and development. Alternatively, it is suggested that a Bayesian approach be used because it will lead to more rapid and more economical drug development without sacrificing good science. However, the use of Bayesian approach in pharmaceutical development is not widely accepted by the regulatory agencies such as the U.S. FDA, although it has been used more in certain therapeutic areas of medical device development. It should be noted that the Bayesian approach is useful for some diseases such as cancer in which there is a burgeoning number of biomarkers available for modelling the disease's progress. These biomarkers will enable a patient's disease progression to be monitored more accurately. Consequently, a more accurate assessment of the patient's outcome can be made. In recent years, trials in early phases of clinical development (e.g., phases I or II) are becoming increasingly Bayesian, especially in the area of oncology. Moreover, strategic planning and portfolio management such as formal utility assessment and decision-making processes in some pharmaceutical companies are becoming increasingly Bayesian. The use of the Bayesian approach in various phases of pharmaceutical development will become evident to the decision makers in the near future.

CHAPTER 11

Clinical Trial Simulation

Clinical trial simulation is a process that uses computers to mimic the conduct of a clinical trial by creating virtual patients and extrapolating (or predicting) clinical outcomes for each virtual patient based on the pre-specified models (Li and Lai, 2003). The primary objective of clinical trial simulation is multi-fold. First, it is to monitor the conduct of the trial, project outcomes, anticipate problems, and recommend remedies before it is too late. Second, it is to extrapolate (or predict) the clinical outcomes *beyond* the scope of previous studies from which the existing models were derived using the model techniques. Third, it is to study the validity and robustness of the trial under various assumptions of study designs. Clinical trial simulation is often conducted to verify (or confirm) the models depicting the relationships between the inputs such as dose, dosing time, patient characteristics, and disease severity and the clinical outcomes such as changes in the signs and symptoms or adverse events within the study domain. In practice, clinical trial simulation is often considered to predict potential clinical outcomes under different assumptions and various design scenarios at the planning stage of a clinical trial for better planning of the actual trial.

Clinical trial simulation is a powerful tool in pharmaceutical development. The concept of clinical trial simulation is very intuitive and easy to implement. In practice, clinical trial simulation is often considered a useful tool for evaluation of the performance of a test treatment under a model with complicated situations. It can achieve the goal with minimum assumptions by controlling type I error rate effectively. It can also be used to visualize the dynamic trial process from patient recruitment, drug distribution, treatment administration, and pharmacokinetic processes to biomarker development and clinical responses. In this chapter, we will review the application of clinical trial simulations in both early and late phases of pharmaceutical development.

In the next section, the framework of a clinical trial simulation is briefly outlined. Section 11.2 provides an overview of commonly employed clinical trial simulations in early phases clinical development, while Section 11.3 discusses some theoretical and practical issues that are commonly encountered when conducting clinical trial simulations in late phases clinical development. Section 11.4 introduces a software product developed by CTriSoft Intl for clinical trial simulation with demonstration. A number of examples concerning early and late phase development are given in Section 11.5. A brief concluding remark is given in the last section.

11.1 Simulation Framework

The framework of clinical trial simulation is rather simple. It consists of trial design, study objectives (hypotheses), model, and statistical tests. For the trial design, critical design features such as (i) a parallel design or a crossover design, (ii) a balanced or unbalanced design, (iii) the number of treatment groups, and (iv) adaptation algorithms need to be clearly specified. For the trial design, hypotheses such as testing for equality, superiority, or non-inferiority/equivalence can then be formulated for achieving the study objectives. A statistical model is necessarily implemented to generate virtual patients and extrapolate (or predict) clinical outcomes. We can then evaluate the performance of the test treatment through the study of statistical properties of the statistical tests derived under the null and alternative hypotheses.

More specifically, we begin a clinical trial simulation by choosing a statistical model under a valid trial design with various assumptions according to the trial setting. We then simulate the trial by creating virtual patients and generating the clinical outcomes for each virtual patient based on the model specifications under the null hypothesis of H_0 for a large number of times (say m times). For each simulation run, we calculate the test statistic. The m test statistic values constitute a distribution of the test statistic numerically. Similarly, we repeat the process to simulate the trial under the alternative hypothesis of H_a m times. The m test statistic values obtained represent the distribution of the test statistic under the alternative hypothesis. These two distributions can be used to determine the critical region for a given α level of significance, p-value for a given data, and the corresponding power for the given critical region. To provide a better understanding, Figure 11.1 provides the flowchart of the general simulation framework.

Note that the computer simulation starts with generating data under the null hypothesis. The data are often generated from a simple distribution such as a normal distribution for continuous variables, a binary distribution for discrete variables, and an exponential distribution for time-to-event data. The generation of simulated data occurs only once per simulation run. The adaptive algorithm is usually applied later for the case of a sequential trial design or an N-adjustable design (sample size re-estimation). In some cases such as response-adaptive

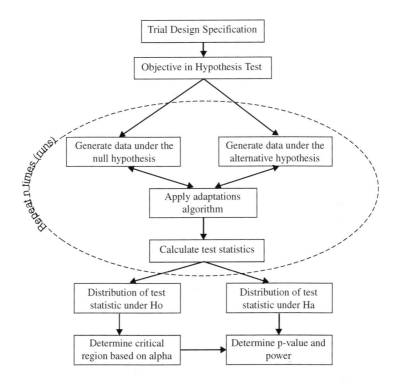

Figure 11.1 Simulation framework.

randomization, the randomization may have to be generated step-by-step. It should be noted that under the above mentioned framework, other operating characteristics such as stopping boundary and conditional probability can also be obtained.

11.2 Early Phases Development

Clinical trial simulation has been widely used in early phases development such as pharmacokinetic and pharmacodynamic (PK/PD) modeling, assessment of QT/QTc prolongation, and optimal dose-finding strategies (Kimko and Duffull, 2003). To illustrate the application of simulation in early phase clinical trials, we will focus on an early phase oncology study (e.g., dose-escalation trial) because (i) typically there are only a very small number of patients involved due to potential high risk of toxicity of the test drug (how to obtain a precise estimation of the dose-toxicity relationship is challenging to the investigator); (ii) the traditional escalation methods are ad hoc and lack scientific or statistical justification (the reliability of the traditional escalation method is always a concern to the investigator); (iii) many approaches based on clinical trial simulation have been proposed in the literature. See, for example, O'Quigley, Pepe, and Fisher (1990), Crowley (2001), CTriSoft Intl (2002), and Babb and Rogatko (2004). Our intention is not only to review or compare these methods and make a recommendation, but also to use several typical methods as vehicles to illustrate the application of clinical trial simulation.

In a typical early phase dose escalation trial, we often begin with a treatment at a low dose that is very likely to be safe. Then, a small number of cohorts of patients are treated at progressively higher doses until drug-related toxicity reaches a pre-determined level. The primary objectives are not only to determine the maximum tolerated dose (MTD), but also to characterize the dose limiting toxicity (DLT) of the test treatment under investigation. In what follows, key study parameters that are necessarily specified when conducting a simulation for dose-escalation trial are briefly described.

11.2.1 Dose limiting toxicity (DLT) and maximum tolerated dose (MTD)

The definitions of dose limiting toxicity (DLT) and maximum tolerable dose (MTD) need to be specified in a simulation for dose-escalation trial. As indicated in Chapter 5, drug toxicity is considered tolerable if the toxicity is acceptable, manageable, and reversible. A dose limiting toxicity (DLT) is defined based on the Common Terminology Criteria (CTC). For example, any AE from the CTC categories of grade 3 or higher related to treatment is considered a DLT. The maximum tolerated dose (MTD) is defined as a dose level at which DLT occurs with at least a certain frequency, e.g., one-third.

11.2.2 Dose-level selection

Next, we need to select initial dose for the simulation. As discussed in Chapter 5, the commonly used starting dose is the dose at which 10% mortality (LD_{10}) occurs in mice. The subsequent dose levels are usually selected based on the following multiplicative set, $x_i = f_{i-1} x_{i-1}$ ($i = 1, 2, \ldots k$), where f_i is the dose-escalation factor. Two commonly used sequences of dose-escalation factors are the Fibonacci numbers (2, 1.5, 1.67, 1.60, 1.63, 1.62, 1.62, ...) and modified Fibonacci numbers (2, 1.65, 1.52, 1.40, 1.33, 1.33, ...). Note that the highest dose level in the trial should be selected such that it covers the biologically active dose.

11.2.3 Sample size per dose level

In principle, the number of patients to be treated per dose level should be small enough to limit any potential safety issues, but large enough to allow the investigators to determine the optimal dose levels. In practice, recommendations may vary between one and eight patients per dose level. It is suggested that three to six patients per lower dose level or a minimum of three per dose level and a minimum of five near the MTD be included. This information is necessarily provided for the conduct of the clinical trial simulation.

11.2.4 Dose-escalation design

For the clinical trial simulation, we need to specify which dose-escalation design will be used. Commonly employed dose-escalation designs include (i) the traditional dose-escalation design and (ii) two-stage dose-escalation design. As indicated in Chapter 5, the traditional dose-escalation design utilizes the traditional escalation rules (TER) or strict traditional escalation rules (STER). Two-stage dose-escalation design utilizes a two-stage escalation algorithm (TSER), where in the first stage, only a single patient is treated at each dose level. When a DLT is observed, the traditional "3 + 3" rule is applied.

If the continual reassessment method (CRM) is to be used, the dose toxicity model and prior distribution of the parameters should be specified. In practice, the logistic model $p(x) = [1 + b \exp(-ax)]^{-1}$ is often utilized, where $p(x)$ is the probability of toxicity associated with dose x, and a and b are positive parameters to be determined. The updated dose toxicity model is then used to determine the dose level for the next patient.

11.3 Late Phases Development

Although clinical trial simulation has been used for several decades, it has not received much attention until recently (Maxwell, Domenet, and Joyce, 1971; Parmigiani, 2002; Kimko and Duffull, 2003). Since clinical trial simulation is useful in evaluating very complicated models with minimum assumptions, it has become a very popular tool for searching for an optimal trial design in late phases clinical development. In this section, we will focus on the simulation for adaptive designs discussed in the previous chapters of this book because statistical theory of an adaptive design could be very complicated with limited analytical solutions under some strong assumptions. Besides, in some complicated adaptive designs, analytical solutions might not exist. Similarly, when conducting a simulation for adaptive trial designs, key adaptation rules are necessarily specified, which are briefly described below.

11.3.1 Randomization rules

In clinical trials, it is desirable to randomize more patients to superior treatment groups. This can be accomplished by increasing the probability of assigning a patient to the treatment group when the evidence of responsive rate increases in a group. The response-adaptive randomization rule can be the randomized-play-the-winner or utility offset model. Response-adaptive randomization requires unblinding the data, which may not feasible at real time. There is often a delayed response, i.e., randomizing the next patient before knowing responses of previous patients. Therefore, it is practical to unblind the data several times during the trial, i.e., group sequential response-adaptive randomization, instead of fully sequential adaptive randomization.

11.3.2 Early stopping rules

It is desirable to stop a trial when the efficacy or futility of the test drug becomes obvious during the trial. To stop a trial prematurely, we provide a threshold for the number of subjects randomized and at least one of the following:

(1) Utility rules: The difference in response rate between the most responsive group and the control group exceeds a threshold, and the corresponding two-sided 95% naive confidence interval lower bound exceeds a threshold.
(2) Futility rules: The difference in response rate between the most responsive group and the control is lower than a threshold, and the corresponding two-sided 90% naive confidence interval upper bound is lower than a threshold.

11.3.3 Rules for dropping losers

In addition to the response-adaptive randomization, you can also improve the efficiency of a trial design by dropping some inferior groups (losers) during the trial. To drop a loser, we provide two thresholds for (1) maximum difference in response rate between any two dose levels, and (2) the corresponding two-sided 90% naive confidence lower bound. We may choose to retain all the treatment groups without dropping a loser and/or to retain the control group with a certain randomization rate for the purpose of statistical comparisons between the active groups and the control.

11.3.4 Sample size adjustment

Sample size determination requires anticipation of the expected treatment effect size defined as the expected treatment difference divided by its standard deviation. It is not uncommon that the initial estimation of the effect size turns out to be too large or small, which consequently leads to an under-powered or over-powered trial. Therefore, it is desirable to adjust the sample size according to the effect size for an on-going trial. The sample size adjustment is determined by a power function of treatment effect size, i.e.,

$$N = N_0 \left(\frac{E_{0\,\max}}{E_{\max}} \right)^a, \tag{11.1}$$

where N is the newly estimated sample size, N_0 the initial sample size, and a a constant. The effect size $E_{\max}$ is defined as

$$E_{\max} = \frac{p_{\max} - p_1}{\sigma^2}; \quad \sigma^2 = \bar{p}(1-\bar{p}); \quad \bar{p} = \frac{p_{\max} + p_1}{2};$$

$p_{\max}$ and p_1 are the maximum response rates, respectively, and the control response rate, and $E_{0\,\max}$ is the initial estimation of $E_{\max}$.

11.3.5 Response–adaptive randomization

Conventional randomization refers to any randomization procedure with a constant treatment allocation probability such as simple randomization. Unlike the conventional randomization, response-adaptive randomization is a randomization in which the probability of allocating a patient to a treatment group is based on the response of the previous patients. The purpose is to improve the overall response rate in the trial. There are many different algorithms such as random-play-the-winner (RPW), the utility-offset model, and the maximum utility model. The generalized randomized-play-the-winner denoted by $RPW(n_1, n_2, \ldots, n_k; m_1, m_2, \ldots, m_k)$ can be described as follows.

- Step 1: Place n_i balls of the ith color (corresponding to the ith treatment) into an urn ($i = 1, 2, \ldots, k$), where k is number of treatment groups. There are initially $N = \sum n_i$ balls in the urn.

Table 11.1 Bias in Rate Due to Adaptive Randomization

Dose Level	1	2	3	4	5
Target rate	0.5	0.1	0.2	0.7	0.55
Number of patients	130	14	23	362	171
Observed rate	0.47	0.08	0.16	0.7	0.53
Standard deviation	0.10	0.08	0.10	0.05	0.08
Bias in rate	0.03	0.02	0.04	0.00	0.02

N = 700; 10,000 simulations.

- Step 2: Randomly choose a ball from the urn. If it is the ith color, assign the next patient to the ith treatment group.
- Step 3: Add m_k balls of the ith color to the urn for each response observed in the ith treatment. This creates more chances for choosing the ith treatment.
- Step 4: Repeat Steps 2 and 3.

When $n_i = n$ and $m_i = m$ for all i, we simply write $RPW(n, m)$ for $RPW(n_1, n_2, \ldots, n_k; m_1, m_2, \ldots, m_k)$.

Note that the commonly used estimators that are based on the assumption of independent samples are often biased due to adaptive randomization RPW(1,1). See Table 11.1.

11.3.6 Utility-offset model

To have a high probability of achieving target patient distribution among the treatment groups, the probability of assigning a patient to a group should be proportional to the corresponding predicted or observed response rate minus the proportion of patients that have been assigned to the group, i.e.,

$$\Pr(i) = \begin{cases} \frac{1}{k}, & S_R = 0, \\ \frac{1}{c} \max\left\{0, \left(\frac{R_i}{S_R} - \frac{n_i}{N}\right)\right\}, & S_R > 0, \end{cases} \quad (11.2)$$

where the normalization factor

$$c = \sum_i \left(\frac{R_i}{S_R} - \frac{n_i}{N}\right),$$

Table 11.2 Comparisons of Simulations Results

N	Dose Level	1	2	3	4	5
	Target rate	0.02	0.07	0.37	0.73	0.52
50	Predicted rate	0.02	0.07	0.40	0.65	0.41
30	Predicted rate	0.02	0.07	0.40	0.63	0.40
20	Predicted rate	0.02	0.07	0.37	0.58	0.38

n_i is the number of patients that have been randomized to the ith group, R_i is the observed response rate for the ith group,

$$S_R = \sum_{i=1}^{k} R_i,$$

k is the number of dose groups and N is the total estimated number of patients in the trial. The maximum utility model for the adaptive-randomization always assigns the next patient to the group that has the highest response rate based on current estimation of either the observed or model-based predicted response rate.

11.3.7 Null-model versus model approach

It is interesting to compare model and null-model approaches. When the sample size is larger than 20 per group, there is no obvious advantage of using the model-based method with respect to the precision and accuracy (Table 11.2). Therefore, a null-model approach will be used in the subsequent simulations.

11.3.8 Alpha adjustment

The α-adjustment is required when (i) there are multiple comparisons with more than two groups involved, (ii) there are interim looks, i.e., early stopping for futility or efficacy, and (iii) there is a response-dependent sampling procedure such as response-adaptive randomization and unblinded sample size re-estimation. When samples or observations from the trial are not independent, the response data are no longer normally distributed. Therefore, the p-value from a normal distribution assumption should be adjusted, or equivalently the alpha should be adjusted if the p-value is not adjusted. For the same reason, the other statistic estimates from normal assumption should also be adjusted.

Table 11.3 Alpha Inflation/Deflation

Randomization	Inflated FWE α	Adjusted α
RPW(1,0)	0.146	0.015
RPW(1,1)	0.143	0.007

Note: Five group with total $N = 100$. H_0 Rate $= 0.5$.

The adjusted alpha can be found easily using simulation (See example, Table 11.3). Run simulations under the null hypothesis H_0 to find the adjusted alpha for the pairwise comparisons such that family-wise error rate $= 0.025$. Then run simulations under the alternative hypothesis H_a using the adjusted alpha to find the power for various sample sizes and other scenarios.

11.4 Software Application

In this section, we will introduce the application of clinical trial simulation through a software ExpDesign Studio® developed by CTriSoft Intl (2002) with demonstration (www.CTriSoft.net).

11.4.1 Overview of ExpDesign Studio

ExpDesign Studio is an integrated environment for designing clinical trials. It is a user-friendly statistical software that consists of five main components. These main components include *Conventional Trial Design* (CTD), *Sequential Trial Design* (STD), *Multi-Stage Trial Design* (MSTD), *Dose-Escalation Trial Design* (DETD), and *Adaptive Trial Design* (ATD). Conventional trial design is probably the most commonly used design in practice. There are over 160 procedures for sample size calculation in CTD for various trial designs. STD covers a broad range of sequential trials including methods for different numbers of experiment groups, different endpoints (e.g., mean, proportion, and survival), different hypotheses (e.g., test for difference and equivalence), and different stopping boundaries. MSTD provides three optimal designs, namely minimax (MinMax) design, MinExp, and maximization of utility (MaxUtility) design. These designs minimize the maximum sample size, the expected sample size, and maximize the utility index, respectively. DETD provides researchers with an efficient way to search the optimal design for dose-escalation trials with different criteria by means of computer simulations. It includes the traditional escalation rules, restricted escalation rules, two-stage escalation algorithms, and customized algorithms with varieties of dose intervals

CLINICAL TRIAL SIMULATION

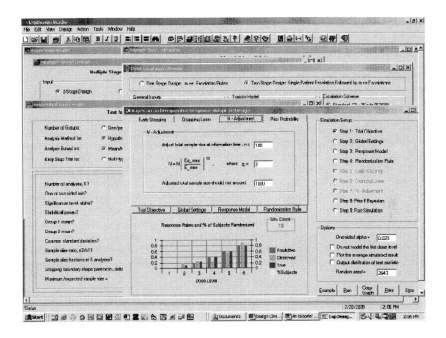

Figure 11.2 The ExpDesign integrated environment.

such as Fibonacci, modified Fibonacci series, and the customized dose interval series. It also provides three different toxicity models. ATD in ExpDesign Studio allows a user to simulate trials under specific adaptive designs. One can use response-adaptive randomization to assign more patients to superior treatment groups or drop the losers (or the inferior groups). One may stop a trial prematurely to claim efficacy or futility based on the observed data. One may also modify sample size based on observed treatment difference. One may also conduct simulations using Bayesian or frequentist modeling approaches or a non-parametric approach. All design reports are generated through an automated procedure.

ExpDesign Studio covers many statistical tools required for designing a trial. It is helpful to get familiar with the functions of the icons on the toolbar. The black-white icons on the left-hand side of the toolbar are standard for all word processors. The first group of the four color icons is the starting point to launch the four different types of designs: *Conventional Trial Design*, *Sequential Trial Design*, *Multi-Stage Trial Design*, and *Dose-Escalation Trial Design* (see Figures 11.2 and 11.3). Alternatively, one may click one of the four buttons in the ExpDesignTM Studio to start the corresponding design. The next set of three color icons are for launching *Design Example*, *Computing Design Parameters*, and

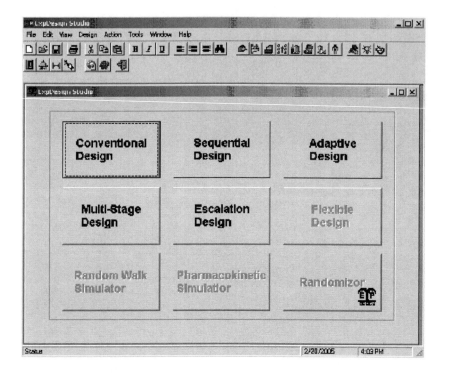

Figure 11.3 ExpDesign start window.

generating *Design Report*. Following these are four color icons for the toolkits including *Graphic Calculator*, *Distribution Calculator*, *Confidence Interval Calculator*, and *TipDay*. One can move the mouse over any icon on the toolbar to see the Tiptext, which describes what the icon is for.

11.4.2 How to design a trial with ExpDesign studio

To get started, we first double-click on ExpDesign Studio icon. Then, on the ExpDesign start window, we select the trial design we wish to implement.

11.4.3 How to design a conventional trial

To design a conventional trial, we simply follow the following steps.

- Step 1: Click *Conventional Trial Design* on the toolbar.
- Step 2: Select the desired option from *Design Option Panel*.

CLINICAL TRIAL SIMULATION

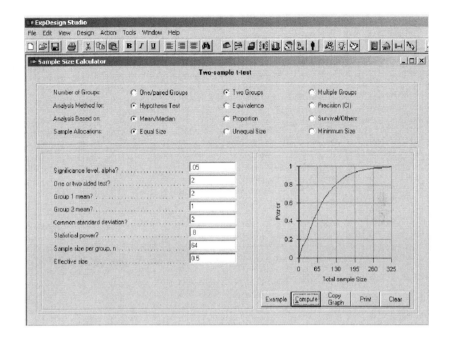

Figure 11.4 The conventional design window.

- Step 3: Select a method from the list of methods available.
- Step 4: Enter appropriate values for the selected design.
- Step 5: Click on *Compute* to calculate the required sample size.
- Step 6: Click on *Report* to view the report of the selected design.
- Step 7: Click on *Print* to print the desired output.
- Step 8: Click on *Copy-Graph* to copy the graph and use *Paste* or *Paste-Special* under *Edit* menu to paste it to other applications (Figure 11.4).

11.4.4 How to design a group sequential trial

To design a group sequential trial, we simply follow the following steps.

- Step 1: Click on *Group Sequential Design* on the toolbar.
- Step 2: Select the desired option from the *Design Option Panel*.
- Step 3: Select a method from the list of methods available.
- Step 4: Enter appropriate values for the selected design.
- Step 5: Click on *Compute* to generate the design.
- Step 6: Click on *Report* to view the design report.

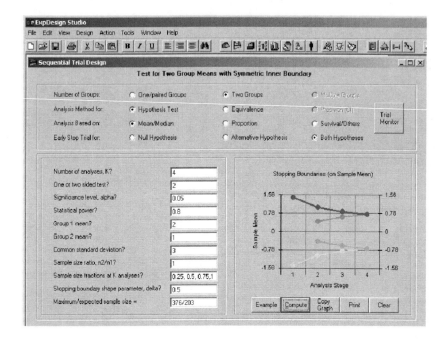

Figure 11.5 Sequential design window.

- Step 7: Click on *Print* to print the desired output.
- Step 8: Click on *Copy-Graph* to copy the graph and use *Paste* or *Paste-Special* under *Edit* menu to paste it to other applications.
- Step 9: Click *Save* to save the design specification or report (Figure 11.5).

11.4.5 How to design a multi-stage trial

To design a multiple-stage design, we simply follow the following steps.

- Step 1: Click on *Multi-Stage Design* on the toolbar.
- Step 2: Select the desired *Option* from the *Multi-Stage Design* window or open an existing design by clicking *Open*.
- Step 3: Enter appropriate values for the selected design in the textboxes.
- Step 4: Click on *Compute* to generate the valid designs.
- Step 5: Click on *Report* to view the report of the selected design.
- Step 6: Click on *Print* to print the desired output.
- Step 7: Click on *Save* to save the design specification or report (Figure 11.6).

CLINICAL TRIAL SIMULATION

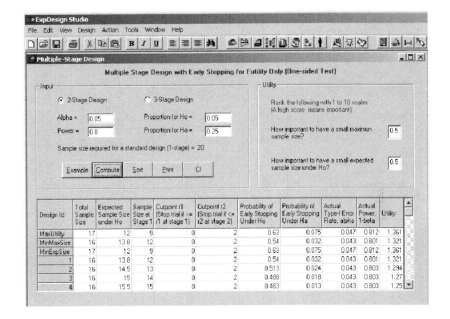

Figure 11.6 Multi-stage design window.

11.4.6 How to design a dose-escalation trial

To design a dose-escalation trial, we simply follow the following steps.

- Step 1: Click *Dose-Escalation Design* on the toolbar.
- Step 2: Enter appropriate values for your design on the *Basic Spec Panel*.
- Step 3: Select *Dose-response Model, Escalation Scheme*, and *Dose Interval Spec* or open an existing design by clicking *Open*.
- Step 4: Click on *Compute* to generate the simulation results.
- Step 5: Click on *Report* to view the design report.
- Step 6: Click on *Print* to print the desired output.
- Step 7: Click on *Save* to save the design specification or report (Figures 11.7 and 11.8).

When clicking on *Customized Design* for the *Escalation Scheme* (see Figure 11.7), a second window will pop up for further selection of the escalation rules. When it is done, click *OK*. It will go back to the *Dose-Escalation Design Window*.

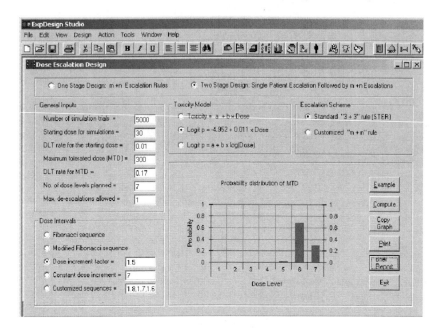

Figure 11.7 Dose-escalation design window.

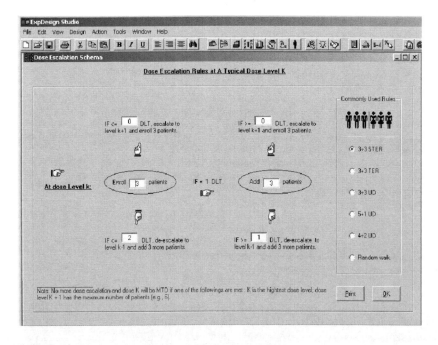

Figure 11.8 Dose-escalation customization window.

CLINICAL TRIAL SIMULATION

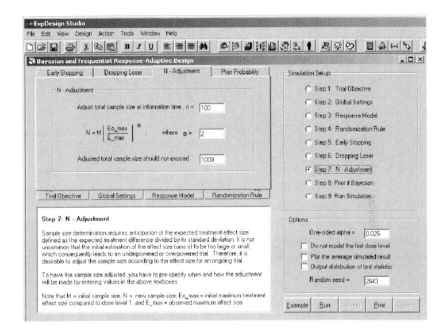

Figure 11.9 The adaptive design window.

11.4.7 How to design an adaptive trial

To design an adaptive trial, we simply follow the following steps.

- Step 1: Click on *Adaptive Design* on the toolbar.
- Step 2: Follow the steps specified in the *Simulation Setup* panel.
- Step 3: Specify parameters in each of the steps.
- Step 4: Click on *Run* to generate the simulation results.
- Step 5: Click on *Report* to view the design report.
- Step 6: Click on *Print* to print the desired output.
- Step 7: Click on *Save* to save the design specification or report (Figure 11.9).

11.5 Examples

In this section, several examples regarding the application of the clinical trial simulations in early and late phases of pharmaceutical development are provided. For early phases development, we will consider phase I oncology study for dose escalation with different traditional

Table 11.4 Simulation Results from TER

Dose Level	1	2	3	4	5	6	7
Dose	30	45	68	101	151	228	342
DLT rate (%)	1	1.2	1.5	2.2	3.7	8.4	25
mean n	3.1	3.1	3.1	3.2	3.5	5.0	5.0
MTD rate (%)	0	0	1	2	6	57	33

escalation rules (TER) and continued re-assessment method (CRM). For late phases development, we will consider phase II oncology trials comparing two treatment groups under different adaptive design setting such as an adaptive group sequential design, an adaptive-randomization design, an N-adjusted design (sample size re-estimation), a drop-the-loser design, and an adaptive dose-response design.

11.5.1 Early phases development

To illustrate the application of clinical trial simulation in early phases of clinical development, we consider the example of dose-escalation trial as described in the previous section. Suppose the study objective is to determine the maximum tolerable dose (MTD) of newly developed test treatment. In what follows, the application of clinical trial simulation for dose escalation with different traditional escalation rules (TER) and continued reassessment method (CRM) are discussed.

Example 11.1 Simulation example using TER and TSER For a planned dose-escalation trial, suppose we are interested in choosing an appropriate dose-escalation algorithm from the traditional escalation rule (TER) and the two-stage escalation rule (TSER) described earlier. Suppose that based on results from pre-clinical studies, it was estimated that the toxicity (DLT rate) is 1% for the starting dose of 30 mg/m^2 (1/10 of the lethal dose). The DLT rate at the MTD was defined as 17% and the MTD was estimated to be 300 mg/m^2. The true dose toxicity was assumed to follow a logistic model, i.e.,

$$Logit(p) = -4.952 + 0.011 Dose,$$

where p is the probability of DLT or DLT rate. There were 7 planned dose levels with a constant dose increment factor of 1.5. Suppose only one dose level de-escalation was allowed. Twenty thousand simulation runs were conducted using ExpDesign Studio (www.CTriSoft.net) for

Table 11.5 Simulation Results from TSER

Dose	30	45	68	101	151	228	342
mean n	1.1	1.1	1.2	1.3	1.5	5.9	5.2
MTD rate (%)	0	0	0	0	2	69	29

each of the two algorithms. The results are summarized in Tables 11.5 through 11.7.

The true MTD is somewhere between dose level 6 and 7. As it can be seen from Tables 11.5 and 11.6, the two-stage design requires fewer patients at the dose levels lower than MTD. Table 11.7 indicates that there is a large gain in the expected sample size with TSER, i.e., 17 compared 26 in TER. On average, both methods cause 2 DLTs each and 5 patients are treated above the MTD. The TSER increases slightly in precision compared to TER (66 versus 70 in dispersion of simulated MTDs). In the given scenario, both TER and TSER underestimate the true MTD (about 13%). This bias can be reduced using continual re-assessment method (CRM), which will be discussed below.

Example 11.2 Simulation example using CRM We repeat the above clinical trial simulation using the Bayesian continual reassessment method (CRM). The logistic model considered to model the dose toxicity relationship is given by

$$\Pr(x = 1) = (1 + 150e^{-ax})^{-1},$$

where parameter a follows a uniform prior distribution over the range of $[0, 0.3]$. The next patient is assigned to the dose level that has the predicted response rate closest to the target DLT rate of 0.17 as defined earlier for the MTD. No response delay is considered. Due to safety concerns, no dose jump is allowed. Ten thousand simulations were conducted using *ExpDesign Studio*® *version 2.0*, where 21 subjects

Table 11.6 Comparison of TER and TSER

Method	MTD	$\overline{MTD}$	σ_{MTD}	N	DLTs	n
3 + 3 TER	300	257	70	26	2	5
Two-stage	300	258	66	17	2	5.2

$\overline{MTD}$ = Simulated MTD, σ_{MTD} = dispersion of MTDs, N = expected sample size, n = patients treated above MTD.

Table 11.7 Simulation Results with CRM

Dose Level	1	2	3	4	5	6	7
Dose	30	45	68	101	151	228	342
$P_{DLT}(\%)$	1	1.2	1.5	2.2	3.7	8.4	25
$\hat{P}_{DLT}(\%)$	.9	1.1	1.4	2.2	4.1	10.3	30
$\sigma_{DLT}(\%)$	1	1	0.3	0.6	1.5	5.2	15
n	1	1	1	1	1.24	9.24	6.5

$P_{DLT} = DLT$ rate, $\hat{P}_{DLT}$ and σ_{DLT} are the predicted rate and its standard deviation, n = number of patients.

were used for each trial or simulation. The results are summarized in Table 11.8.

In this example, the CRM produces excellent predictions for the DLT rates. We can see that one of the advantages with CRM is that it produces the posterior parameter distribution and predicted probability of DLT for each dose level (any dose) and allows us to select an unplanned dose level as the MTD. In the current case, the true MTD is 300 mg/m² with a DLT rate $P_{DLT} = 0.17$, which is an unplanned dose level. As long as the dose-response model is appropriately selected, bias can be avoided. This is an advantage compared to TER or TSER discussed in the previous example. The simulations also indicate that the number of DLTs per trial is 2.5. The number of patients treated with dose higher than MTD is 6.5 per trial. These numbers are larger than those in TER and TSER, which can be viewed as a trade-off for bias reduction.

11.5.2 Late phases development

To investigate the effect of the adaptations, we will compare the classic, group sequential, and adaptive designs with regards to their operating

Table 11.8 Group Sequential Design

Dose Level	Control	Active
Number of patients	244	244
Response rate	0.2	0.3
Observed rate	0.198	0.303
Standard deviation	0.028	0.033

characteristics using computer simulations. In what follows, each example represents a different trial design. Examples 3 through 6 assume a phase II oncology trial with two treatment groups. The primary endpoint is tumor response (PR and CR), and the estimated response rates for the two groups are 0.2 and 0.3, respectively. We use simulation to calculate the sample size required, given that one-sided alpha = 0.05 and power = 80%. Note that a classical fixed sample size design with 600 subjects will have a power of 81.4% at one-sided $\alpha = 0.025$. The total number of responses per trial is 150 based on 10,000 simulations.

Example 11.3 Flexible design with sample size re-estimation In practice, since the power of a trial depends upon the estimated effect size, it is desirable to have a design that allows modification of the sample size at some points of time during the conduct of the trial. Let us design a trial that allows a sample size re-estimation and evaluate the robustness of the design. In order to control the family-wise error rate (FWE) at 0.025, the alpha must be adjusted to 0.023, which can be done by computer simulation under the null hypothesis. The average sample size is 960 under the null hypothesis. Using the algorithm for sample size re-estimation (1), where $E_{0\,\max} = 0.1633$ and $a = 2$, the design has 92% power with an average sample size of 821.5. Now assume that the initial effect sizes are not 0.2 versus 0.3 for the two treatment groups. Instead, they are 0.2 and 0.28, respectively. We want to know what power the flexible design will have. Keep everything the same (also keep $E_{0\,\max} = 0.1633$), but change the response rates to 0.2 and 0.28 for the two dose levels and run the simulation again. It turns out that the design has 79.4% power with an average sample size of 855. Given the two response rates 0.2 and 0.28, the design with a fixed sample size of 880 has a power of 79.4%. We can see that there is a saving of 25 patients by using the flexible design. If the response rates are 0.2 and 0.3, for 92.1% power, the required sample size is 828 with the fixed sample size design, which means that the flexible design saves 6–7 subjects. A flexible design increases power when observed effect size is less than expected, while a traditional design with a fixed sample size either increases or decreases the power regardless of the observed effect size when the sample increases.

Example 11.4 Design with play-the-winner randomization To randomize more patients to the superior treatment group using response-adaptive randomization, the same example with a sample size of 600 subjects is used. The commonly used response-adaptive randomization is RPW(1,1), i.e., one initial ball for each group and one additional ball with the corresponding color for each response. The data will be unblinded for every 100 new patients. The adjusted alpha is found to be 0.02. The design has 77.3% power with an average sample size of 600. On average, there are 223 subjects in dose level 1 and 377 in dose level 2. The expected number of responses is 158. Comparing this to the classical design, the RPW design gains 8 responses, but loses 4% in power.

Example 11.5 Group sequential design with one Interim analysis Group sequential design is very popular in clinical trials. For the two-arm trial, the adjusted alpha is found to be 0.024. The maximum number of subjects is 700. The trial will stop if 350 or more patients are randomized and one of the following criteria is met: (1) The efficacy (utility) stopping criterion: The maximum difference in response rate between any dose and the control is larger than 0.1 with the lower bound of the two-sided 95% naive confidence interval greater than or equal to 0.0; or (2) The futility stopping criterion: The maximum difference in response rate between any dose and dose level 1 is less than 0.05 with the upper bound of the one-sided 95% naive confidence interval less than 0.1.

The average total number of subjects for each trial is 488. The total number of responses per trial is 122. The probability of correctly predicting the most responsive dose level is 0.988 based on observed rates. Under the alternative hypothesis, the probability of early stopping for efficacy is 0.505, and the probability of early stopping for futility is 0.104. The power for testing the treatment difference is 0.825.

Example 11.6 Adaptive design permitting early stopping and sample size re-estimation Sometimes it is desirable to have a design permitting both early stopping and sample size modification.

With an initial sample size of 700 subjects, a grouping size of 350, and a maximum sample size of 1000, the one-sided adjusted alpha is found to be 0.05. The simulation results are presented as follows:

The maximum sample size is 700. The trial will stop if 350 patients or more are randomized and one of the following criteria is met: (1) The efficacy (utility) stopping criterion: The maximum difference in response rate between any dose and the control is larger than 0.1 with the lower bound of the two-sided 95% naive confidence interval greater than or equal to 0.0; or (2) The futility stopping criterion: The maximum difference in response rate between any dose and the control is less than 0.05 with the upper bound of the one-sided 95% naive confidence interval less than 0.1. The sample size will be re-estimated when 350 subjects have been randomized. When the null hypothesis is true ($p_1 = p_2 = 0.2$), the average total number of subjects for each trial is 398.8. The probability

Table 11.9 Design with Early Stopping and n-Re-estimation

Dose Level	Control	Active
Number of patients	271	272
Response rate	0.2	0.3
Observed rate	0.198	0.303
Standard deviation	0.028	0.032

of early stopping for efficacy is 0.0096. The probability of early stopping for futility is 0.9638.

When the alternative hypothesis is true ($p_1 = 0.2$, $p_2 = 0.3$), the average total number of subjects for each trial is 543.5. The total number of responses per trial is 136 (Table 11.9). The probability of correctly predicting the most responsive dose level is 0.985 based on observed rates. The probability of early stopping for efficacy is 0.6225. The probability of early stopping for futility is 0.1546. The power for testing the treatment difference is 0.842. Examples 11.7 through 11.9 are for the same scenario as the six-arm study with response rates of 0.5, 0.4, 0.5, 0.6, 0.7, and 0.55 for the 6 dose levels from doses 1 through 6, respectively.

Example 11.7 Conventional design with multiple treatment groups With 800 subjects, a 0.5 response rate under H_0, and a grouping size of 100, we found the one-sided adjusted α to be 0.0055. The total number of responses per trial is 433. The probability of correctly predicting the most responsive dose level is 0.951 based on observed rates. The power for testing the maximum effect comparing any dose level to the control is 80%. The powers for comparing each of the 5 dose levels to the control are 0, 0.008, 0.2, 0.796, and 0.048, respectively.

Example 11.8 Response-adaptive design with multiple treatment groups To further investigate the effect of Random-Play-the-Winner randomization RPW(1,1), a design with 800 subjects, a grouping

Table 11.10 Design with RPW(1,1) under H_0

Dose Level	1	2	3	4	5	6
Response rate	0.5	0.5	0.5	0.5	0.5	0.5
Observed rate	0.50	0.49	0.49	0.49	0.49	0.49

Table 11.11 Design with RPW(1,1) Under H_a

Dose Level	1	2	3	4	5	6
No. of subjects	200	74	100	133	176	116
Response rate	0.5	0.4	0.5	0.6	0.7	0.55
Observed rate	0.50	0.39	0.49	0.59	0.7	0.54

size of 100, and a response rate of 0.2 under the null hypothesis is simulated (Table 11.10). The one-sided adjusted α is found to be 0.016. Using this adjusted alpha and response rates 0.5, 0.4, 0.5, 0.6, 0.7, and 0.55 for dose levels 1 through 6, respectively, the simulation indicates that the designed trial has 86% power and 447 responders per trial on average (Table 11.11). In comparison to 80% power and 433 responders for the design with simple randomization RPW(1,0), the adaptive randomization is superior in both power and number of responders. The simulation results also indicate that there are biases in the estimated mean response rates in all dose levels except dose level 1, where a fixed randomization rate is used.

The average total number of subjects for each trial is 800. The total number of responses per trial is 446.8. The probability of correctly predicting the most responsive dose level is 0.957 based on observed rates. The power for testing the maximum effect comparing any dose level to the control (dose level 1) is 0.861 at a one-sided significance level (alpha) of 0.016. The powers for comparing each of the 5 dose levels to the control are 0, 0.008, 0.201, 0.853, and 0.051, respectively.

Example 11.9 Adaptive design with dropping the losers Implementing the mechanism of dropping losers can also improve the efficiency of a design. With 800 subjects, a grouping size of 100, a response rate of 0.2 under the null hypothesis, and a fixed randomization rate in dose level 1 at 0.25, an inferior group (loser) will be dropped if the maximum difference in response between the most effective group and the least effective group (loser) is greater than 0 with the lower bound of the one-sided 95% naive confidence interval greater than or equal

Table 11.12 Bias in Rate with Dropping Losers Under H_0

Dose Level	1	2	3	4	5	6
Response rate	0.5	0.5	0.5	0.5	0.5	0.5
Observed rate	0.50	0.46	0.46	0.46	0.46	0.46

Table 11.13 Bias in Rate with Dropping Losers under H_a

Dose Level	1	2	3	4	5	6
No. of subjects	200	26	68	172	240	95
Response rate	0.5	0.4	0.5	0.6	0.7	0.55
Observed rate	0.50	0.37	0.46	0.57	0.69	0.51

to 0. Using the simulation, the adjusted alpha is found to be 0.079. From the simulation results in Tables 11.12 and 11.13, biases can be observed with this design. The design has 90% power with 467 responders. The probability of correctly predicting the most responsive dose level is 0.965 based on observed rates. The powers for comparing each of the 5 dose levels to the control (dose level 1) are 0.001, 0.007, 0.205, 0.889, and 0.045, respectively. The design is superior to both RPW(1,0) and RPW(1,1).

Example 11.10 Dose-response trial design The trial objective is to find the optimal dose with the highest response rate. There are 5 dose levels and 30 planned subjects in each simulation (Table 11.14). The hyper-logistic model is defined with the parameters $a_3 \in [20, 100]$ and $a_4 \in [0, 0.05]$. The $RPW(1, 1)$ is used for the randomization. The simulation results show that the probability of correctly predicting the most responsive dose level is 0.992 by the model and only 0.505 based on observed rates.

11.6 Concluding Remarks

From classic design to group sequential design to adaptive design, each step forward increases in complexity and at the same time improves the efficiency of clinical trials as a whole. Adaptive designs can increase the

Table 11.14 Dose-Response Trial Design

Dose Level	1	2	3	4	5
No. of subjects	15	30	50	85	110
Response rate	0.2	0.3	0.6	0.7	0.5
Observed rate	0.193	0.294	0.593	0.691	0.489
Predicted rate	0.098	0.181	0.406	0.802	0.379
σ_{obs}	0.185	0.209	0.221	0.204	0.226
σ_{prd}	0.074	0.073	0.104	0.151	0.056

number of responses in a trial and provide more benefits to the patient in comparison to the classic design. With sample size re-estimation, an adaptive design can preserve the power even when the initial estimations of treatment effect and its variability are inaccurate. In the case of a multiple-arm trial, dropping inferior arms or response-adaptive randomization can improve the efficiency of a design dramatically. Finding analytic solutions for adaptive designs is theoretically challenging. However, computer simulation makes it easier to achieve an optimal adaptive design. It allows a wide range of test statistics as long as they are monotonic functions of treatment effects. Adjusted alpha and p-values due to response-adaptive randomization and other adaptations with multiple comparisons can be determined easily using computer simulations. Unbias in point estimations with adaptive designs has not been completely resolved by using computer simulations. However, the bias can be ignored in practice by using a proper grouping size (cluster) such that there are only a limited number of adaptations (<8).

Simulations have many applications in clinical trials. In early phases of the clinical development with many uncertainties (variables), clinical trial simulation can be used to assess the impacts of the variables. Clinical trial simulation with the Bayesian approach could produce certain desirable operating characteristics that can answer questions raised in the early development phase such as posterior distribution of toxicity. There are a few things we should caution about with regard to clinical trial simulation. The quality of simulation results is very much dependent on the quality of the pseudo-random number. We should be aware that most built-in random number generators in computer languages and software tools are poor in quality; therefore it should not be used directly if we are not sure about the algorithm. Implementing a high-quality of random number generator is as simple as a dozen of lines of computer code (Press et al., 2002; Gentle, 1998) as implemented by ExpDesign Studio®. The common steps for conducting a clinical trial simulation include defining the objectives, analyzing the problem, assessing the scope of the work and proposing time and resources required to complete the task, examining the assumptions, obtaining and validating the data source if applicable, nailing down evaluation criteria for various trial designs/scenarios, selecting an appropriate software tool, outlining the computer algorithms for the simulation, implementing and validating the algorithms, proposing scenarios to simulate, conducting simulations, interpreting results and making recommendations, and last but not least, addressing the limitations of the performed simulations.

We have demonstrated that clinical trial simulation can be used for various complex designs. By comparing the operating characteristics of each design provided by clinical trial simulation, we are able to choose an optimal design or development strategy. Computer simulation is commonly seen in statistics literature related to clinical trials, most of them for power calculations and data analyses. We will see more pharmaceutical companies using clinical trial simulation for their clinical development planning to streamline the drug process, increase the probability of success, and reduce the cost and time-to-market. Ultimately, clinical trial simulation will bring the best treatment to the patients. When conducting clinical trial simulation for an adaptive design, the following is recommended in order to protect the integrity of the trial: Specify in the trial protocol (i) the type of adaptive design, (ii) details of the adaptations to be used, (iii) the estimator for treatment effect, and (iv) the hypotheses and the test statistics. Run the simulation under the null hypothesis and construct the distribution of the test statistic. To estimate the sample size for the adaptive design, run the simulation under the alternative hypothesis and construct the distribution of the test statistic. Sensitivity analyses are suggested to simulate potential major protocol deviations that would impact the validity of the trial simulations. To achieve an optimal design, a Bayesian or frequentist-Bayesian hybrid adaptive approach should be used. There are several simulation tools available on the Web. For adaptive designs discussed in this section, the ExpDesign Studio® can be used.

CHAPTER 12

Case Studies

As indicated earlier, the adaptation or modification made to a clinical trial includes prospective adaptation (by design), concurrent or on-going adaptation (ad hoc), and retrospective adaptation (at the end of the trial and prior to database lock or unblinding). Different adaptation or modification could lead to different adaptive designs with different levels of complexity. In practice, it is suggested that by design prospective adaptation be considered at the planning stage of a clinical trial (Gallo et al., 2006), although it may not reflect real practice in the conduct of clinical trials. Li (2006) pointed out that the use of adaptive design methods (either by design adaptation or ad hoc adaptation) provides a second chance to re-design the trial after seeing data internally or externally at interim. However, it may introduce so-called operational biases such as selection bias, method of evaluations, early withdrawal, and modification of treatments. Consequently, the adaptation employed may inflate type I error rate. Uchida (2006) also indicated that these biases could be translated to information (assessment) biases, which may include (i) patient enrollment, (ii) differential dropouts in favor of one treatment, (iii) crossover of the other treatment, (iv) protocol deviation due to additional medications/treatments, and (v) differential assessment of the treatments. As a result, it is difficult to interpret the clinically meaningful effect size for the treatments under study (see also, Quinlan, Gallo, and Krams, 2006).

In the next section, basic considerations when implementing adaptive design methods in clinical trials are given. Successful experience for the implementation of adaptive group sequential design (see, e.g., Cui, Hung, and Wang, 1999), adaptive dose-escalation design (see, e.g., Chang and Chow, 2005), and adaptive seamless phase II/III trial design (see, e.g., Maca et al., 2006) are discussed in Section 12.2, Section 12.3, and Section 12.4, respectively.

12.1 Basic Considerations

As discussed in early chapters of this book, the motivation behind the use of adaptive design methods in clinical trials includes (i) the flexibility in modifying trial and statistical procedures for identifying best clinical benefits of a compound under study and (ii) the efficiency in shortening the development time of the compound. In addition, adaptive designs provide the investigator a second chance to re-design the trial with more relevant data observed (internally) or clinical information available (externally) at interim. The flexibility and efficiency are very attractive to investigators and/or sponsors. However, major adaptation may alter trial conduct and consequently result in a biased assessment of the treatment effect. Li (2006) suggested a couple of principles when implementing adaptive designs in clinical trials: (i) adaptation should not alter trial conduct and (ii) type I error should be preserved. Following these principles, some studies with complicated adaptation may be more successful than others. In what follows, some basic considerations when implementing adaptive design methods in clinical trials are discussed.

12.1.1 Dose and dose regimen

Dose selection is an integral part of clinical development. An inadequate selection of dose for a large confirmatory trial could lead to a failure of the development of the compound under study. Traditional dose-escalation and/or dose de-escalation studies are not efficient. The objective of dose or dose regimen selection is not only to select the best dose group but also to drop the least efficacious or unsafe dose group with limited number of patients available. Under this consideration, adaptive designs with appropriate adaptation in selection criteria and decision rules are useful.

12.1.2 Study endpoints

Maca et al. (2006) suggested that well-established and well-understood study endpoints or surrogate markers be considered when implementing adaptive design methods in clinical trials, especially when the trial is to learn about the primary endpoints to be carried forward into later phase clinical trials. An adaptive design would not be feasible for clinical trials without well-established or well-understood study endpoints due to (i) uncertainty of the treatment effect and (ii) the fact that a clinically meaningful difference cannot be determined.

12.1.3 Treatment duration

For a given study endpoint, treatment duration is critical in order to reach the optimal therapeutic effect. If the treatment duration is short relative to the time needed to enroll all patients planned for the study, then an adaptive design such as response-adaptive randomization design is feasible. On the other hand, if the treatment duration is too long, too many patients would be randomized during the period, which could result in unacceptable inefficiencies. In this case, it is suggested that an adaptive biomarker design be considered.

12.1.4 Logistical considerations

Logistical considerations relative to the feasibility of adaptive designs in clinical trials include, but are not limited to, (i) drug management, (ii) site management, and (iii) procedural consideration. For costly and/or complicated dose regimens drug packaging and drug supply could be a challenge to the use of adaptive design methods in clinical trials, especially when the adaptive design allows dropping the inferior dose groups. Site management is the selection of qualified study sites and patient recruitment for the trial. For some adaptive designs, recruitment rate is crucial to the success of the trial, especially when the intention of the trial is to shorten the time of development. Procedural considerations are decision processes and dissemination of information in order to maintain the validity and integrity of the trial.

12.1.5 Independent data monitoring committee

When implementing an adaptive design in a clinical trial, an independent data monitoring committee (DMC) is necessarily considered for maintaining the validity and integrity of the clinical trial. A typical example is the implementation of an adaptive group sequential design which cannot only allow stopping a trial early due to safety and/or futility/efficacy, but also address sample size re-estimation based on the review of unblinded data. In addition, DMC conveys some limited information to investigators or sponsors about treatment effects, procedural conventions, and statistical methods with recommendations so that the adaptive design methods can be implemented with less difficulty.

12.2 Adaptive Group Sequential Design

12.2.1 Group sequential design

Group sequential design is probably one of the most commonly used clinical trial designs in clinical research and development. As indicated in Chapter 6, the primary reasons for conducting interim analyses of accrued data are probably due to (i) ethical consideration, (ii) administrative reasons, and (iii) economic constraints. Group sequential design is very attractive because it allows stopping a trial early due to (i) safety, (ii) futility, and/or (iii) efficacy. Moreover, it also allows adaptive sample size adjustment at interim either blinding or unblinding through an independent data monitoring committee (DMC).

12.2.2 Adaptation

Basic adaptation strategy for an adaptive group sequential design is that one or more interim analyses may be planned. In practice, it is desirable to stop a trial early if the test compound is found to be ineffective or not safe. However, it is not desirable to terminate a trial early if the test compound is promising. To achieve these goals, data safety monitoring and interim analyses for efficacy are necessarily performed. Note that how to control the overall type I error rate and how to determine treatment effect that the trial should be powered at the time of interim analyses would be the critical issues for this adaptation.

At each interim analysis, an adaptive sample size adjustment based on unblinded interim results and/or external clinical information available at interim may be performed. In practice, at the planning stage of a clinical trial, a pre-study power analysis is usually conducted based on some initial estimates of the within or between patient variation and the clinically meaningful difference to be detected. This crucial information is usually not available or it is available (e.g., data from small pilot studies) with a high degree of uncertainty (Chuang-Stein, et al., 2006). Lee, Wang, and Chow (2006) showed that sample size obtained based on estimates from small pilot studies is highly unstable. Thus, there is a need to adjust sample size adaptively at interim. Mehta and Patel (2003) and Offen et al. (2006) also discussed other situations where sample size re-estimation at interim is necessary. The use of an independent data monitoring committee (DMC) would be the critical issue for this adaptation.

Other adaptations such as adaptive hypotheses from a superiority trial to a non-inferiority trial may be considered. In practice, interim results may indicate that the trial will never achieve statistical significance at the end of the trial. In this case, the sponsors may consider changing the hypotheses or study endpoints to increase the probability of success of the trial. A typical example is to switch from superiority hypotheses to non-inferiority hypotheses. At the end of the trial, final analysis will be performed for testing non-inferiority rather than superiority. Note that superiority can still be tested after the non-inferiority has been established without paying any statistical penalty due to closed testing procedure. Note that the determination of non-inferiority margin would be the challenge for this adaptation.

12.2.3 Statistical methods

For the adaptation of interim analyses, statistical methods as described in Chapter 6 for controlling overall type I error rate are useful. For the adaptation of sample size re-estimation, the methods proposed by Cui, Hung, and Wang (1999), Fisher's combination of p-values, error-function method, inverse normal method, or linear combination of p-values can be used. For the adaptation of switching hypotheses, statistical methods discussed in Chapter 4 are useful. As indicated by Chuang-Stein et al. (2006), since the weighting of the normal statistics will not, in general, be proportional to the sample size for that stage, the method does not use the sufficient statistics (the unweighted mean difference and estimated standard deviation from combined stages) for testing, and is therefore less efficient (Tsiatis and Mehta, 2003). Additional discussion on efficiency can be found in Burman and Sonesson (2006) and Jennison and Turnbull (2006a).

12.2.4 Case study — an example

For illustration purposes, consider the example given in Cui, Hung, and Wang (1999). This example considers a phase III two-arm trial for evaluating the effect of a new drug for prevention of myocardial infection (MI) in patients undergoing coronary artery bypass graft surgery. It was estimated that a sample size of 300 patients per group would give a 95% power for detecting a 50% reduction in incidence rate from 22% to 11% at the one-sided significance level of $\alpha = 0.025$. Although the sponsor was confident about the incidence rate of 11% in the control group, they were not sure about the 11% incidence rate in the test group. Thus, an interim analysis was planned to allow for sample size re-estimation based on observed treatment difference. The interim analysis was scheduled when 50% of the patients were enrolled and had their efficacy assessment. The adaptive group sequential using the method of Fisher's combination of stage-wise p-values was considered. The decision rules were: at stage 1, stop for futility if the stage-wise p-value $p_1 > \alpha_0$ and stop for efficacy if $p_1 \leq \alpha_1$; at the final stage, if $p_1 p_2 \leq C_\alpha$, claim efficacy; otherwise claim futility. The stopping boundary was chosen from Table 7.4. The futility boundary $\alpha_0 = 0.5$, the efficacy stopping boundary $\alpha_1 = 0.0102$ at stage 1 and $C_\alpha = 0.0038$ at the final stage. The upper limit of the sample size is $N_{max} = 800$ per group. The futility boundary was used to stop the trial in the case of very small effect size because in such a case, to continue the trial would result in an unrealistic large sample size or N_{max} with insufficient power. The adaptive group sequential design would have a 99.6% power when the incidence rates were 22% and 11%, and an 80% power when the incidence rates were 22% and 16.5%.

At interim analysis based on data from 300 patients, it was observed that the test group had an incidence rate of 16.5% and 11% in the control group. If these incidence rates were the true incidence rates, the power for the classical design would be about 40%. Under the adaptive group sequential design, the sample size was re-estimated to be 533 per group. If the 16.5% and 11% are the true incidence rates, the conditional power is given by 88.6%.

Remarks Note that the trial was originally designed not allowing for sample size re-estimation. The sponsor requested sample size re-estimation and was rejected by the FDA. The trial eventually failed to demonstrate statistical significance. In practice, it is recommended that the adaptation for sample size re-estimation be considered in the study protocol and an independent data monitoring committee (DMC) be established to perform sample size re-estimation based on the review of unblinded date at interim to maintain the validity and integrity of the trial.

12.3 Adaptive Dose-Escalation Design

12.3.1 Traditional dose-escalation design

As discussed in Chapter 5, the traditional "3 + 3" escalation rule is commonly considered in phase I dose-escalation trials for oncology. The "3 + 3" rule is to enter three patients at a new dose level and then enter another three patients when dose limiting toxicity is observed. The assessment of the six patients is then performed to determine whether the trial should be stopped at the level or to increase the dose. The goal is to find the maximum tolerated dose (MTD). The traditional "3 + 3" rule (TER) is not efficient with respect to the number of dose limiting toxicities and the estimation of MTD. There is a practical need to have a better design method that will reduce the number of patients and number of DLTs, and at the same time have a more precise estimation of MTD. We will use Bayesian continual reassessment method (CRM) to achieve our goals.

12.3.2 Adaptation

The basic adaptation strategy for an adaptive dose-escalation trial design is change in traditional escalation rule (TER). As discussed in Chapter 5, the traditional 3 + 3 dose-escalation rule is not efficient. As a result, a m + n dose-escalation rule may be considered with some pre-specified selection criteria based on the dose limiting toxicity (DLT). Other adaptations that are commonly considered include the application of adaptation to the design characteristics such as the selection of starting dose, the determination of dose levels, prior information on the maximum tolerable dose (MTD), dose toxicity model (Figure 12.1), stopping rules, and statistical methods.

12.3.3 Statistical methods

As indicated earlier, many methods such as the assessment of dose response using multiple-stage designs (Crowley, 2001) and the continued re-assessment method (CRM) are available in the literature for assessment of dose-escalation trials. For the method of CRM, the dose-response relationship is continually re-assessed based on accumulative data collected from the trial. The next patient who enters the trial is then assigned to the potential MTD level. This approach is more efficient than that of the usual TER with respect to the allocation of the MTD. However, the efficiency of CRM may be at risk due to delayed response and/or a constraint on dosejump in practice (Babb and Rogatko, 2004). Chang and Chow (2005) proposed an adaptive method that combines CRM and utility-adaptive randomization (UAR) for multiple-endpoint trials. The proposed UAR is an extension of the response-adaptive randomization (RAR). Note that the CRM could be a Bayesian, a frequentist, or a hybrid frequentist-Bayesian–based approach. As pointed out by Chang and Chow (2005), this method has the advantage of achieving the optimal design by means of the adaptation to the accrued data of an on-going trial. In addition, CRM could provide a better prediction of dose-response relationship by selecting an appropriate model as compared to the method simply based on the observed response.

12.3.4 Case study — an example

A trial is designed to establish the dose toxicity relationship and to identify maximum tolerable dose (MTD) for a compound in treatment of patients with metastatic androgen independent prostate cancer. Based on pre-clinical data, the estimated MTD is about 400 mg/m^2. The modified

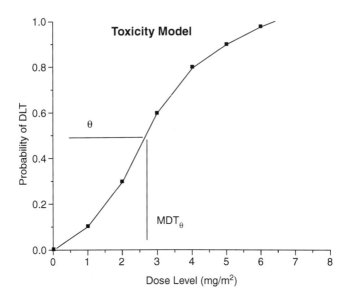

Figure 12.1 Example of dose-toxicity model.

Fibonacci series is chosen for the dose levels (Table 12.1). Eight dose levels are considered in this trial with the option of adding more dose levels if necessary. The initial dose level is chosen to be 30 mg/m^2, at which about 10% of deaths (MELD10) occur in mice after the verification that no lethal and no life-threatening effects were seen in another species. The toxicity rate (i.e., the DLT rate) at MTD defined for this indication/population is 17%.

We compare the operating characteristics between the traditional escalation rule (TER) design and the CRM design. In CRM, the following logistic model is used:

$$p = \frac{1}{1 + 150\exp(-ax)},$$

where the prior distribution for parameter a is flat over (0,0.12).

Using ExpDesign Studio®, the simulation results are presented as follows. The TER predicts the MTD at dose level 7 (lowest dose level to the true MTD) with a probability of 75%. The CRM predicted the MTD at dose level 7 with a probability of 100% (5000 out of 5000 simulations). The TER requires average 18.2 patients and 2.4 DLTs per trial. CRM requires only 12 patients with 4 DLTs per trial.

Remarks Dose-escalation trial is an early phase trial with flexible adaptation for dose selection using CRM. It is suggested that the protocol

CASE STUDIES 247

Table 12.1 Dose Levels and DLT Rates

Dose Level	1	2	3	4	5	6	7	8
dose	30	60	99	150	211	280	373	496
DLT rate	0.010	0.012	0.017	0.026	0.042	0.071	0.141	0.309

should be submitted to the Regulatory Agencies for review and approval prior to the initiation of the trial. The design characteristics such as starting dose, dose levels, prior information on the MTD, dose toxicity model, escalation rule, and stopping rule should be clearly stated in the study protocol. In practice, there may be a situation that the next patient has enrolled before the response from the previous patient is obtained. In this case, the efficiency of the TER and CRM may be reduced. There may also have been limitation for dose escape which may also reduce the efficiency of the CRM. To investigate this, a simulation was conducted using ExpDesign Studio with cluster randomization of size 3 patients (i.e., 2 patients have enrolled before the response is obtained). In the simulation, we allow for one level of dose escape. Under this scenario, the CRM requires only 12 patients with 1.8 DLTs. It can be seen that with the limitation of dose escalation, the average DLTs per trial is reduced from 4 to 2 without sacrificing the precision. This is because with 12 patients there is enough precision to eliminate the precision loss due to the delayed response. Note that when we use CRM, we need to do the modeling or simulation at real time such that the next dose level can be determined quickly.

12.4 Adaptive Seamless Phase II/III Design

12.4.1 Seamless phase II/III design

A seamless phase II/III trial design is a design that combines a traditional phase IIb trial and a traditional phase III trial into a single trial. As a result, the study objectives of a seamless design are the combination of the objectives which have been traditionally addressed in separate trials. This type of design closes the gap of the time that would have occurred between the two trials which are traditionally conducted separately. Maca et al. (2006) defines an adaptive seamless phase II/III design as a seamless phase II/III design that would use data from patients enrolled before and after the adaptation in the final analysis. Thus, the feasibility and/or efficiency of an adaptive seamless phase II/III trial design depend upon the adaptation employed. In practice, it is possible to combine studies into a seamless design within or across phases of clinical development. Seamless designs are useful in early clinical development since there are opportunities in the seamless transition between phase IIb (learning phase) and phase III (confirming phase).

12.4.2 Adaptation

The basic adaptation strategy for a seamless phase II/III trial design is to drop the inferior arms (or drop the losers) based on some pre-specified criteria at the learning phase. The best arms and the control arm will be retained and advanced to the confirming phase. Other commonly employed adaptations include (i) enrichment process at the learning phase of the trial and (ii) change in treatment allocation at the confirming phase. The enrichment process is commonly employed to identify sub-populations, which are most likely to respond to the treatment or to suffer from adverse events based on some pre-specified criteria on genomic biomarkers. Change in treatment allocation at the confirming phase is not only to have more patients to be assigned to superior arms but also to increase the probability of success of the trial. In practice, it is not uncommon to apply an adaptation on the primary study endpoint. For example, at the learning phase, the treatment effect may be assessed based on a short-term primary efficacy endpoint (or a surrogate endpoint or some biomarkers), while a long-term primary study endpoint is considered at the confirming phase. It should be noted that the impact on statistical inference should be carefully evaluated when implementing an adaptation to a seamless trial design.

12.4.3 Methods

For an adaptive seamless phase II/III trial design, if the trial is not stopped for lack of efficacy after the first stage, we proceed into the second stage. At the end of the second stage, we may calculate the second stage p-value based upon the disjoint sample of the second stage only. The final analysis is conducted by combining the two p-values into a single test statistic using a pre-defined combination function. The method proposed by Sampson and Sill (2005) for dropping the losers in normal case and the contrast test with p-value combination method suggested by Chang, Chow, and Pong (2006) are useful. Note that a data-dependent combination rule should not be used after the first stage. It is suggested that a prior be considered at the planning phase.

CASE STUDIES   249

Thall, Simon, and Ellenberg (1989) proposed a two-stage design for trials with binary outcomes. In their proposed two-stage design, the first stage is used to select the best treatment, and the second stage includes just the selected treatment together with the control. As indicated by Thall, Simon, and Ellenberg (1989), the inclusion of the control in the first stage is crucial because it allows results from that stage to be pooled with the data observed in the second stage. On the other hand, Schaid, Wieand, and Therneau (1990) considered a time-to-event endpoint. Their design not only allows stopping the trial early for efficacy after the first stage, but also allows more than one treatment to continue into the second stage. Stallard and Todd (2003) generalized these designs to allow for the possibility of more than two stages by using error-spending functions. The design is applicable for general endpoint such as normal, binary, ordinal, or survival time. These methods are useful for adaptive seamless phase II/III trial designs.

Remarks Note that the methods considered above are based on the same primary endpoint. As an alternative, Todd and Stallard (2005) considered an adaptive group sequential design that incorporates treatment selection based upon a short-term endpoint, followed by a confirmation stage comparing the selected treatment with control in terms of a long-term primary endpoint.

12.4.4 Case study — some examples

In what follows, several examples are provided to illustrate the implementation of adaptive seamless phase II/III trial designs in clinical trials. The first three examples are adopted from Maca et al. (2006).

Example 12.1 Adaptive Treatment Selection Similar to the study design described in Bauer and Kieser (1999), an adaptive seamless phase II/III two-stage design is considered to evaluate the efficacy and safety of a compound when given in combination with methotrexate to patients with active rheumatoid arthritis (RA) who have had two or more inadequate responses to anti-TNF therapy (Maca et al., 2006). The objectives of this trial include treatment selection and efficacy confirmation. The primary clinical endpoint is ACR-20 (American College of Rheumatology 20 score) at 6 months. The first stage will be used for dose selection, while the second stage is for efficacy confirmation. At the end of the second stage, data obtained from the second stage and the relevant data from the first stage will be combined for final analysis using Fisher's combination test at the significance level of 0.025. In this adaptive seamless phase II/III two-stage design, early stopping is allowed for futility, but not for efficacy.

Qualified subjects will be randomly assigned to five treatment arms (4 active and 1 placebo) in equal ratio. At the end of the first stage, a planned interim analysis will be conducted. The best active treatment arm and the placebo arm will be retained and advanced to the second stage for efficacy confirmation. The best treatment arm will be selected based on a set of pre-defined efficacy, safety, and immunogenicity criteria. Based on interim results, the decisions that (i) the best treatment group (safe and efficacious) will be advanced to the second stage, (ii) the least efficacious and/or unsafe treatment groups will be dropped, and (iii) the futility requirement will be evaluated will be made based upon the clinical endpoint in conjunction with information obtained from early endpoint. To ensure the validity and integrity of the trial design, two committees will be established: one is an external independent data monitoring committee (DMC) and the other one is an internal Executive Decision Committee (EDC).

Example 12.2 Confirming Treatment Effect A seamless phase II/III trial design is employed to confirm substantial treatment effect in patients with neuropathic pain (Maca et al., 2006). The primary endpoint considered in this trial is the PI-NRS score change from baseline to the 8th week of treatment. Qualified patients will be randomly assigned to four treatment groups (three active doses and one placebo) at equal ratio. An adaptation for having two interim analyses is planned prior to the end of the enrollment period. Another adaptation to select best dose and change treatment allocation at first interim is also made. Note that patients are initially equally randomized to three doses of the new compound and placebo. Two interim analyses are planned before the end of the enrollment period. At the second interim, one dose will be selected to continue for confirmation of treatment effect. Final analysis will use a p-value combination test to confirm the superiority of the selected dose over placebo.

As compared to the traditional approach of a phase IIb trial with three doses and placebo based on a short-term endpoint (e.g., 2 weeks change from baseline) followed by a confirmatory phase III trial with a long-term (e.g., 8 week) endpoint, this adaptive design combines the two trials in one study with a single protocol and uses information on the long-term endpoint from patients in the first (learning) and the second (confirmatory) phases of the study. Note that a longitudinal model for the primary endpoint in time (i.e., at 2 weeks, 4 weeks, 6 weeks, and 8 weeks) can be used to improve the estimate of the sustained treatment effect.

Example 12.3 Confirming Efficacy in Sub-population Maca et al. (2006) presented an example concerning a clinical trial using a two-stage adaptive design trial for patients with metastatic breast cancer. This trial has two objectives. First, it is to select patient population at the first stage. Second, it is to confirm the efficacy based on the hazard ratio between treatment and control at the second stage. In addition, a genomic biomarker (expression level) was used. Patients were initially randomized into three treatment arms (two actives and one control) in equal ratio. One interim analysis was planned for this study when the trial reached approximately 60% of the targeted events. During the interim analysis, two sub-populations were defined based on whether the biomarker expression level of each subject of that population exceeded a pre-defined cutoff value. Data were analyzed for efficacy evaluation and safety assessment for both populations. A decision was made based on patients advanced to the second stage. Moreover, a futility was also assessed at this interim analysis. The final analysis was performed using the inverse normal p-value combination test for the selected population to confirm the superiority of the selected dose over control. In contrast to a conventional design with one phase IIb for population selection followed by a confirmatory phase III study, this trial design was able to achieve the same objectives.

Example 12.4 The objective of this trial in patients with asthma is to confirm sustained treatment effect, measured as FEV1 change from baseline to the 1 year of treatment. Initially, patients are equally randomized to four doses of the new compound and placebo. Based on early studies, the estimated FEV1 changes at 4 weeks are 6%, 13%, 15%, 16%, and 17% (with pooled standard deviation 18%) for the placebo (dose level 0), dose level 2, 3, and 4, respectively. One interim analysis is planned when 50% of patients have their short-term efficacy assessment (4-week change from baseline). The interim analysis will lead to either picking the winner (arm with best observed response) or early stopping for futility with a very conservative stopping boundary. The selected dose and placebo will be used at the stage 2. The final analysis will use a sum of the stage-wise p-values from both stages. (Note that the Fisher's combination of p-values was not used because it does not provide a design with futility stopping only. In other work, Fisher's combination is not efficient for adaptive design with no early efficacy stopping.) The stopping boundaries are shortened from Table 7.7: $\alpha_1 = 0$, $\beta_1 = 0.25$, $\alpha_2 = 0.2236$. The decision rule will be: if $p_1 > \beta_1$, stop the trial; if $p_1 \leq \beta_1$, proceed to the second stage. At the final analysis, if $p_1 + p_2 \leq 0.2236$, claim efficacy, otherwise claim futility. The p_1 is the p-value from a contrast test based on sub-sample from stage 1 (See Table 12.2 for contrasts).

With the maximum sample size of 120 per group, the power is 91.2% at overall one-sided α−level of 0.025. The expected total sample size is

Table 12.2 Seamless Design

Arms	0	1	2	3	4
4-week FEV1 change	0.06	0.12	0.13	0.14	0.15
Contrasts	−0.54	0.12	0.13	0.14	0.15

240 and 353 under the null hypothesis and the alternative hypothesis, respectively. As mentioned earlier, the method controls the type I error under global null hypothesis.

12.4.5 Issues and recommendations

Adaptive seamless trial designs are very attractive to the sponsors in pharmaceutical development. They help in identifying best treatment in a more efficient way with certain accuracy and reliability within a relatively short time frame. In practice, the following issues are commonly encountered when implementing a seamless trial design.

Clinical development time

As indicated earlier, the primary rationale behind the use of an adaptive seamless trial design is to shorten the time of development. Thus, it is important to consider whether a seamless development program would accomplish the goal for reducing the development time. In practice, it is clear if the seamless trial is the only pivotal trial required for regulatory submission. However, if the seamless trial is one of the two pivotal trials required for registration, the second pivotal trial should be completed in a timely fashion, which can shorten the overall development time. During the planning stage, the additional time required for the second seamless trial must be included in the evaluation of the overall clinical development time.

Statistical inference

As indicated by Maca et al. (2006), data analysis for seamless trials may be problematic due to bias induced by the adaptation employed. This bias of the maximum likelihood estimate of the effect of the selected treatment over the control could lead to an inaccurate coverage for the associated confidence interval. As a result, it is suggested that the test comparing the selected treatment with the control must be adjusted to give a correct type I error rate. Estimates of treatment effect must also be adjusted to avoid statistical bias and produce confidence intervals with correct coverage probability. Brannath, Koening, and Bauer (2003) derived a set of repeated confidence intervals by exploiting the duality of hypothesis tests and confidence intervals. This approach, however, is strictly conservative if the trial stops at the interim analysis. Alternatively, Posch et al. (2005) proposed a more general approach: to use for each null hypothesis a different combination test. Stallard and Todd (2005) evaluated the bias of the maximum likelihood estimate and proposed a bias-adjusted estimate. Using a stage-wise ordering of the sample space, they also constructed a confidence region for the selected treatment effect.

Decision process

Seamless Phase II/III trials usually involve critical decision making at the end of the learning phase. A typical approach is to establish an independent data monitoring committee (DMC) to monitor ongoing trials. For an adaptive seamless phase II/III trial design, the decision process may require additional expertise not usually represented on DMCs, which may require a sponsor's input or at least a sponsor's ratification on DMC's recommendation. Maca et al. (2006) pointed out several critical aspects that are relevant to the decision process in seamless phase II/III designs. These critical aspects include (i) composition of the decision board, (ii) process for producing analysis results, (iii) sponsor representation, (iv) information inferable from the selection decision, and (v) regulatory perspectives.

For the composition of the decision board, it is not clear whether all of the study objectives or adaptation of a seamless trial at the learning phase should be addressed by the same board or by separate boards. There seems to be no universal agreement on which approach is correct. Maca et al. (2006) suggested that if it is decided that a single board would suffice, then at a minimum, it should be strongly considered whether the composition of the board should be broadened to include individuals not normally represented on a DMC who have proper perspective and experience in making the selection decision; for example, individuals with safety monitoring expertise may not have relevant experience in dose selection. On the other hand, if separate boards are used, then the members of the board making the selection decision should in general only review unblinded data at the selection point and should only see results relevant to the decision they are charged to make. For the process of producing analysis results, results should be produced by an independent statistician and/or programmer who should provide the results directly to the appropriate DMC for review.

For sponsor representation, as indicated in a recent FDA guidance, the following principles should be followed (FDA, 2005):

- Sponsor representatives who will participate in the recommendation, or be allowed to ratify the recommendation, are adequately distanced from trial activities, i.e., they do not have other trial responsibilities, and should have limited direct contact with people who are involved in the day-to-day management of the trial.
- Sponsor representation is minimal to meet the needs, i.e., the smallest number of sponsor representatives which can provide the necessary perspective is involved, these individuals see the minimum amount of unblinded information needed to participate in the decision process, and only at the decision point.
- Appropriate protections and firewalls are in place to ensure that knowledge is appropriately limited; e.g., procedures and responsibilities are clearly documented and understood by all parties involved, confidentiality agreements reflecting these are produced, secure data access and transfer processes are in place, etc.

For information inferable from the selection decision, as a general principle, knowledge regarding which treatment groups continue into the confirming phase should be perceived to provide only minimal information without potentially biasing the conduct of the trial. There should be caution to limit the information to personnel who may infer from a particular selection decision. For regulatory perspectives, it is strongly recommended that a regulatory reviewer be consulted when implementing adaptive seamless trial designs in appropriate clinical development programs in order to maintain the validity and integrity of the trial.

Bibliography

Arbuck, S. G. (1996). Workshop on phase I study design. *Annals of Oncology*, 7, 567–573.

Atkinson, A. C. (1982). Optimum biased coin designs for sequential clinical trials with prognostic factors. *Biometrika*, 69, 61–67.

Atkinson, A. C. and Donev, A. N. (1992). *Optimum Experimental Designs*. Oxford University Press, New York, New York.

Babb, J. S. and Rogatko, A. (2001). Patient specific dosing in a cancer phase I clinical trial. *Statistics in Medicine*, 20, 2079–2090.

Babb, J. S. and Rogatko, A. (2004). Bayesian methods for cancer phase I clinical trials. In *Advances in Clinical Trial Biostatistics*, Geller, Nancy L. (ed.). Marcel Dekker, New York, New York.

Babb, J., Rogatko, A., and Zacks, S. (1998). Cancer phase I clinical trials. Efficient dose escalation with overdose control. *Statistics in Medicine*, 17, 1103–1120.

Bandyopadhyay, U. and Biswas, A. (1997). Some sequential tests in clinical trials based on randomized play-the-winner rule. *Calcutta. Stat. Assoc. Bull.*, 47, 67–89.

Banerjee, A. and Tsiatis, A. A. (2006). Adaptive two-stage designs in phase II clinical trials. *Statistics in Medicine*, in press.

Bauer, P. (1999). Multistage testing with adaptive designs (with discussion). *Biometrie und Informatik in Medizin und Biologie*, 20, 130–148.

Bauer, P. and Kieser, M. (1999). Combining different phases in development of medical treatments within a single trial. *Statistics in Medicine*, 18, 1833–1848.

Bauer, P. and Köhne, K. (1994). Evaluation of experiments with adaptive interim analysis. *Biometrics*, 50, 1029–1041.

Bauer, P. and Köhne, K. (1996). Evaluation of experiments with adaptive interim analyses. *Biometrics*, 52, 380 (Correction).

Bauer, P. and König, F. (2006). The reassessment of trial perspectives from interim data – A critical view. *Statistics in Medicine*, 25, 23–36.

Bauer, P. and Röhmel, J. (1995). An adaptive method for establishing a dose-response relationship. *Statistics in Medicine*, 14, 1595–1607.

Bechhofer, R. E., Kiefer, J., and Sobel, M. (1968). *Sequential Identification and Ranking Problems*. University of Chicago Press, Chicago, Illinois.

Berry, D. A. (2005). Introduction to Bayesian methods III: Use and interpretation of Bayesian tools in design and analysis. *Clinical Trials*, 2, 295–300.

Berry, D. A. and Eick, S. G. (1995). Adaptive assignment versus balanced randomization in clinical trials: A decision analysis. *Statistics in Medicine*, 14, 231–246.

Berry, D. A. and Fristedt, B. (1985). *Bandit Problems: Sequential Allocation of Experiments*. Chapman and Hall, London.

Berry, D. A., Müller, P., Grieve, A. P., Smith, M., Parke, T., Blazek, R., Mitchard, N., and Krams, M. (2002). Adaptive Bayesian designs for dose-ranging drug trials. In *Case Studies in Bayesian Statistics V*. Lecture Notes in Statistics. Springer, New York, 162–181.

Berry, D. A. and Stangl, D. K. (1996). *Bayesian Biostatistics*. Marcel Dekker, New York, New York.

Birkett, N. J. (1985). Adaptive allocation in randomized controlled trials. *Controlled Clinical Trials*, 6, 146–155.

Bischoff, W. and Miller, F. (2005). Adaptive two-stage test procedures to find the best treatment in clinical trials. *Biometrika*, 92, 197–212.

Blackwell, D. and Hodges, J. L. Jr. (1957). Design for the control of selection bias. *Annal. of Mathematical Statistics*, 28, 449–460.

Brannath, W., Koening, F., and Bauer, P. (2003). Improved repeated confidence bounds in trials with a maximal goal. *Biometrical Journal*, 45, 311–324.

Brannath, W., Posch, M., and Bauer, P. (2002). Recursive combination tests. *Journal of American Statistical Association*, 97, 236–244.

Branson, M. and Whitehead, W. (2002). Estimating a treatment effect in survival studies in which patients switch treatment. *Statistics in Medicine*, 21, 2449–2463.

Bretz, F. and Hothorn, L. A. (2002). Detecting dose-response using contrasts: Asymptotic power and sample size determination for binary data. *Statistics in Medicine*, 21, 3325–3335.

Bronshtein, I. N., Semendyayev, K. A., Musiol, G., and Muehlig, H. (2004). *Handbook of Mathematics*. Springer-Verlag, Berlin, Heidelberg.

Brophy, J. M. and Joseph, L. (1995). Placing trials in context using Bayesian analysis. GUSTO revisited by reverend Bayes [see comments]. *Journal of American Medical Association*, 273, 871–875.

Burman, C. F. and Sonesson, C. (2006). Are flexible designs sound? *Biometrics*, in press.

Chaloncr, K. and Larntz, K. (1989). Optimal Bayesian design applied to logistic regression experiments. *Journal of Planning and Inference*, 21, 191–208.

Chang, M. (2005). Bayesian adaptive design with biomarkers. Presented at IBC's Second Annual Conference on *Implementing Adaptive Designs for Drug Development*, November 7–8, 2005, Nassau Inn, Princeton, New Jersey.

Chang, M. (2005). A simple n-stage adaptive design, submitted.

Chang, M. (2005). Adaptive design based on sum of stagewise p-values, submitted.

Chang, M. and Chow, S. C. (2005). A hybrid Bayesian adaptive design for dose response trials. *Journal of Biopharmaceutical Statistics*, 15, 667–691.

Chang, M. and Chow, S. C. (2006a). Power and sample size for dose response studies. In *Dose Finding in Drug Development*, N. Ting (ed.). Springer, New York, New York.

Chang, M. and Chow, S. C. (2006b). An innovative approach in clinical development - Utilization of adaptive design methods in clinical trials, submitted.

Chang, M., Chow, S. C., and Pong, A. (2006). Adaptive design in clinical research - Issues, opportunities, and recommendations. *Journal of Biopharmaceutical Statistics*, 16, 299–309.

Chang, M. N. (1989). Confidence intervals for a normal mean following group sequential test. *Biometrics*, 45, 249–254.

Chang, M. N. and O'Brien, P. C. (1986). Confidence intervals following group sequential test. *Controlled Clinical Trials*, 7, 18–26.

Chang, M. N., Wieand, H. S., and Chang, V. T. (1989). The bias of the sample proportion following a group sequential phase II trial. *Statistics in Medicine*, 8, 563–570.

Chen, J. J., Tsong, Y., and Kang, S. (2000). Tests for equivalence or non-inferiority between two proportions, *Drug Information Journal*, 34, 569–578.

Chen, T. T. (1997). Optimal three-stage designs for phase II cancer clinical trials. *Statistics in Medicine*, 16, 2701–2711.

Chen, T. T. and Ng, T. H. (1998). Optimal flexible designs in phase II cancer clinical trials. *Statistics in Medicine*, 17, 2301–2312.

Chevret, S. (1993). The continual reassessment method in cancer phase I clinical trials: A simulation study. *Statistics in Medicine*, 12, 1093–1108.

Chow, S. C. (2005). Randomized trials stopped early for benefit. Presented at Journal Club, Infectious Diseases Division, Duke University School of medicine, Durham, North Carolina.

Chow, S. C. (2006). Adaptive design methods in clinical trials. *International Chinese Statistical Association Bulletin*, January 2006, 37–41.

Chow, S. C., Chang, M., and Pong, A. (2005). Statistical consideration of adaptive methods in clinical development. *Journal of Biopharmaceutical Statistics*, 15, 575–591.

Chow, S. C. and Liu, J. P. (2003). *Design and Analysis of Clinical Trials*, 2nd ed. John Wiley and Sons, New York, New York.

Chow, S. C. and Shao, J. (2002). *Statistics in Drug Research*. Marcel Dekker, New York, New York.

Chow, S. C. and Shao, J. (2005). Inference for clinical trials with some protocol amendments. *Journal of Biopharmaceutical Statistics*, 15, 659–666.

Chow, S. C. and Shao, J. (2006). On margin and statistical test for non-inferiority in active control trials. *Statistics in Medicine*, 25, 1101–1113.

Chow, S. C., Shao, J., and Hu, Y. P. (2002). Assessing sensitivity and similarity in bridging studies. *Journal of Biopharmaceutical Statistics*, 12, 385–400.

Chow, S. C., Shao, J., and Wang, H. (2003). *Sample Size Calculation in Clinical Research*. Marcel Dekker, New York, New York.

Chuang-Stein, C. and Agresti, A. (1997). A review of tests for detecting a monotone dose-response relationship with ordinal response data. *Statistics in Medicine*, 16, 2599–2618.

Chuang-Stein, C., Anderson, K., Gallo, P., and Collins, S. (2006). Sample size re-estimation, submitted.

Coad, D. S. and Rosenberger, W. F. (1999). A comparison of the randomized play-the-winner and the triangular test for clinical trials with binary responses. *Statistics in Medicine*, 18, 761–769.

Coburger, S. and Wassmer, G. (2003). Sample size reassessment in adaptive clinical trials using a bias corrected estimate. *Biometrical Journal*, 45, 812–825.

Cohen, A. and Sackrowitz, H. B. (1989). Exact tests that recover interblock information in balanced incomplete block design. *Journal of American Statistical Association*, 84, 556–559.

Conaway, M. R. and Petroni, G. R. (1996). Designs for phase II trials allowing for a trade-off between response and toxicity. *Biometrics*, 52, 1375–1386.

Cox, D. R. (1952). A note of the sequential estimation of means. *Proc. Camb. Phil. Soc.*, 48, 447–450.

Cox, D. R. and Oakes, D. (1984). *Analysis of Survival Data*. Monographs on Statistics and Applied Probability, Chapman and Hall, London.

Crowley, J. (2001). *Handbook of Statistics in Clinical Oncology*. Marcel Dekker, New York, New York.

CTriSoft Intl. (2002). Clinical Trial Design with ExpDesign Studio, www.ctrisoft.net.

Cui, L., Hung, H. M. J., and Wang, S. J. (1999). Modification of sample size in group sequential trials. *Biometrics*, 55, 853–857.

DeMets, D. L. and Ware, J. H. (1980). Group sequential methods for clinical trials with a one-sided hypothesis. *Biometrika*, 67, 651–660.

DeMets, D. L. and Ware, J. H. (1982). Asymmetric group sequential boundaries for monitoring clinical trials. *Biometrika*, 69, 661–663.

Dent, S. F. and Fisenhauer, F. A. (1996). Phase I trial design: Are new methodologies being put into practice? *Annals of Oncology*, 6, 561–566.

Dunnett, C. W. (1955). A multiple comparison procedure for comparing several treatments with a control. *Journal of American Statistical Association*, 50, 1076–1121.

Efron, B. (1971). Forcing a sequential experiment to be balanced. *Biometrika*, 58, 403–417.

Efron, B. (1980). Discussion of "Minimumchi-square, not maximum likelihood." *Annal of Statistics*, 8, 469–471.

Ellenberg, S. S., Fleming, T. R., and DeMets, D. L. (2002). *Data Monitoring Committees in Clinical Trials – A Practical Perspective*. John Wiley and Sons, New York, New York.

EMEA (2002). Point to Consider on *Methodological Issues in Confirmatory Clinical Trials with Flexible Design and Analysis Plan*. The European Agency for the Evaluation of Medicinal Products Evaluation of Medicines for Human Use. CPMP/EWP/2459/02, London, UK.

EMEA (2004). Point to Consider on the *Choice of Non-inferiority Margin*. The European Agency for the Evaluation of Medicinal Products Evaluation of Medicines for Human Use. London, UK.

EMEA (2006). Reflection paper on *Methodological Issues in Confirmatory Clinical Trials with Flexible Design and Analysis Plan*. The European Agency for the Evaluation of Medicinal Products Evaluation of Medicines for Human Use. CPMP/EWP/2459/02, London, UK.

Ensign, L. G., Gehan, E. A., Kamen, D. S., and Thall, P. F. (1994). An optimal three-stage design for phase II clinical trials. *Statistics in Medicine*, 13, 1727–1736.

Faries, D. (1994). Practical modification of the continual reassessment method for phase I cancer clinical trials. *Journal of Biopharmaceutical Statistics*, 4, 147–164.

FDA (1988). Guideline for *Format and Content of the Clinical and Statistical Sections of New Drug Applications*. The United States Food and Drug Administration, Rockville, Maryland.

FDA (2000). Guidance for *Clinical Trial Sponsors On the Establishment and Operation of Clinical Trial Data Monitoring Committees*. The United States Food and Drug Administration, Rockville, Maryland.

FDA (2005). Guidance for *Clinical Trial Sponsors. Establishment and Operation of Clinical Trial Data Monitoring Committees (Draft)*. The United States Food and Drug Administration, Rockville, Maryland. http://www.fda.gov/cber/qdlns/clintrialdmc.htm.

Follman, D. A., Proschan, M. A., and Geller, N. L. (1994). Monitoring pairwise comparisons in multi-armed clinical trials. *Biometrics*, 50, 325–336.

Friedman, B. (1949). A simple urn model. *Comm. Pure Appl. Math.*, 2, 59–70.

Gallo, P., Chuang-Stein, C., Dragalin, V., Gaydos, B., Krams, M., and Pinheiro, J. (2006). Adaptive design in clinical drug development - An executive summary of the PhRMA Working Group (with discussions). *Journal of Biopharmaceutical Statistics*, 16, 275–283.

Gasprini, M. and Eisele, J. (2000). A curve-free method for phase I clinical trials. *Biometrics*, 56, 609–615.

Gelman, A., Carlin, J. B., and Rubin, D. B. (2003). *Bayesian Data Analysis*, 2nd ed. Chapman and Hall/CRC, New York, New York.

Gillis, P. R. and Ratkowsky, D. A. (1978). The behaviour of estimators of the parameters of various yield-density relationships. *Biometrics*, 34, 191–198.

Goodman, S. N. (1999). Towards evidence-based medical statistics I: The p-value fallacy. *Annals of Internal Medicine*, 130, 995–1004.

Goodman, S. N. (2005). Introduction to Bayesian methods I: Measuring the strength of evidence. *Clinical Trials*, 2, 282–290.

Goodman, S. N., Lahurak, M. L., and Piantadosi, S. (1995). Some practical improvements in the continual reassessment method for phase I studies. *Statistics in Medicine*, 5, 1149–1161.

Gould, A. L. (1992). Interim analyses for monitoring clinical trials that do not materially affect the type I error rate. *Statistics in Medicine*, 11, 55–66.

Gould, A. L. (1995). Planning and revising the sample size for a trial. *Statistics in Medicine*, 14, 1039–1051.

Gould, A. L. (2001). Sample size re-estimation: Recent developments and practical considerations. *Statistics in Medicine*, 20, 2625–2643.

Gould, A. L. and Shih, W. J. (1992). Sample size re-estimation without unblinding for normally distributed outcomes with unknown variance. *Communications in Statistics - Theory and Methodology*, 21, 2833–2853.

Hallstron, A. and Davis, K. (1988). Inbalance in treatment assignments in stratified blocked randomization. *Controlled Clinical Trials*, 9, 375–382.

Hardwick, J. P. and Stout, Q. F. (1991). Bandit strategies for ethical sequential allocation. *Computing Science and Stat.*, 23, 421–424.

Hardwick, J. P. and Stout, Q. F. (1993). Optimal allocation for estimating the product of two means. *Computing Science and Stat.*, 24, 592–596.

Hardwick, J. P. and Stout, Q. F. (2002). Optimal few-stage designs. *Journal of Statistical Planning and Inference*, 104, 121–145.

Hawkins, M. J. (1993). Early cancer clinical trials: Safety, numbers, and consent. *Journal of the National Cancer Institute*, 85, 1618–1619.

Hedges. L. V. and Olkin, I. (1985). *Statistical Methods for Meta-analysis*. Academic Press, New York, New York.

Hellmich, M. (2001). Monitoring clinical trials with multiple arms. *Biometrics*, 57, 892–898.

Hochberg, Y. (1988). A sharper Bonferroni's procedure for multiple tests of significance. *Biometrika*, 75, 800–803.

Holmgren, E. B. (1999). Establishing equivalence by showing that a specified percentage of the effect of the active control over placebo is maintained. *Journal of Biopharmaceutical Statistics*, 9, 651–659.

Hommel, G. (2001). Adaptive modifications of hypotheses after an interim analysis. *Biometrical Journal*, 43, 581–589.

Hommel, G. and Kropf, S. (2001). Clinical trials with an adaptive choice of hypotheses. *Drug Information Journal*, 33, 1205–1218.

Hommel, G., Lindig, V., and Faldum, A. (2005). Two stage adaptive designs with correlated test statistics. *Journal of Biopharmaceutical Statistics*, 15, 613–623.

Horwitz, R. I. and Horwitz, S. M. (1993). Adherence to treatment and health outcomes. *Annals of Internal Medicine*, 153, 1863–1868.

Hothorn, L. A. (2000). Evaluation of animal carcinogenicity studies: Cochran-Armitage trend test vs. Multiple contrast tests. *Biometrical Journal*, 42, 553–567.

Hughes, M. D. (1993). Stopping guidelines for clinical trials with multiple treatments. *Statistics in Medicine*, 12, 901–913.

Hughes, M. D. and Pocock, S. J. (1988). Stopping rules and estimation problems in clinical trials. *Statistics in Medicine*, 7, 1231–1242.

Hung, H. M. J., Wang, S. J., Tsong, Y., Lawrence, J., and O'Neil, R. T. (2003). Some fundamental issues with non-inferiority testing in active controlled trials. *Statistics in Medicine*, 22, 213–225.

Hung, H. M. J., Cui, L, Wang, S. J., and Lawrence, J. (2005). Adaptive statistical analysis following sample size modification based on interim review of effect size. *Journal of Biopharmaceutical Statistics*, 15, 693–706.

ICH (1996). International Conference on Harmonization Tripartite Guideline for Good Clinical Practice.

ICH E9 Expert Working Group (1999). Statistical principles for clinical trials (ICH Harmonized Tripartite Guideline E9). *Statistics in Medicine*, 18, 1905–1942.

Inoue, L. Y. T., Thall, P. F. and Berry, D. A. (2002). Seamlessly expanding a randomized phase II trial to phase III. *Biometrics*, 58, 823–831.

Ivanova, A. and Flournoy, N. (2001). A birth and death urn for ternary outcomes: Stochastic processes applied to urn models. In *Probability and Statistical Models with Applications*. Charalambides, C. A., Koutras, M. V., and Balakrishnan, N. (eds.). Chapman and Hall/CRC Press, Boca Raton, Florida, 583–600.

Jennison, C. and Turnbull, B. W. (1990). Statistical approaches to interim monitoring of medical trials: A review and commentary. *Statistics in Medicine*, 5, 299–317.

Jennison, C. and Turnbull, B. W. (2000). *Group Sequential Method with Applications to Clinical Trials*. Chapman and Hall/CRC Press, New York, New York.

Jennison, C. Turnbull, B. W. (2003). Mid-course sample size modification in clinical trials based on the observed treatment effect. *Statistics in Medicine*, 22, 971–993.

Jennison, C. and Turnbull, B. W. (2006a). Adaptive and non-adaptive group sequential tests. *Biometrika*, 93, in press.

Jennison, C. and Turnbull, B. W. (2006b). Efficient group sequential designs when there are several effect sizes under consideration. *Statistics in Medicine*, 25, in press.

Jennison, C. and Turnbull, B. W. (2005). Meta-analysis and adaptive group sequential design in the clinical development process. *Journal of Biopharmaceutical Statistics*, 15, 537–558.

Johnson, N. L., Kotz, S., and Balakrishnan, N. (1994). *Continuous Univariate Distributions*, Vol. 1. John Wiley and Sons, New York, New York.

Kalbeisch, J. D. and Prentice, R. T. (1980). *The Statistical Analysis of Failure Time Data*. Wiley, New York, New York.

Kelly, P. J., Sooriyarachchi, M. R., Stallard, N., and Todd, S. (2005). A practical comparison of group-sequential and adaptive designs. *Journal of Biopharmaceutical Statistics*, 15, 719–738.

Kelly, P. J., Stallard, N., and Todd, S. (2005). An adaptive group sequential design for phase II/III clinical trials that select a single treatment from several. *Journal of Biopharmaceutical Statistics*, 15, 641–658.

Kieser, M., Bauer, P., and Lehmacher, W. (1999). Inference on multiple endpoints in clinical trials with adaptive interim analyses. *Biometrical Journal*, 41, 261–277.

Kieser, M. and Friede, T. (2000). Re-calculating the sample size in internal pilot study designs with control of the type I error rate. *Statistics in Medicine*, 19, 901–911.

Kieser, M. and Friede, T. (2003). Simple procedures for blinded sample size adjustment that do not affect the type I error rate. *Statistics in Medicine*, 22, 3571–3581.

Kim, K. (1989). Point estimation following group sequential tests. *Biometrics*, 45, 613–617.

Kimko, H. C. and Duffull, S. B. (2003). *Simulation for Designing Clinical Trials*. Marcel Dekker, New York, New York.

Kramar, A., Lehecq, A., and Candalli, E. (1999). Continual reassessment methods in phase I trials of the combination of two drugs in oncology. *Statistics in Medicine*, 18, 1849–1864.

Lachin, J. M. (1988). Statistical properties of randomization in clinical trials. *Controlled Clinical Trials*, 9, 289–311.

Lan, K. K. G. (2002). Problems and issues in adaptive clinical trial design. Presented at New Jersey Chapter of the American Statistical Association, Piscataway, New Jersey, June 4, 2002.

Lan, K. K. G. and DeMets, D. L. (1983). Discrete sequential boundaries for clinical trials. *Biometrika*, 70, 659–663.

Lan, K. K. G. and DeMets, D. L. (1987). Group sequential procedures: calendar versus information time. *Statistics in Medicine*, 8, 1191–1198.

Lee, Y., Wang, H., and Chow, S. C. (2006). A bootstrap-median approach for stable sample size determination based on information from a small pilot study, submitted.

Lehmacher, W., Kieser, M., and Hothorn, L. (2000). Sequential and multiple testing for dose-response analysis. *Drug Information Journal*, 34, 591–597.

Lehmacher, W. and Wassmer, G. (1999). Adaptive sample size calculations in group sequential trials. *Biometrics*, 55, 1286–1290.

Lehmann, E. L. (1975). *Nonparametric: Statistical Methods Based on Ranks*. Holden-Day, San Francisco.

Lehmann, E. L. (1983). *The Theory of Point Estimation*. Wiley, New York, New York.

Li, H. I. and Lai, P. Y. (2003). Clinical trial simulation. In *Encyclopedia of Biopharmaceutical Statistics*, Chow, S. C. (ed.). Marcel Dekker, New York, New York, 200–201.

Li, N. (2006). Adaptive trial design - FDA statistical reviewer's view. Presented at the CRT 2006 Workshop with the FDA, Arlington, Virginia, April 4, 2006.

Li, W. J., Shih, W. J., and Wang, Y. (2005). Two-stage adaptive design for clinical trials with survival data. *Journal of Biopharmaceutical Statistics*, 15, 707–718.

Lilford, R. J. and Braunholtz, D. (1996). For debate: The statistical basis of public policy: A paradigm shift is overdue. *British Medical Journal*, 313, 603–607.

Lin, Y. and Shih, W. J. (2001). Statistical properties of the traditional algorithm-based designs for phase I cancer clinical trials. *Biostatistics*, 2, 203–215.

Liu, Q. (1998). An order-directed score test for trend in ordered 2xK Tables. *Biometrics*, 54, 1147–1154.

Liu, Q. and Chi, G. Y. H. (2001). On sample size and inference for two-stage adaptive designs. *Biometrics*, 57, 172–177.

Liu, Q. and Pledger, G. W. (2005). Phase 2 and 3 combination designs to accelerate drug development. *Journal of American Statistical Association*, 100, 493–502.

Liu, Q., Proschan, M. A., and Pledger, G. W. (2002). A unified theory of two-stage adaptive designs. *Journal of American Statistical Association*, 97, 1034–1041.

Lokhnygina, Y. (2004). Topics in design and analysis of clinical trials. Ph.D. Thesis, Department of Statistics, North Carolina State Univeristy. Raleigh, North Carolina.

Louis, T. A. (2005). Introduction to Bayesian methods II: Fundamental concepts. *Clinical Trials*, 2, 291–294.

Maca, J., Bhattacharya, S., Dragalin, V., Gallo, P., and Krams, M. (2006). Adaptive seamless phase II/III designs - Background, operational aspects, and examples, submitted.

Marubini, E. and Valsecchi, M. G. (1995). *Analysis Survival Data from Clinical Trials and Observational Studies*. John Wiley and Sons, New York, New York.

Maxwell, C., Domenet, J. G., and Joyce, C. R. R. (1971). Instant experience in clinical trials: A novel aid to teaching by simulation. *J. Clin. Pharmacol.*, 11, 323–331.

Melfi, V. and Page, C. (1998). Variability in adaptive designs for estimation of success probabilities. In New Developments and Applications in Experimental Design, *IMS Lecture Notes Monograph Series*, 34, 106–114.

Mendelhall, W. and Hader, R. J. (1985). Estimation of parameters of mixed exponentially distributed failure time distributions from censored life test data. *Biometrika*, 45, 504–520.

Mehta, C. R. and Tsiatis, A. A. (2001). Flexible sample size considerations using information-based interim monitor. *Drug Information Journal*, 35, 1095–1112.

Mehta, C. R. and Patel, N. R. (2005). Adaptive, group sequential and decision theoretic approaches to sample size determination, submitted.

Montori, V. M., Devereaux, P. J., Adhikari, N. K. J., Burns, K. E. A. et al. (2005). Randomized trials stopped early for benefit - A systematic review. *Journal of American Medical Association*, 294, 2203–2209.

Müller, H. H. and Schäfer, H. (2001). Adaptive group sequential designs for clinical trials: Combining the advantages of adaptive and classical group sequential approaches. *Biometrics*, 57, 886–891.

Neuhauser, M. and Hothorn, L. (1999). An exact Cochran-Armitage test for trend when dose-response shapes are a priori unknown. *Computational Statistics & Data Analysis*, 30, 403–412.

Offen, W. W. (2003). Data Monitoring Committees (DMC). In *Encyclopedia of Biopharmaceutical Statistics*, Chow, S. C. (ed.) Marcel Dekker, New York, New York.

Offen, W., Chuang-Stein, C., Dmitrienko, A., Littman, G., Maca, J., Meyerson, L., Muirhead, R., Stryszak, P., Boddy, A., Chen, K., Copley-Merriman, K., Dere, W., Givens, S., Hall, D., Henry, D., Jackson, J. D., Krishen, A., Liu, T., Ryder, S., Sankoh, A. J., Wang, J., and Yeh, C. H. (2006). Multiple co-primary endpoints: Medical and statistical solutions. *Drug Information Journal*, in press.

O'Quigley, J., Pepe, M., and Fisher, L. (1990). Continual reassessment method: A practical design for phase I clinical trial in cancer. *Biometrics*, 46, 33–48.

O'Quigley, J. and Shen, L. (1996). Continual reassessment method: A likelihood approach. *Biometrics*, 52, 673–684.

Parmigiani, G. (2002). *Modeling in Medical Decision Making*. John Wiley and Sons, West Sussex, England.

Paulson, E. (1964). A selection procedure for selecting the population with the largest mean from k normal populations. *Annal of Mathematical Statistics*, 35, 174–180.

Pocock, S. J. (2005). When (not) to stop a clinical trial for benefit. *Journal of American Medical Association*, 294, 2228–2230.

Pocock, S. J. and Simon, R. (1975). Sequential treatment assignment with balancing for prognostic factors in the controlled clinical trials. *Biometrics*, 31, 103–115.

Pong, A. and Luo, Z. (2005). Adaptive design in clinical research. A special issue of the *Journal of Biopharmaceutical Statistics*, 15, No. 4.

Posch, M. and Bauer, P. (1999). Adaptive two stage designs and the conditional error function. *Biometrical Journal*, 41, 689–696.

Posch, M. and Bauer, P. (2000). Interim analysis and sample size reassessment. *Biometrics*, 56, 1170–1176.

Posch, M., Bauer, P., and Brannath, W. (2003). Issues in designing flexible trials. *Statistics in Medicine*, 22, 953–969.

Posch, M., König, F., Brannath, W., Dunger-Baldauf, C., and Bauer, P. (2005). Testing and estimation in flexible group sequential designs with adaptive treatment selection. *Statistics in Medicine*, 24, 3697–3714.

Proschan, M. A. and Hunsberger, S. A. (1995). Designed extension of studies based on conditional power. *Biometrics*, 51, 1315–1324.

Proschan, M. A. (2005). Two-stage sample size re-estimation based on a nuisance parameter: A review. *Journal of Biopharmaceutical Statistics*, 15, 539–574.

Proschan, M. A., Leifer, E., and Liu, Q. (2005). Adaptive regression. *Journal of Biopharmaceutical Statistics*, 15, 593–603.

Proschan, M. A. and Wittes, J. (2000). An improved double sampling procedure based on the variance. *Biometrics*, 56, 1183–1187.

Proschan, M. A., Follmann, D. A., and Waclawiw, M. A. (1992). Effects of assumption violations on type I error rate in group sequential monitoring. *Biometrics*, 48, 1131–1143.

Proschan, M. A., Follmann, D. A., and Geller, N. L. (1994). Monitoring multi-armed trials. *Statistics in Medicine*, 13, 1441–1452.

Quinlan, J. A., Gallo, P., and Krams, M. (2006). Implementing adaptive designs: Logistical and operational consideration, submitted.

Ravaris, C. L., Nies, A., Robinson, D. S., and Ives, J. O. (1976). Multiple dose controlled study of phenelzine in depression anxiety states. *Areh Gen Psychiatry*, 33, 347–350.

Robins, J. M. and Tsiatis, A. A. (1991). Correcting for non-compliance in randomized trials using rank preserving structural failure time models. *Communications in Statistics – Theory and Methods*, 20, 2609–2631.

Rom, D. M. (1990). A sequentially rejective test procedure based on a modified Bonferroni inequality. *Biometrika*, 77, 663–665.

Rosenberger, W. F. and Lachin, J. (2002). *Randomization in Clinical Trials.* John Wiley and Sons, New York, New York.

Rosenberger, W. F. and Seshaiyer, P. (1997). Adaptive survival trials. *Journal of Biopharmaceutical Statistics,* 7, 617–624.

Rosenberger, W. F., Stallard, N., Ivanova, A., Harper, C. N., and Ricks, M. L. (2001). Optimal adaptive designs for binary response trials. *Biometrics,* 57, 909–913.

Sampson, A. R. and Sill, M. W. (2005). Drop-the-loser design: Normal case (with discussions). *Biometrical Journal,* 47, 257–281.

Sargent, D. J. and Goldberg, R. M. (2001). A flexible design for multiple armed screening trials. *Statistics in Medicine,* 20, 1051–1060.

Schaid, D. J., Wieand, S., and Therneau, T. M. (1990). Optimal two stage screening designs for survival comparisons. *Biometrika,* 77, 659–663.

Shao, J., Chang, M., and Chow, S. C. (2005). Statistical inference for cancer trials with treatment switching. *Statistics in Medicine,* 24, 1783–1790.

Shen, Y. and Fisher, L. (1999). Statistical inference for self-designing clinical trials with a one-sided hypothesis. *Biometrics,* 55, 190–197.

Shih, W. J. (2001). Sample size re-estimation - A journey for a decade. *Statistics in Medicine,* 20, 515–518.

Shirley, E. (1977). A non-parametric equivalent of Williams' test for contrasting increasing dose levels of treatment. *Biometrics,* 33, 386–389.

Siegmund, D. (1985). *Sequential Analysis: Tests and Confidence Intervals.* Springer, New York, New York.

Simon, R. (1979). Restricted randomization designs in clinical trials. *Biometrics,* 35, 503–512.

Simon, R. (1989). Optimal two-stage designs for phase II clinical trials. *Controlled Clinical Trials,* 10, 1–10.

Sommer, A. and Zeger, S. L. (1991). On estimating efficacy from clinical trials. *Statistics in Medicine,* 10, 45–52.

Sonnemann, E. (1991). Kombination unabhängiger Tests. In *Biometrie in der chemisch-pharmazeutischen Industrie 4, Stand und Perspektiven,* Vollmar, J. (ed.). Stuttgart: Gustav-Fischer.

Spiegelhalter, D. J., Abrams, K. R, and Myles, J. P. (2004). *Bayesian Approach to Clinical Trials and Health-care Evaluation.* John Wiley and Sons, Ltd., The Atrium, Southern Gate, Chrichester, West Sussex P019 8SQ, England.

Stallard, N. and Todd, S. (2003). Sequential designs for phase III clinical trials incorporating treatment selection. *Statistics in Medicine,* 22, 689–703.

Stallard, N. and Todd, S. (2005). Point estimates and confidence regions for sequential trials involving selection. *Journal of Statistical Planning and Inference,* 135, 402–419.

Stewart, W. and Ruberg, S. J. (2000). Detecting dose response with contrasts. *Statistics in Medicine,* 19, 913–921.

Susarla, V. and Pathala, K. S. (1965). A probability distribution for time of first birth. *Journal of Scientific Research,* Banaras Hindu University, 16, 59–62.

Taves, D. R. (1974). Minimization - A new method of assessing patients and control groups. *Clinical Pharmacol. Ther.*, 15, 443–453.

Temple, R. (2005). How FDA currently make decisions on clinical studies. *Clinical Trials*, 2, 276–281.

Thall, P. F., Simon, R., and Ellenberg, S. S. (1989). A two-stage design for choosing among several experimental treatments and a control in clinical trials. *Biometrics*, 45, 537–547.

Todd, S. (2003). An adaptive approach to implementing bivariate group sequential clinical trial designs. *Journal of Biopharmaceutical Statistics*, 13, 605–619.

Todd, S. and Stallard, N. (2005). A new clinical trial design combining Phases 2 and 3: Sequential designs with treatment selection and a change of endpoint. *Drug Information Journal*, 39, 109–118.

Tsiatis, A. A and Mehta, C. (2003). On the inefficiency of the adaptive design for monitoring clinical trials. *Biometrika*, 90, 367–378.

Tsiatis, A. A., Rosner, G. L., and Mehta, C. R. (1984). Exact confidence interval following a group sequential test. *Biometrics*, 40, 797–803.

Tukey, J. W. and Heyse, J. F. (1985). Testing the statistical certainty of a response to increasing doses of a drug. *Biometrics*, 41, 295–301.

Uchida, T. (2006). Adaptive trial design - FDA view. Presented at the CRT 2006 Workshop with the FDA, Arlington, Virginia, April 4, 2006.

Wald, A. (1947). *Sequential Analysis*. Dover Publications, New York, New York.

Wang, S. J. and Hung, H. M. J. (2005). Adaptive covariate adjustment in clinical trials. *Journal of Biopharmaceutical Statistics*, 15, 605–611.

Wang, S. K. and Tsiatis, A. A. (1987). Approximately optimal one-parameter boundaries for a sequential trials. *Biometrics*, 43, 193–200.

Wassmer, G. (1998), A comparison of two methods for adaptive interim analyses in clinical trials. *Biometrics*, 54, 696–705.

Wassmer, G., Eisebitt, R., and Coburger, S. (2001). Flexible interim analyses in clinical trials using multistage adaptive test designs. *Drug Information Journal*, 35, 1131–1146.

Wei, L. J. (1977). A class of designs for sequential clinical trials. *Journal of American Statistical Association*, 72, 382–386.

Wei, L. J. (1978). The adaptive biased-coin design for sequential experiments. *Annal of Statistics*, 9, 92–100.

Wei, L. J. and Durham, S. (1978). The randomized play-the-winner rule in medical trials. *Journal of American Statistical Association*, 73, 840–843.

Wei, L. J., Smythe, R. T., and Smith, R. L. (1986). K-treatment comparisons with restricted randomization rules in clinical trials. *Annal of Statistics*, 14, 265–274.

Weinthrau, M., Jacox, R. F., Angevine, C. D., Atwater, E. C. (1977). Piroxicam (CP 16171) in rheumatoid arthritis: A controlled clinical trial with novel assessment features. *J Rheum*, 4, 393–404.

White, I. R., Babiker, A. G., Walker, S., and Darbyshire, J. H. (1999). Randomisation-based methods for correcting for treatment changes:

Examples from the Concorde trial. *Statistics in Medicine*, 18, 2617–2634.

White, I. R., Walker, S., and Babiker, A. G. (2002). Randomisation-based efficacy estimator. *Stata Journal*, 2, 140–150.

Whitehead, J. (1993). Sample size calculation for ordered categorical data. *Statistics in Medicine*, 12, 2257–2271.

Whitehead, J. (1994). Sequential methods based on the boundaries approach for the clinical comparison of survival times (with discussions). *Statistics in Medicine*, 13, 1357–1368.

Whitehead, J. (1997). Bayesian decision procedures with application to dose-finding studies. *International Journal of Pharmaceutical Medicine*, 11, 201–208.

William, D. A. (1971). A test for difference between treatment means when several dose levels are compared with a zero dose control. *Biometrics*, 27, 103–117.

William, D. A. (1972). Comparison of several dose levels with a zero dose control. *Biometrics*, 28, 519–531.

Williams, G., Pazdur, R., and Temple, R. (2004). Assessing tumor-related signs and symptoms to support cancer drug approval. *Journal of Biopharmaceutical Statistics*, 14, 5–21.

Woodcock, J. (2005). DFA introduction comments: Clinical studies design and evaluation issues. *Clinical Trials*, 2, 273–275.

Zelen, M. (1974). The randomization and stratification of patients to clinical trials. *Journal of Chronic Diseases*, 28, 365–375.

Zucker, D. M., Wittes, J. T., Schabenberger, O., and Brittain, E. (1999). Internal pilot studies II: Comparison of various procedures. *Statistics in Medicine*, 19, 901–911.

Index

A

Accelerated failure time model, 174
Accidental bias, 70
Accrual bias, 70
Accrued data, 9, 18, 45, 90, 245
   adaptations based on, 2, 5
   analysis, 93
   design modifications based on, 6
   determination of non-inferiority margin based on, 88
   interim analysis based on, 109
   modification of hypothesis based on, 15, 75
   sample size adjustment based on, 137, 158
Active-control
   agent, 76, 77, 80
   parallel-group, 18
Adaptation(s), 3, 5, 16, 19, 64, 90, 242–243
   ad hoc, 2, 5, 239
   after final analysis, 17, 161
   algorithms, 212
   basic strategy, 242, 245
   biomarkers and, 6
   of design characteristics, 245
   dose-escalation trial, 245
   effect on clinical trials, 2, 240
   effects of, 2, 230, 240
   examples, 2, 242
   flexibility, 12
   of interim analyses, 243
   population, 165
   prospective, 2, 239
   retrospective, 2, 5, 239
   rule, 41, 42, 45, 216
   of sample size, 146, 243
   for seamless phase II/II trial designs, 248
   of switching hypotheses, 243
Adaptive design(s)
   basic considerations when implementing, 239–241
   bias and, 19
   biomarker, 6
   computer simulation and, 236
   defined, 3–6
   disadvantages, 16, 45
   dose-escalation, 244–247
   for dose-response trials, 19
   drop-the-loser, 167–170, 234–235
   four-stage specifications, 129
   group sequential, 5, 15–16, 107–136, 228, 241–244, 249
      adaptation, 242–243
      case study, 243–244
      commonly used, 20
      implementation, 20, 239, 241–244
      statistical, 243
   hybrid frequentist-Bayesian, 15, 93–100
   key issue, 7
   methods, 3, 5, 8
      advantages of, 19, 45
      basic considerations when implementing, 239–241
      Bayesian approach, 195
      disadvantages of, 19, 21
      for dose-response curves, 90
      impact of, 13
      theoretical basis for, 11
   multiple, 6, 17
   n-stage, 123
   overall type I error rate, 16
   permitting early stopping and sample size re-estimation, 232
   response, 233
   seamless phase II/III, 247–254
   selection, 205
   statistical theory, 215
   two-stage, 16
   window, 227

Adaptive dose-escalation trial, 12, 15, 89–105, 245
Adaptive group sequential design, 5, 15–16, 107–136, 228, 249
  adaptation, 242–243
  case study, 243–244
  commonly used, 20
  implementation, 20, 239, 241–244
  statistical, 243
Adaptive hypothesis design, 6, 166
Adaptive model(s), 93
  for ordinal and continuous outcomes, 68–69
  response, 68
Adaptive randomization, 2, 12, 13–14, 47–73
  bias and, 218
  design, 5
  definition of, 5–6
  procedures, 14, 20
Adaptive sample size adjustment, 12, 16–17, 137–159
  at interim, 242
Adaptive seamless phase II/III design, 5, 17, 161–171
  benefits and drawbacks, 171
  case studies, 247–254
  traditional approach vs., 162
Adaptive stratification, 55
Adaptive treatment switching, 12, 18, 173–193
  biomarker response, 182
  design, 5, 6
  simulation approach, 189
Adjusted p-value, 125, 128, 150, 152, 156
Allocation probability, 47, 54, 217
  for covariate-adaptive randomization, 55
  defined, 53
  equal, 49
  fixed, 48
  varied, 52
Allocation rule
  in Atkinson optimal model, 58
  balanced randomization, 73
  bandit, 61, 64
  in Efron's biased coin model, 53
  in Friedman-Wei's Efron's urn model, 54, 70, 72
  Lachin's, 70, 72
  stratified, 70, 72

  in Pocock-Simon's model, 57
  in truncated binomial model, 70, 72
Alpha spending function, 122–123, 136
Alternative hypothesis, 77
  conditional power and, 133
  sample size adjustment and, 35, 115, 122, 138
  simulation and, 212–213
  true, 233
  two-stage design and, 203
Analysis of covariance (ANCOVA), 51
Asthma, 42–43, 251
Atkinson optimal model, 55, 58

B

Balance design, 35
  perfect, 54
Balanced randomized design, 65, 68
Bandit allocation rule, 61, 64
Bandit model, 58, 61–68
  for finite population, 64–68
Bauer and Köhne's method, 14, 137, 146–248, 151, 168, 249
Bayes rule, 196–200
Bayesian adaptive design, 15, 195
  for dose-response trials, 90
  hybrid frequentist, 15, 93–100
Bayesian approach, 18, 92, 195–210
  advantages, 209–210
  bandit allocation rule as, 61
  basic concepts, 195–201
  hybrid-frequentist, 98–99
  predictive power as, 131
  prior probability and, 97
  simulation with, 236
Bayesian optimal design, 205–209
Bias
  accidental, 70
  accrual, 70
  adaptation and, 10
  adaptive design and, 19
  adaptive randomization and, 218
  expected factor, 71
  group size and, 236
  minimization, 2
  operational, 239
  potential risks for, 44
  in rate with dropping losers, 234, 235

reduction, 229, 230
selection, 55, 71
statistical, 239
Biased coin design, 53
Binary endpoint, 118, 155, 164
Bioequivalence, 77
Biological efficacy, 18, 173
Biomarker-adaptive design, 5, 6
Block randomization, 52–53
permuted, 13
Boundary scales, 109–110

C

Cancer trials, 18, 68, 77, 201. *See also* Oncology
biomarkers and, 182, 210
breast, 251
optimal/flexible multiple-stage design, 110
ovarian, 57
parallel-group active control randomization, 173
prostatic, 245
responding to early beneficial trends in, 132
treatment-switch in, 181
two-stage design in phase II, 202
Case studies, 19–20, 239–254
Chow and Shao's approach, 79
Clinical trial simulation, 12, 19, 211–237
early phase, 228–230
considerations, 213–215
dose-escalation design, 215
dose-level selection, 214
dose limiting toxicity and maximum tolerated dose, 214
sample size per dose level, 215
examples, 227–230
with CRM, 229–230
with TER and TSER, 228–229
examples, 227–235
framework, 212–213
late phase, 230–235
considerations, 215–220
alpha adjustment, 219–220
early stopping rules, 216
null-model *vs.* model approach, 219
randomization rules, 216
response-adaptive randomization, 217–218
rules for dropping losers, 216–217

sample size adjustment, 217
utility-offset model, 218–219
examples, 230–235
adaptive design permitting early stopping, 232–233
adaptive design with dropping the losers, 234–235
conventional design with multiple treatments, 233
design with play-the-winner randomization, 231–232
dose-response trial design, 235
flexible design with sample size re-estimation, 231
group sequential design, 232
responsive-adaptive design with multiple treatments, 233–234
software application, 220–227
designing with, 222–227
adaptive trial, 227
conventional trial, 222–223
dose-escalation trial, 225–226
group sequential trial, 223–224
multi-stage trial, 224
overview, 220–222
Closed testing procedure, 78, 243
Cluster randomization, 47, 48, 51–52, 247
Combined adaptive design, 17
Common toxicity criteria, 91
Comparing means, 108, 133–134
Comparing proportions, 108, 134–135
Complete randomization, 13, 47, 48. *See also* Simple randomization
accidental bias, 70
urn procedure and, 55
Complete randomization design, 55
Conditional inference, 39–40
Conditional power, 131, 133–135, 142, 203, 244
Confidence interval, 4, 8, 11, 79, 169, 252
asymptotic, 180
final, 136
naive, 100, 131, 216
simulation, 222
Constancy condition, 84, 86
Continual reassessment method (CRM), 15, 89, 90, 215, 228, 244
in reduction of bias, 229
Conventional randomization, 48–52, 217
Convergence strategy, 71

Covariate-adaptive randomization, 55–58
Covariate-adjustment, 38–43
Cox's proportional hazard model, 177, 179
CRM. See Continual reassessment method (CRM)
CTriSoft, 103, 212, 220, 228
Cui-Hui-Wang method, 137, 140–142

D

Data monitoring committee, 76, 109, 128–131, 158, 241, 253
Data safety monitoring board, 75
DLT. See Dose limiting toxicity (DLT)
DMC. See Data monitoring committee
Dose, 212
    adjustment, 2
    assignment based on minimization/maximization of function, 90
    efficacious, 15, 89
    maximum tolerable, 6, 89, 214
    optimal, strategies for finding, 213
    reduction, 8
    toxicity and, 91
Dose de-escalation, 89
Dose-efficiency response study, 15, 89
Dose-escalation design, 5, 20, 239, 244–247
Dose escalation factor, 92, 214
Dose-escalation trial, 213
    adaptive, 12, 15, 89–105, 245
    design, 225
    simulation for, 214, 220
Dose-level selection, 92
Dose limiting toxicity (DLT), 89, 92, 214, 244
    selection criteria based on, 245
Dose regimen, 2, 39, 42, 77, 108, 240
Dose response, 15, 89
    study, 15, 17
        curves, 90
        model, 99
        using multiple-stage designs, 90
Dose-toxicity modeling, 91–92
Dose-toxicity study, 15, 89
Drop the loser design, 5, 167–170
Dropping losers, 12, 77, 162, 234, 248
    rules, 100, 101, 216

E

Early efficacy-futility stopping, 119–122
Early efficacy stopping, 114–116, 156, 251
Early futility stopping, 116–119, 156, 162
Early phases development, 213–215
Early stopping boundaries, 114–122
Effect size, 8, 115, 198, 239
    clinically meaningful, 16
    sample size and, 140, 217
    sensitivity index and, 24
Efficacy, 42, 89, 107
    biological, 18, 173, 174
    Chow and Shao's approach, 79
    comparisons, 48
    early (See Early efficacy)
    early stopping for, 114, 161, 162
    endpoints, 42, 60, 77, 118, 128, 251
    evaluation, 18
    lack of, 17
    premature termination of trial and, 5, 221
    unbiased and fair assessment, 47
Efron's biased coin model, 53
EM algorithm, 139
EMEA. See European Agency for the Evaluation of Medicinal Products
Equal randomization, 65
Error inflation, 109
Ethical consideration, 18, 48, 77, 107, 110, 173, 201, 242
European Agency for the Evaluation of Medicinal Products, 6, 34
Expected bias factor, 71
Extrapolate, 211, 212

F

Family experiment-wise, 151
FEV1 change, as endpoint parameter, 42, 128, 251
Flexible design, 4, 7, 231
    with sample size re-estimation, 231
Flexible trials, 15
Force expiratory volume per second. See FEV1 change, as endpoint parameter
Friedman-Wei's urn model, 54–55
    accidental bias, 70
    selection bias, 72

INDEX

Futility, 2
  assessment, 108, 250
  based on interim analyses, 5
  early stopping for, 15, 88
  rules, 100, 216
Futility design, 112
Futility index, 131
Futility inner stopping boundary, 118

G

GCP. See Good Clinical Practices
Genomic markers, 6, 166
Gittins lower bound, 63–64
Good Clinical Practices, 9, 108
Group sequential design
  adaptive, 5, 15–16, 107–136, 228, 249
    adaptation, 242–243
    case study, 243–244
    commonly used, 20
    implementation, 20, 239, 241–244
    statistical, 243
  based on independent p-values, 123–125
  five-arm, 166
  general approach for, 112–114
  with one interim analyses, 232
  sample size adjustment in, 137

H

Heart failure, 132
HIV/AID, 18, 132, 173
Homogeneity, 13, 35, 50, 164
Hybrid, 15, 89
Hybrid frequentist-Bayesian adaptive design, 15, 93–100
Hyper-logistic function, 91, 96, 104
Hypothesis test, 123, 148, 187–189, 213
  global, 149
  null, 149

I

Imbalance minimization model, 57–58
Inclusion/exclusion criteria, 2, 3, 7, 11, 38
  modification, 9
Individual p-value, 151
Inferential analysis, 71–72

Interactive parameter estimation (IPE), 176–177
IPE. See Interactive parameter estimation (IPE)

K

k-stage design, 125–126

L

Lachin's urn model, 53–54
Lan-DeMets-Kim functions, 110, 122–123
Late phases development, 215–220
Latent event times, 174–177
Latent hazard rate, 177–181
Linear combination of p-values, 150, 243
Log-likelihood function, 29, 30, 31, 139
Log-rank test, 155
Long-term treatment, 131

M

Marginal distribution, 196, 197
Maximum likelihood estimates (MLE), 28–31, 139, 181, 186, 190
Maximum likelihood estimator, 136
Maximum tolerable dose, 6, 15, 89, 90, 214, 228, 244
  based on dose response model, 93
  defined, 214
  expression of, 92
  in simulation studies, 214
Median survival time, 18, 77, 120, 181
Median unbiased estimator, 136
Method of individual p-values (MIP), 151–152, 156, 157, 162
Method of products of p-values (MPP), 153, 156
Method of sum of p-values (MSP), 152, 156, 162
MIP. See Method of individual p-values (MIP)
Mixed exponential model, 173, 181–193
Mixed normal distribution, 28
MLE. See Maximum likelihood estimates (MLE); Maximum likelihood estimator (MLE)
Moving target patient population, 12–13, 25, 31, 44, 159
MPP. See Method of products of p-values (MPP)

MSP. See Method of sum of p-values (MSP)
Muller-Schafer method, 146
Multiple adaptive design, 6, 17
Multiple-endpoint oriented, 105
Multiple stage design, 110, 224
    for single-arm trial, 201–205
Multiple testing, 14–15

N

N-adjustable design, 5, 213
Naive p-value, 163–165
National Cancer Institute, 91
Non-inferiority, 165
    hypothesis, 76
    margin, 34, 36, 75, 78–84, 243
    switch from superiority to, 2, 78–87
    test for, 34, 36, 212
Non-informative priors, 101, 102, 103
Nonparametric method, 185, 187–188
Normal endpoint, 17, 115, 155, 164
Normal outcome, 69
Null hypothesis, 17, 72, 109
    hazard rates under, 188
    interchange between alternative hypothesis and, 77
    one-sided, 43
    under population model, 72
    rejection of, 34, 78, 133, 143, 191
    in simulation framework, 213
    test, 149
    test statistic and, 33

O

O'Brien and Fleming's test, 115, 133, 136
O'Brien-Fleming boundary, 110, 130, 205, 207, 209
O'Brien-Fleming error spending functions, 122
O'Brien-Fleming group sequential procedure, 136
O'Brien-Fleming test, 115, 133
Oncology, 8
    trials, 15, 18 (*See also* Cancer trials)
        mixed exponential model, 181
        phase I, 89, 91–93, 227
            dose-escalation, 244
            dose-level selection, 92
            dose-toxicity modeling, 91–92

reassessment of model parameters, 92–93
phase II, 228
two-arm comparative, 126, 155
Operating characteristics, 102, 155–156, 203, 207
    of adaptive methods, 128
    comparisons, 236, 246
    desirable, 236
    of various designs, 129
Optimal allocation, 60, 61
Optimal/flexible multiple-stage designs, 110–111
Optimal randomized play-the-winner model, 60–61
Optimal two-stage design, 110–111, 202–203
Ordinal outcome, 68–69

P

Parallel group, 18, 174, 198
Patient population
    actual, 4, 6, 10, 23–26
    genomic markers, 166
    homogenous, 13
    selection, 251
    target, 2, 3, 8–10, 31
        conclusions for, 13
        moving, 12–13, 25, 159
        shift in, 30
        for stratified randomization, 50, 107
        subgroups of, 181
Permutation test, 71–72
Pharmacodynamics, 213
Pharmacokinetics, 211, 213
Phase I oncology study. See Oncology, trials, phase I
PhRMA Working Group, 3–4, 6
Play-the-winner model, 58–59
Pocock, 136, 158, 159
Pocock boundary, 110, 131, 205, 208, 209
Pocock error spending functions, 122
Pocock-Simon's model, 56–57
Pocock's test, 115, 133
Population model, 13, 71, 72
Posterior distribution, 64, 92, 195, 230
    of toxicity, 236
Posterior means, 62
Power, 64, 118
    analysis, 9, 13, 17, 51, 77, 187
    pre-study, 242

conditional, 130, 131, 133–135, 244
for detection of clinically important
  effect, 45
function, 91
insufficient, 11, 244
optimal, 49
predictive, 130, 131, 203
protocol amendments on, 23
statistical, 14, 48, 51, 73
stealing, 162
test for equivalence, 37
test for non-inferiority/superiority, 36
Predictive power, 130, 131, 203
Prior distribution, 61, 62, 101, 195, 196,
  215, 246
Bayesian approach and, 92
binomial, 203
of parameter tensor, 97
uniform, 67, 229
Product of p-values, 150, 151, 153–155
Proportional hazard model, 177–181
Proschan-Hunsberger's method, 137,
  142–145
Prospective trials, 2
adaptation, 5, 239
stratification, 55
Protocol amendment(s), 5, 23–46, 95, 108
actual patient population, 23–26
estimation of shift and scale
  parameters, 26–31
sample size adjustment, 35–38
statistical inference, 31–34
statistical inference with covariate
  adjustment, 38–43

Q

QTc prolongation, 213

R

Randomization
cluster, 51–52, 247
model, 13, 47, 71, 72, 99
  accidental bias, 70
simple, 48–50
stratified, 50–51
Randomized play-the-winner model, 59,
  216, 217
Reassessment method, 101
continual, 15, 89, 90, 215, 228, 229, 244
Relative efficiency, 36, 37, 38, 49, 50

Repeated confidence interval, 131
Reproducibility, 19, 159
Response-adaptive randomization, 14,
  47–48, 58–70, 90, 92, 165, 216,
  236, 241
defined, 58
Retrospective adaptation, 2, 5, 239
Robustness, 19, 211, 231

S

Sample size
adjustment, 12, 15, 16–17, 35–38,
  137–159
calculation, 90, 112, 114
change, 3
fixed, 119
insufficient, 64
maximum, 116, 118
power analysis, for calculation, 13, 20,
  23, 77
power and, 72–73
pre-selected, 75
re-assessment, 4
saving in, 108
Sample size ratio, 49–50, 112
maximum, 100
Sample size re-estimation, 2, 5, 9, 20,
  123, 130, 212, 228
flexible design with, 231
unblinded, 219
without unblinding, 138–140
Sampling distribution, 40, 196
Scale parameter, 23, 26, 29
Seamless design, 161–171
comparisons, 165–167
contrast test and naive p-value,
  163–165
drop-the-loser adaptive design,
  167–170
efficiency, 161–162
objectives, 247
step-wise test and adaptive procedures,
  162–163
Seamless phase II/III design, 161–171,
  247–254
Selection bias, 19, 71, 239
expected factors, 72
sample size and, 55
Sensitivity
analyses, 19, 45, 84, 237
index, 23

changes in, 25
  estimation of, 27
  indication of, 24
Sequential methods, 108–112
  basic concepts, 109–112
Shift parameter, 23, 29
Short-term treatment, 132
  efficacy, 248, 251
  endpoints, 249
  long-term treatment vs., 131
Simon's two-stage design, 110, 202
Simple randomization, 48–50, 217, 234
  for two-arm parallel group, 49
Statistical analysis plan, 4, 7, 11
Statistical inference, 2, 10–11, 31–34, 84–86
  conclusions from, 9
  with covariate adjustment, 38–43
  impact of protocol amendments on, 23
  valid, 45
  validity, 7
Statistical procedures, 2, 3
  defined, 9
  documentation, 7, 11
  for identifying best clinical benefit, 239–240
  modifications, 20, 23, 45, 239–240, 444
  for sample size re-estimation, 137
Step-wise test, 162–163
STER. See Strict traditional escalation rule (STER)
Stopping boundary, 109, 110, 131, 213, 243
  for efficacy, 114, 120, 207, 208, 243
  for futility, 118, 120, 207
Stopping rule(s), 100, 149, 163, 245
  choice of, 136
  clear statement of, 247
  early, 216
  in first stage, 144, 203
  as guide, 128
  in second stage, 203
Stratified randomization, 47, 50–51
Strict traditional escalation rule (STER), 89–90, 215
Sum of p-values, 152–153
Superiority margin, 34, 36, 80
  switch to non-inferiority margin, 2, 78–87
Survival endpoint, 120, 155, 164
Survival outcome, 69

Switch from superiority to non-inferiority, 2, 78–87
Switching effect, 173, 182
  Cox's proportional hazard model with, 179
  in statistical analyses, 191
Symmetric boundary, 118, 119

T

Target patient population, 8–10
  defining, 2
  moving, 12–13, 25, 31, 44, 159
  statistical inference and, 31
  for stratified randomization, 50
  subgroups, 181
TER. See Traditional escalation rules (TER)
Test for equality, 33, 35
Test for equivalence, 34, 37
Test for non-inferiority/superiority, 34, 36
Tests without historical data, 87
Time-dependent covariate, 177
Time-to-event analysis, 112
Traditional escalation rules (TER), 89–90, 215
Treatment-adaptive randomization, 14, 47–48, 52–55
Treatment imbalance, 48, 57
  impact of, 50
  reducing, 54
  of stratified randomization, 50
Treatment switching, 5
  adaptive, 6, 12, 18, 173–193
  in cancer trials, 18
Trial procedure, 24
Triangular boundary, 118
Truncated-binomial randomization, 52
  accidental bias, 70
Truncation, defined, 63
Two-arm bandit, 61, 66
Two-stage design, 108, 125–126, 142, 146–147
  classical approach for, 202–203
  optimal, 110
  patient population for, 229
  for trials with binary outcomes, 249
Type I error rate, 14, 16, 75, 109, 124, 127, 141
  control of, 159, 162, 209, 211, 242
  family experiment-wise, 151
  inflation of, 239

U

Unadjusted p-value, 150
Unbalanced design, 49, 212
Unconditional inference, 40–42, 40–43
Uniform bandit, 63
Uniformly most powerful unbiased, 169
United States National Cancer Institute, 91
Urn design, 54
  Wei's marginal, 57
Utility-adaptive randomization, 90, 93, 99–100, 101, 245
Utility-based unified CRM adaptive approach, 94
Utility function, 90, 99
  construction of, 94–95
Utility index, 91, 96, 100, 205, 220
Utility-offset model, 100, 101, 217, 218–219

V

Variance-adaptive randomization, 52
Variation, 1, 24
  coefficient of, 180, 186
  controlling and eliminating sources of, 10
  patient, 242
  statistical procedures and, 10
Virtual patients, 211, 212

W

Wang-Tsiatis' boundary, 118
Wei's marginal urn design, 57
Whitehead triangle boundaries, 130
Wilcoxon rank-sum test, 72
Without unblinding, 138–140

Z

Zelen's model, 56